Heart Disease (Clinical Cases in Cardiology)

Heart Disease (Clinical Cases in Cardiology)

Editor: Mitchell Burton

AMERICAN
MEDICAL PUBLISHERS
www.americanmedicalpublishers.com

AMERICAN
MEDICAL PUBLISHERS
www.americanmedicalpublishers.com

Cataloging-in-Publication Data

Heart disease (clinical cases in cardiology) / edited by Mitchell Burton.
p. cm.
Includes bibliographical references and index.
ISBN 979-8-88740-640-4
1. Heart--Diseases. 2. COVID-19 (Disease). 3. COVID-19 (Disease)--Complications.
4. Cardiology. I. Burton, Mitchell.
RC681 .H43 2023
616.12--dc23

American Medical Publishers,
41 Flatbush Avenue,
1st Floor, New York,
NY 11217, USA

ISBN 979-8-88740-640-4 (Hardback)

Contents

Preface

Over the recent decade, advancements and applications have progressed exponentially. This has led to the increased interest in this field and projects are being conducted to enhance knowledge. The main objective of this book is to present some of the critical challenges and provide insights into possible solutions. This book will answer the varied questions that arise in the field and also provide an increased scope for furthering studies.

Heart diseases, also called cardiac diseases, refer to conditions that affect the heart. The most common types of heart diseases include atherosclerosis, congenital heart defects, heart infections, arrhythmia, coronary artery disease (CAD), and cardiomyopathy. The major causes of heart disease include genetics, medications, lifestyle, infections, and other diseases. Lifestyle habits like smoking, and medical conditions like high blood pressure and high cholesterol are the major risk factors for heart diseases. Depending on the type of heart disease that a patient has, several treatment options may be used. However, some common strategies for managing heart conditions include lifestyle changes, surgery, and medications. Exercising regularly, avoiding or quitting smoking, eating a balanced diet, limiting alcohol intake, maintaining a moderate body weight, and managing the underlying conditions are few examples of lifestyle changes that can help reduce the risk of developing heart diseases. This book provides comprehensive insights into the field of cardiology. For all readers who are interested in cardiology, the case studies included in this book will serve as an excellent guide to develop a comprehensive understanding.

I hope that this book, with its visionary approach, will be a valuable addition and will promote interest among readers. Each of the authors has provided their extraordinary competence in their specific fields by providing different perspectives as they come from diverse nations and regions. I thank them for their contributions.

Editor

1

Elevated CA-125 as Humoral Biomarker of Congestive Heart Failure: Illustrative Cases and a Short Review of Literature

Attila Frigy,[1] **Boglárka Belényi**,[1] **Ádám Kirchmaier**,[1] **Nándor Fekete**,[1] **and István Adorján Szabó**[2]

[1]*Department of Internal Medicine IV, G.E, Palade University of Medicine, Pharmacy, Science and Technology of Tirgu Mures, Tirgu Mures, Romania*
[2]*Department of Physiopathology, G.E. Palade University of Medicine, Pharmacy, Science and Technology of Tirgu Mures, Tirgu Mures, Romania*

Correspondence should be addressed to Attila Frigy; afrigy68@gmail.com

Academic Editor: Ertugrul Ercan

Despite the recent, remarkable achievements in cardiology, heart failure (HF) remains a major public health problem due to its increasing prevalence, frequent hospitalizations, and significant mortality. Humoral biomarkers in HF are capable to reflect different aspects of the cardiac morpho-functional changes and the related pathophysiological processes and could have important diagnostic, prognostic, and therapeutical roles. CA-125 is a well-known tumor marker (mainly for ovarian cancer), and also a useful, but less applied cardiac biomarker. Practical aspects, possible pitfalls related with increased CA-125 levels are illustrated by two cases, both with HF, with the biomarker determined for other reasons and having high levels in the context of the cardiac decompensation. The paper presents a short review of the main biochemical, pathophysiological, and clinical data linked to CA-125, with special accent on its utility in patients with HF.

1. Introduction

Heart failure (HF) affects nearly 26 million patients worldwide, being associated with excessive morbidity and mortality. In Europe and in the US, HF is the third largest cause of cardiovascular mortality, provoking more than 1 million hospitalizations annually [1].

The complex pathophysiology of HF involves different—subcellular-molecular, cellular, neurohumoral (local and systemic), inflammatory, etc.—mechanisms. These pathological and adaptive processes induce changes in the production of specific biochemical compounds, called cardiac (humoral) biomarkers. These substances can be used in the diagnosis of HF, in the evaluation of disease evolution, for follow-up and prognosis, and for guiding therapy [1, 2].

Morrow and de Lemos [3] stated, that relevant, new cardiac biomarkers should have the following properties: the assay should be precise, accurate, and rapidly available to the clinician at a relatively low cost, should provide additional information, and should help in clinical decision making. Humoral biomarkers in HF can be classified according to the pathophysiological processes they are related (and could monitor) more closely. In this regard, they can be arranged into the following subcategories: markers of (1) myocardial stretch and injury (e.g., natriuretic peptides and troponins), (2) neurohumoral (renin-angiotensin-aldosterone system, sympathetic nervous system) activation, (3) remodeling (inflammation, hypertrophy, fibrosis, oxidative stress, and apoptosis), and (4) comorbidities (e.g., renal damage, malnutrition) [2, 4, 5].

CA-125 is a well-known tumor marker [6] and has been investigated as a potential cardiac biomarker since the early 2000s, despite the fact that it does not fit well into the main categories presented above [7].

In the followings, we present two cases with congestive HF, which illustrate the pitfalls related to the interpretation of elevated CA-125 levels.

2. Case Report

The patients signed an informed consent at admission regarding anonymous data collection for scientific purposes. Data handling and publication respected the Declaration of Helsinki, also having the approval (3865/01.03.2016) of the Ethical Committee of Clinical County Hospital Mureş.

2.1. Case No. 1. D.I., a 73 years old female, without a significant medical history, was admitted with a large pericardial effusion causing resting dyspnea and severe fatigue. Physical examination showed tachycardia, hypotension, and the presence of right basal pleural effusion. The transthoracic echocardiography revealed a large quantity of pericardial fluid (predominantly near to the right ventricle and right atrium—Figure 1) associated with typical signs of cardiac tamponade; hence, an urgent pericardiocentesis was performed with a good clinical result. The liquid was hemorrhagic, rising a possible tumoral etiology. To establish the etiology, complex imaging and laboratory evaluation was started. Thoraco-abdominal computed tomography (CT), with pulmonary angiography, showed a diffuse, inhomogeneous opacity in the right inferior lobe (Figure 2) and a right-sided ovarian (tumoral) mass. Bronchoscopy was negative, and the gynecological examination revealed a cystic type right ovarian tumor. The tumor marker panel included the determination of CA-125, which was found highly increased (247,5 IU/ml), supporting the suspicion of ovarian cancer with possible pericardial and pulmonary metastases. However, the magnetic resonance imaging described only right ovarian cysts, and the repeated CA-125 (at two weeks) had normal value, practically disclosing this suspicion. The highly elevated level of CA-125 was interpreted in the context of congestive HF caused by cardiac tamponade. Also, the pericardial involvement could have a direct contribution to the elevated CA-125.

Histopathological examination of the pericardial fluid confirmed primary lung cancer with pericardial metastases.

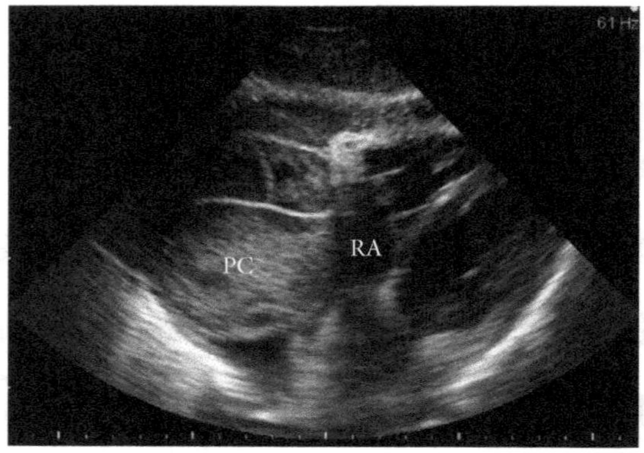

Figure 1: Echocardiography—subcostal four-chamber view. PC—encapsulated pericardial effusion with fibrinous septa compressing the right atrium (RA).

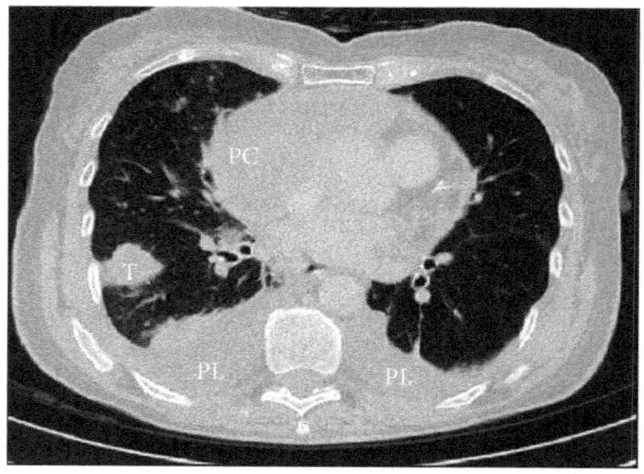

Figure 2: Computed tomography of the chest. PC—encapsulated pericardial effusion; PL—bilateral pleural effusion; T—tumoral mass in the right inferior lobe.

2.2. Case No. 2. P.N., a 68-year-old female, was admitted due to an episode of acute, predominantly right-sided HF, presenting severe fatigue, markedly increased abdominal circumference, and ankle edema. She had a nine years history of valve replacement (mechanical prosthesis) for rheumatic mitral valve disease. Routine transthoracic echocardiographic examination revealed dilated right heart cavities and severe tricuspid regurgitation with severe pulmonary hypertension (systolic pulmonary arterial pressure about 120 mmHg, Figure 3). The valvular prosthesis was normally functioning. The abdominal ultrasound examination showed a large quantity of ascites. To exclude a malignant process as substrate of abdominal fluid collection, CT imaging of the abdomen and thorax, and a tumor marker screening, including CA-125 were performed. CT examination confirmed the large intra-abdominal collection (Figure 4) and a right pleural effusion. The level of CA-125 was found to be highly elevated (357,6 IU/ml); however, the gynecologic examination and the abdominal CT did not demonstrate the presence of any pelvic tumoral mass. The increase of CA-125 level, based on the clinical and imaging data, was interpreted in the context of the severely decompensated right HF with ascites and pleural effusion.

3. Discussion

CA-125 (cancer antigen 125, carcinoma antigen 125 or carbohydrate antigen 125), also known as mucin 16 (MUC 16), is a soluble, high molecular weight (220 kD), heavily glycolisated transmembrane molecule with two parts: an intracytoplasmic-transmembrane part made of protein and an extracellular domain made of O- and N-linked oligosaccharide chains. This molecule is considered to be normally expressed in different tissues such as pleura, pericardium, peritoneum, fallopian tubes, endometrium, endocervix, lung, conjunctiva, and prostate. The role of CA-125 is to hydrate, lubricate, and protect from physical stress the epithelial luminal surfaces. The physiologic half-life of CA-125 is

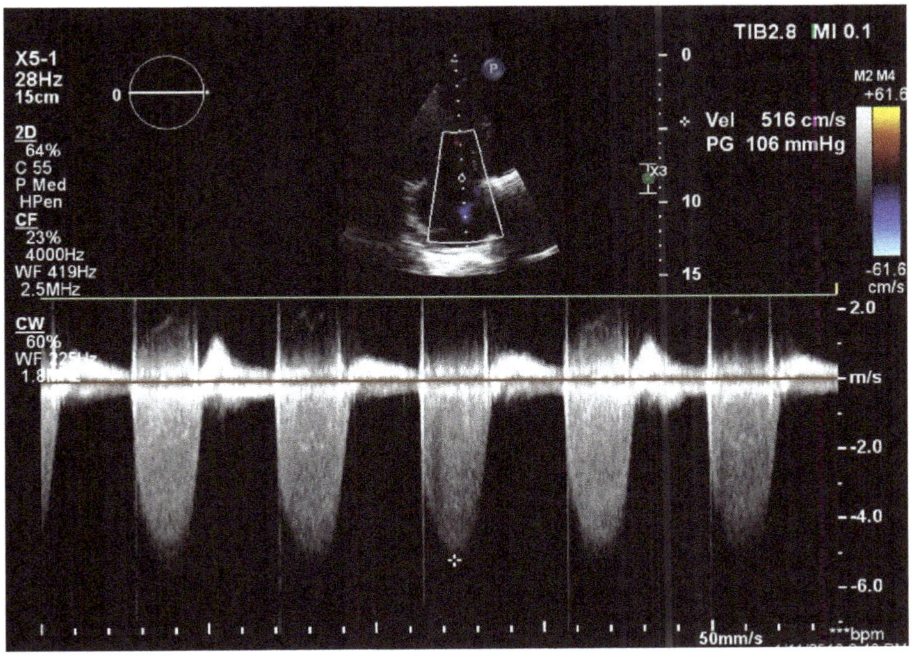

FIGURE 3: Continuous-wave Doppler interrogation of tricuspid regurgitation. Systolic gradient of 106 mmHg between the right ventricle and right atrium, revealing severe pulmonary hypertension.

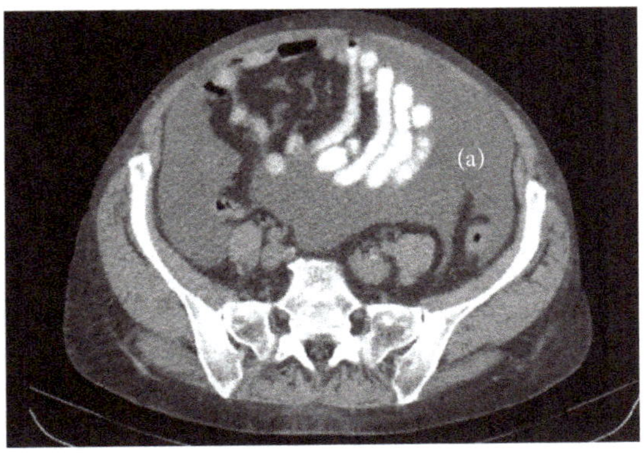

FIGURE 4: Abdominal computed tomography showing a large quantity of ascites (a).

approximately 5 days. Serum levels of CA-125 can be measured with standard immunochemical methods. The commercially available AxSYM CA-125 assay (Abbott Laboratories, IL) uses microparticle enzyme immunoassay technology. The range of normal values is 0-35 U/ml [8, 9].

Serum levels of CA-125 become elevated under certain physiologic conditions (menstruation, early pregnancy) and in certain, malignant and nonmalignant, pathological conditions, mainly in the case of epithelial ovarian cancer. Increased levels of CA-125 were found also in benign pelvic tumors, pelvic inflammatory diseases, lung cancer, peritoneal trauma, ascites, and liver cirrhosis [10].

A peculiar etiology of elevated serum levels of CA-125 is represented by congestive HF, with significant volume overload and effusions, as a rule [11]. Two hypotheses exist concerning the (over) production of the molecule in the setting of HF: (1) mesothelial cells are stimulated by tissue stretching/mechanical stress induced by serosal fluid accumulations (pleural effusion, ascites, pericardial effusion—even in the case of subclinical forms); (2) the overproduction of CA-125 in mesothelial cells is the result of the action of the inflammatory cytokine network (interleukin-1, tumor necrosis factor-α, lipopolysaccharides) activation, characteristic for HF [12, 13].

The link between CA-125 and HF was first described in 1999 by Nagele et al. in a group of patients with chronic HF undergoing heart transplantation. Several tumor markers were measured before and after transplantation, and only the level of CA-125 has normalized after the intervention, reflecting properly the hemodynamic improvement [14].

The studies dealing with the role of this biomarker in HF have proven that serum levels of CA-125 correlate well with the clinical status (including the presence of effusions with diverse localizations), the hemodynamic and echocardiographic parameters and with prognosis. Also, CA-125 could serve as a potent biomarker for guiding therapy [15, 16]. The results of the most important studies in this field are presented in Table 1.

An important issue is the relationship between CA-125 and natriuretic peptides, the gold standard of humoral biomarkers in HF. Several studies have shown that there is a significant correlation between the levels of CA-125, natriuretic peptides, and the severity of heart failure. In the diagnosis of heart failure, NTproBNP and CA-125 have a similar positive predictive value. Also, the sensitivity of BNP and the specificity of CA-125 are high in diagnosing acute heart failure. For the presence of effusions, CA-125 is more specific and more sensitive than BNP [19].

Table 1: Studies on CA-125 in the setting of diverse clinical forms of heart failure.

Heart failure type	Authors/year	No. of patients	Main findings
Chronic HF	D'Aloia A. et al., 2003. [17]	286	(i) CA-125 is correlated with clinical status, NYHA functional class and hemodynamic variables (right atrial pressure, pulmonary capillary wedge pressure, left ventricular systolic and diastolic dysfunction) (ii) Proposal for using CA-125 for evaluation of treatment efficacy
	Vizzardi E. et al., 2012. [18]	102	(i) CA-125 is a strong predictor of long term mortality
	Ordu S. et al., 2012. [19]	102	(i) CA-125 and NT-proBNP have similar accuracy in predicting major adverse events and death (ii) Independent prognostic value of CA-125
Acute HF	Nunez J. et al., 2010. [20]	1111	(i) The elevation of CA-125 (≥60 U/mL) and BNP (≥350 pg/mL) levels are significant in patients with NYHA class III and IV (ii) CA-125 levels are correlated with the severity of congestion (fluid retention)
	Nunez J. et al., 2016 [21] CHANCE-HF trial	380	(i) The CA-125 guided therapy reduces the rate of rehospitalizations
	Nunez J. et al., 2014 [22]	1389	(i) Levels of CA-125 combined with BUN (blood urea nitrogen) are predictive for mortality in patients receiving high dose diuretics at hospital discharge
Advanced heart failure	Monteiro S. et al., 2009. [23]	88	(i) CA-125 is a useful prognostic marker and permits a better risk stratification

4. Conclusions

CA-125 is a well-known tumor marker, routinely used for screening, diagnosis, and treatment follow-up of ovarian malignancy. In HF, there is also an overproduction of CA-125, a phenomenon triggered by both mechanical (fluid overload and tissue stretching) and inflammatory (cytokine activation) stimuli, which are mainly the consequences of cardiac decompensation. CA-125 proved to be a potent humoral biomarker in HF, with important prognostic, risk stratification, monitoring, and therapy guiding role. Its wider use has to be encouraged in this setting.

In both cases presented, the increase of CA-125 levels occurred in the context of congestive HF. It is important to mention, that in women undergoing ovarian tumor screening, comorbid congestive HF has to be taken into account when high CA-125 levels are interpreted.

Authors' Contributions

Attila Frigy and Boglárka Belényi contributed equally to this work.

Acknowledgments

The article was elaborated as part of the grant nr. 524/17.01.2017, with private financing, of the University of Medicine and Pharmacy of Tîrgu Mureş, Tîrgu Mureş, Romania.

References

[1] P. Ponikowski, A. A. Voors, S. D. Anker et al., "2016 ESC Guidelines for the diagnosis and treatment of acute and chronic heart failure: the task force for the diagnosis and treatment of acute and chronic heart failure of the European Society of Cardiology (ESC). Developed with the special contribution of the Heart Failure Association (HFA) of the ESC," *European Heart Journal*, vol. 37, no. 27, pp. 2129–2200, 2016.

[2] C. W. Yancy, M. Jessup, B. Bozkurt et al., "2017 ACC/AHA/HFSA focused update of the 2013 ACCF/AHA guideline for the management of heart failure: a report of the American College of Cardiology/American Heart Association Task Force on Clinical Practice Guidelines and the Heart Failure Society of America," *Circulation*, vol. 136, no. 6, pp. e137–e161, 2017.

[3] D. A. Morrow and J. A. de Lemos, "Benchmarks for the assessment of novel cardiovascular biomarkers," *Circulation*, vol. 115, no. 8, pp. 949–952, 2007.

[4] M. Lichtenauer, P. Jirak, B. Wernly et al., "A comparative analysis of novel cardiovascular biomarkers in patients with chronic heart failure," *European Journal of Internal Medicine*, vol. 44, pp. 31–38, 2017.

[5] M. Correale, I. Monaco, N. D. Brunetti, M. di Biase, and M. Metra, "Redefining biomarkers in heart failure," *Heart Failure Reviews*, vol. 23, no. 2, pp. 237–253, 2018.

[6] T. Muinao, H. P. Deka Boruah, and M. Pal, "Diagnostic and prognostic biomarkers in ovarian cancer and the potential roles of cancer stem cells - an updated review," *Experimental Cell Research*, vol. 362, no. 1, pp. 1–10, 2018.

[7] P. Faggiano, A. D'Aloia, L. Brentana et al., "Serum levels of different tumour markers in patients with chronic heart failure," *European Journal of Heart Failure*, vol. 7, no. 1, pp. 57–61, 2005.

[8] M. Felder, A. Kapur, J. Gonzalez-Bosquet et al., "MUC16 (CA125): tumor biomarker to cancer therapy, a work in progress," *Molecular Cancer*, vol. 13, no. 1, p. 129, 2014.

[9] S. Das and S. K. Batra, "Understanding the unique attributes of MUC16 (CA125): potential implications in targeted therapy," *Cancer Research*, vol. 75, no. 22, pp. 4669–4674, 2015.

[10] C. Miralles, M. Orea, P. España et al., "Cancer antigen 125 associated with multiple benign and malignant pathologies," *Annals of Surgical Oncology*, vol. 10, no. 2, pp. 150–154, 2003.

[11] E. Vizzardi, A. D'Aloia, A. Curnis, and L. Dei Cas, "Carbohydrate antigen 125," *Cardiology in Review*, vol. 21, no. 1, pp. 23–26, 2013.

[12] F. Huang, J. Chen, Y. Liu, K. Zhang, J. Wang, and H. Huang, "New mechanism of elevated CA125 in heart failure: the mechanical stress and inflammatory stimuli initiate CA 125 synthesis," *Medical Hypotheses*, vol. 79, no. 3, pp. 381–383, 2012.

[13] G. Miñana, J. Núñez, J. Sanchis, V. Bodí, E. Núñez, and A. Llàcer, "CA125 and immunoinflammatory activity in acute heart failure," *International Journal of Cardiology*, vol. 145, no. 3, pp. 547-548, 2010.

[14] H. Nagele, M. Bahlo, R. Klapdor, D. Schaeperkoetter, and W. Rödiger, "CA 125 and its relation to cardiac function," *American Heart Journal*, vol. 137, no. 6, pp. 1044–1049, 1999.

[15] J. Nunez, G. Minana, E. Nunez, F. J. Chorro, V. Bodi, and J. Sanchis, "Clinical utility of antigen carbohydrate 125 in heart failure," *Heart Failure Reviews*, vol. 19, no. 5, pp. 575–584, 2014.

[16] J. Zhuang, P. Faggiano, Q. Li et al., "Insights into the clinical implications of carbohydrate antigen 125 as a biomarker of heart failure," *Journal of Cardiovascular Medicine*, vol. 15, no. 12, pp. 864–872, 2014.

[17] A. D'Aloia, P. Faggiano, G. Aurigemma et al., "Serum levels of carbohydrate antigen 125 in patients with chronic heart failure," *Journal of the American College of Cardiology*, vol. 41, no. 10, pp. 1805–1811, 2003.

[18] E. Vizzardi, A. D'aloila, N. Pezzali, S. Bugatti, A. Curnis, and L. Dei Cas, "Long-Term Prognostic Value of CA 125 Serum Levels in Mild to Moderate Heart Failure Patients," *Journal of Cardiac Failure*, vol. 18, no. 1, pp. 68–73, 2012.

[19] S. Ordu, H. Ozhan, R. Alemadar et al., "Carbohydrate antigen-125 and N-terminal pro-brain natriuretic peptide levels: compared in heart-failure prognostication," *Texas Heart Institute Journal*, vol. 39, no. 1, pp. 30–35, 2012.

[20] J. Núñez, J. Sanchis, V. Bodí et al., "Improvement in risk stratification with the combination of the tumour marker antigen carbohydrate 125 and brain natriuretic peptide in patients with acute heart failure," *European Heart Journal*, vol. 31, no. 14, pp. 1752–1763, 2010.

[21] J. Núñez, P. Llàcer, V. Bertomeu-González, M. J. Bosch, P. Merlos, and S. García-Blas, "Carbohydrate Antigen-125–Guided Therapy in Acute Heart Failure: CHANCE-HF: A Randomized Study," *JACC: Heart Failure*, vol. 4, no. 11, pp. 833–843, 2016.

[22] J. Núñez, E. Núñez, G. Miñana et al., "Differential mortality association of loop diuretic dosage according to blood urea nitrogen and carbohydrate antigen 125 following a hospitalization for acute heart failure," *Journal of Critical Care*, vol. 14, no. 9, pp. 974–984, 2012.

[23] S. Monteiro, F. franco, S. Costa et al., "Prognostic value of CA125 in advanced heart failure patients," *International Journal of Cardiology*, vol. 140, no 1, pp. 115–118, 2010.

2

Case Report of an Acute Myocardial Infarction as a Result of Spontaneous Coronary Artery Dissection in a Patient with Fibromuscular Dysplasia

A. Kalinskaya, D. Skrypnik, A. Kostin, E. Vasilieva, and A. Shpektor

Moscow State University of Medicine and Dentistry Named After A.I. Evdokimov, Clinical Hospital Named After I.V. Davidovsky, Moscow, Russia

Correspondence should be addressed to A. Kostin; kostilok@yandex.ru

Academic Editor: Kuan-Rau Chiou

Background. Spontaneous coronary artery dissection (SCAD) is an underdiagnosed and rare cause of myocardial infarction (MI). SCAD is defined as the separation of the coronary artery wall by hemorrhage with or without intimal tear. It causes acute coronary syndrome in 1.7% to 4% of cases. *Case Summary.* We report a case of a patient with acute MI caused by SCAD with marked progression of dissection within 4 days and spontaneous healing in 2 months. Fibromuscular dysplasia (FMD) of the arteries is an associated condition of SCAD that was found in our patient. *Conclusion.* In young women admitted to the clinic with signs of acute myocardial infarction, SCAD should be suspected. FMD as an associated condition that should be ruled out in every SCAD patient. Conservative treatment of SCAD is the most preferable strategy.

1. Introduction

Spontaneous coronary artery dissection (SCAD) is an underdiagnosed and rare cause of myocardial infarction (MI). SCAD is defined as the separation of the coronary artery wall by hemorrhage with or without intimal tear. SCAD causes acute coronary syndrome in 1.7% to 4% of cases [1]. We report a case of a patient with acute MI caused by SCAD with marked progression of dissection within 4 days and spontaneous healing in 2 months.

2. Case Report

A 47-year-old woman with a 4-day history of chest pain, which had begun directly after emotional stress (air travel), was transferred to our clinic from another hospital. The patient was normosthenic, had practiced gymnastics in youth, and had no signs of joint hypermobility syndrome or other connective tissue disorder. She had smoked for a long time and had arterial hypertension grade 2. She had never experienced chest pain before and was very active in her everyday life.

An electrocardiogram upon admission to our clinic revealed a sinus rhythm with a 2 mm ST elevation in leads II, III, aVF, V3-V5, "-" and T V3-V5 (Figure 1). On echocardiography, an apex dyskinesis was found; the left ventricle ejection fraction was 56%. The level of cardiac troponin-I was 13.2 ng/mL, confirming the development of acute myocardial infarction. We analysed the first angiogram, which had been performed in another clinic. It revealed 70–75% smooth extended narrowing in the middle segment of the left anterior descending artery, and no signs of atherosclerosis in the proximal segment of LAD or the remaining arteries were found. Side branches were absolutely normal as well (Figure 2). It looked like a subintimal hematoma. We repeated the coronary angiography upon admission on day 4; the extension of the culprit lesion to the distal segment of the LAD was observed (Figure 3). Because of the high risk of intima rupture, intravascular visualization was not performed. This finding on the second angiogram confirmed our initial suspicion and corresponded to SCAD type 2.

Considering that the association of SCAD and FMD is a well-known fact, we performed angiography of the renal and carotid arteries [2]. In the mid and distal portions of

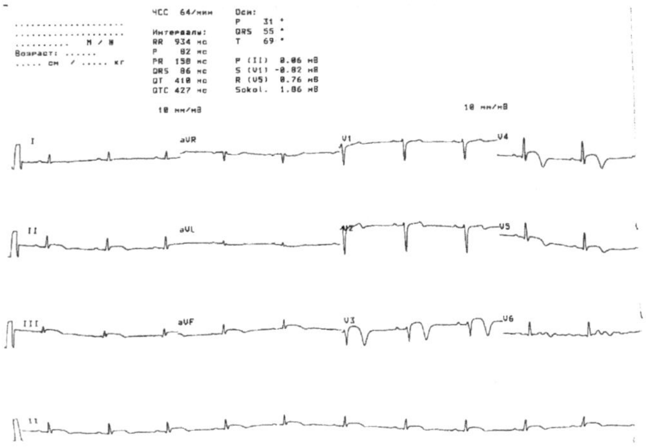

FIGURE 1: Electrocardiogram revealed a sinus rhythm with a 2 mm ST elevation in leads II, III, aVF, V3-V5, "-" and T V3-V5.

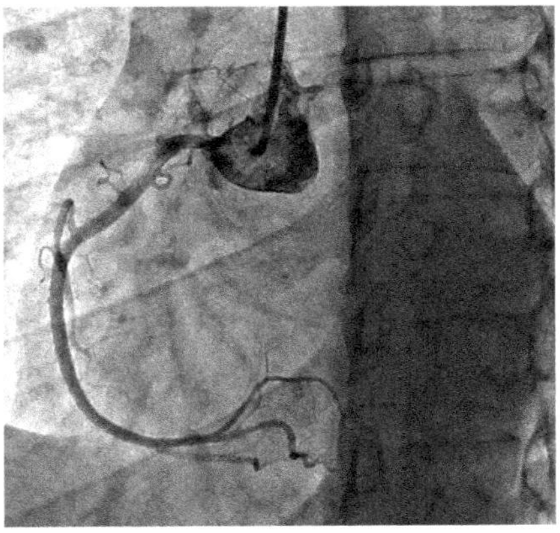

(a)

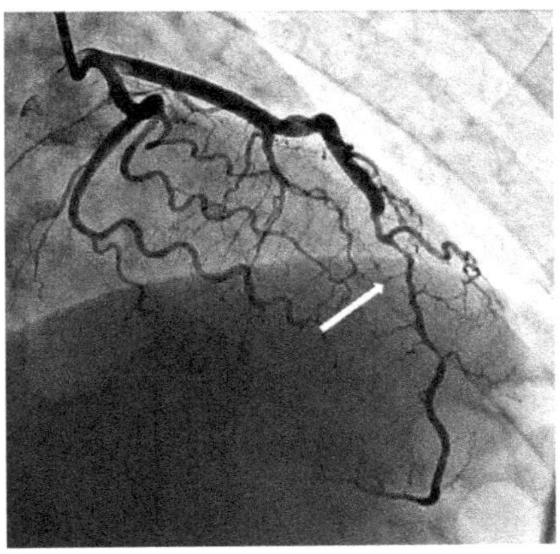

(b)

FIGURE 2: The first coronary angiography revealed a long segment disease of the LAD artery. Right coronary artery is normal.

the renal arteries, alternating dilatation and constriction (string-of-beads) were observed (Figure 4), confirming a diagnosis of fibromuscular dysplasia (FMD). The patient received conservative treatment only (metoprolol 25 mg/day and aspirin 75 mg/day). In two months, a follow-up visit took place. The patient had no episodes of chest pain or dyspnea.

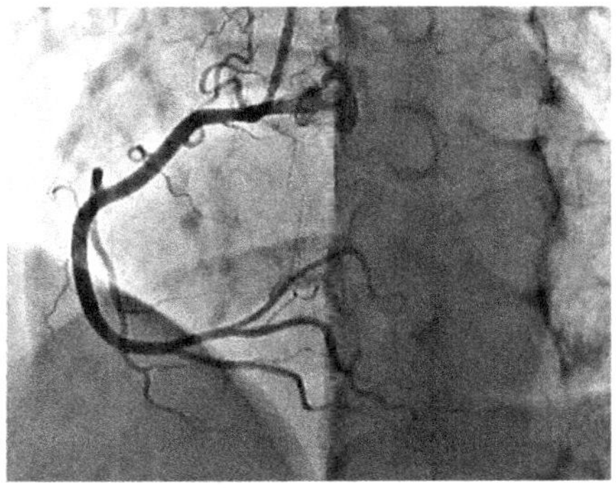

(a)

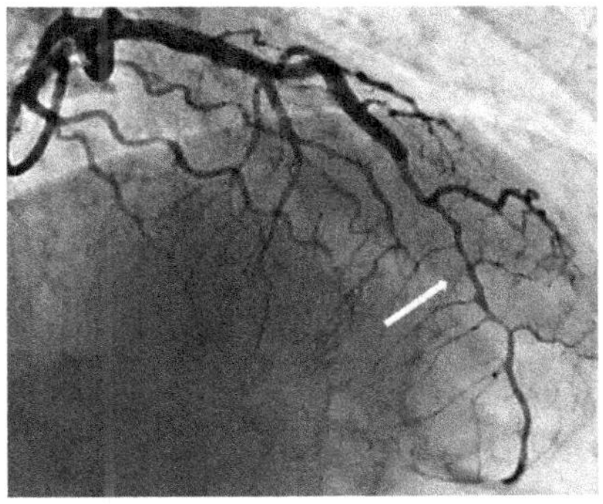

(b)

FIGURE 3: Coronary angiography view 4 days after admission with dissection of the LAD.

Repeated coronary angiography revealed absolutely normal coronary arteries (Figure 5).

3. Discussion

The patient developed acute MI without any signs of atherosclerosis. SCAD, defined as the separation of the coronary artery wall by hemorrhage, is a rare underlying cause of acute coronary syndrome [3, 4]. There are three known types of SCAD. Type 1 is characterized by the appearance of a double lumen under contrast staining of the arterial wall. Type 2 appears as diffuse (typically 20 to 30 mm) and smooth narrowing that can vary in severity (due to intramural hematoma). Type 3 appears as focal or tubular stenosis that mimics atherosclerosis and can be confirmed only under intravascular visualization [1, 5].

SCAD is often underdiagnosed and mistaken for atherosclerosis. In order to establish the challenging diagnosis of SCAD, the specific flowchart was developed [6]. This flowchart includes clinical and angiographic features of SCAD. In 2017, Motreff et al. identified the specific five angiographic features of SCAD: (1) absence of atheroma on other coronary arteries; (2) radiolucent flap(s); (3) contrast dye staining of the arterial wall; (4) starting and/or ending of the angiographic ambiguity on a side branch; and (5) long narrowing of the lumen calibre: smooth and linear, or stenosis of varying severity mimicking a "stick insect" or "radish" aspect [7]. In this case, we found the following: (1) typical smooth narrowing of the coronary artery, (2) progress of artery dissection in the distal direction in 4 days, (3) no signs of

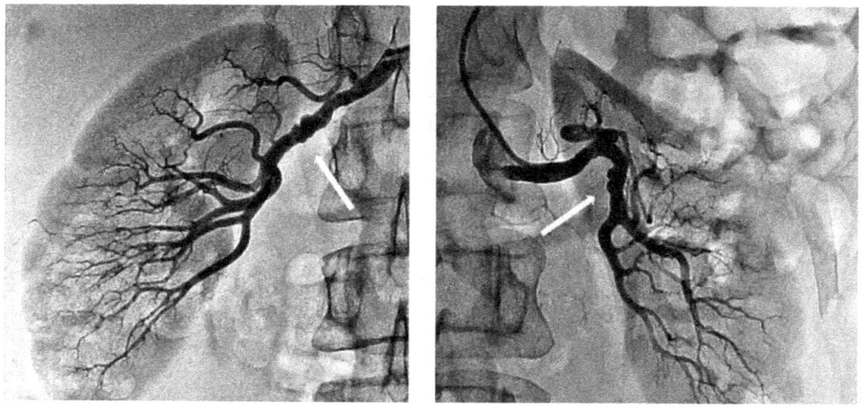

(a) (b)

FIGURE 4: Arteriogram with contrast showing fibromuscular dysplasia of the middle right and left renal arteries.

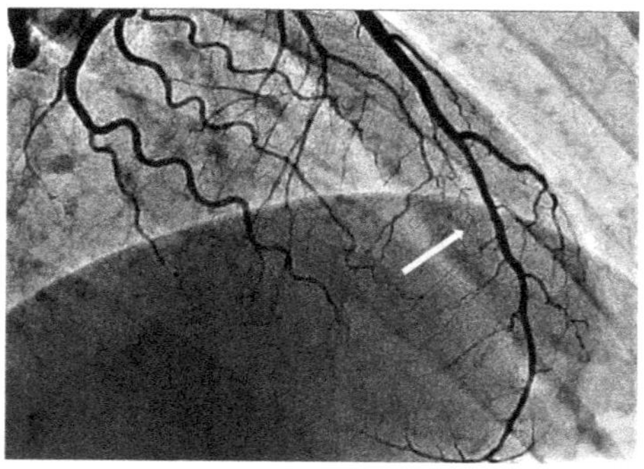

FIGURE 5: The last coronary angiography shows near-normal left coronary artery.

atherosclerosis in the remaining arteries, and (4) dissection ended on a side branch. All these findings were conclusive for SCAD. This case demonstrates the rapid progression of SCAD leading to acute MI.

The acute and long-term management of SCAD is not well developed, as there have been no randomized trials assessing the optimal strategy. According to observational studies, most SCAD lesions heal spontaneously [8]. For this reason, the preferred strategy in SCAD treatment is conservative [4]. We chose medical treatment as well. According to data in the literature, the full resolution of SCAD occurs in 12 to 40 months [9, 10]. Our patient was doing well after 2 months; that is why we decided to repeat the control angiography well before 12 months. It revealed a healed coronary artery.

SCAD is often accompanied by FMD (in 62–86% of cases) [11]. The recent published study showed that SCAD may have a genetic link to FMD. There is an increased risk for both SCAD and FMD in patients carrying the rs9349379-A allele of PHACTR1/EDN1 genetic locus (chromosome 6q24) [2].

FMD is a nonatherosclerotic vascular disease that results in occlusion, aneurysm, or dissection of the artery. The most commonly affected vascular bed is the renal or carotid arteries (65% of cases) [12]. The exact frequency of FMD of coronary arteries is still unknown, as the diagnosis of coronary FMD is rather challenging. The string-of-beads appearance is rarely seen. In most cases, we can see distal tapering, nonatherosclerotic stenosis, or dissection of the artery [13]. To confirm the diagnosis of coronary FMD, the visualization of another vascular bed is necessary. In our case, we found the typical string-of-beads in renal arteries.

4. Conclusion

In young women admitted to the clinic with signs of acute myocardial infarction, SCAD should be suspected. FMD as an associated condition should be ruled out in every SCAD patient. Conservative treatment of SCAD is the most preferable strategy.

Authors' Contributions

AK, DS, AK, EV, and AS contributed equally to the care of this patient. AK and AK wrote the manuscript. All the authors read and approved the final manuscript.

Acknowledgments

All interventions and lab tests were done in Moscow State Clinical Hospital Named After I.V. Davidovsky. Clinical Hospital Named After I.V. Davidovsky provided all the funding.

References

[1] J. Saw, K. Humphries, E. Aymong et al., "Spontaneous coronary artery dissection," *Journal of the American College of Cardiology*, vol. 70, no. 9, pp. 1148–1158, 2017.

[2] D. Adlam, T. M. Olson, N. Combaret et al., "Association of the PHACTR1/EDN1 genetic locus with spontaneous coronary artery dissection," *Journal of the American College of Cardiology*, vol. 73, no. 1, pp. 58–66, 2019.

[3] T. Nishiguchi, A. Tanaka, Y. Ozaki et al., "Prevalence of spontaneous coronary artery dissection in patients with acute coronary syndrome," *European Heart Journal: Acute Cardiovascular Care*, vol. 5, no. 3, pp. 263–270, 2016.

[4] D. Buccheri, G. Zambelli, F. Alfonso, and B. Cortese, "Pulse on spontaneous coronary artery dissections: experience-based survey," *JACC: Cardiovascular Interventions*, vol. 10, no. 14, pp. 1469–1471, 2017.

[5] S. Aziz, "Spontaneous coronary artery dissection," *E-Journal of Cardiology Practice*, vol. 14, no. 38, 2017.

[6] L. E. L. Gort, S. A. Romani, C. R. R. Carreras, and F. J. F. Portales, "Score system approach to diagnose and manage spontaneous coronary artery dissection," *Revista Española de Cardiología*, vol. 69, no. 9, pp. 879-880, 2016.

[7] P. Motreff, G. Malcles, N. Combaret et al., "How and when to suspect spontaneous coronary artery dissection: novel insights from a single-centre series on prevalence and angiographic appearance," *EuroIntervention*, vol. 12, no. 18, pp. e2236–e2243, 2017.

[8] F. Alfonso, M. Paulo, V. Lennie et al., "Spontaneous coronary artery dissection: long-term follow-up of a large series of patients prospectively managed with a "conservative" therapeutic strategy," *JACC: Cardiovascular Interventions*, vol. 5, no. 10, pp. 1062–1070, 2012.

[9] F. Alfonso, M. Paulo, N. Gonzalo et al., "Diagnosis of spontaneous coronary artery dissection by optical coherence tomography," *Journal of the American College of Cardiology*, vol. 59, no. 12, pp. 1073–1079, 2012.

[10] S. J. DeMaio Jr, S. H. Kinsella, and M. E. Silverman, "Clinical course and long-term prognosis of spontaneous coronary artery dissection," *The American Journal of Cardiology*, vol. 64, no. 8, pp. 471–474, 1989.

[11] J. Saw, D. Ricci, A. Starovoytov, R. Fox, and C. E. Buller, "Spontaneous coronary artery dissection," *JACC: Cardiovascular Interventions*, vol. 6, no. 1, pp. 44–52, 2013.

[12] J. W. Olin, J. Froehlich, X. Gu et al., "The United States Registry for Fibromuscular Dysplasia: results in the first 447 patients," *Circulation*, vol. 125, no. 25, pp. 3182–3190, 2012.

[13] G. E. Pate, R. Lowe, and C. E. Buller, "Fibromuscular dysplasia of the coronary and renal arteries?," *Catheterization and Cardiovascular Interventions*, vol. 64, no. 2, pp. 138–145, 2005.

3

Prosthetic Valve *Candida* Endocarditis: A Case Report with 18F-FDG-PET/CT as Part of the Diagnostic Workup

Soile Pauliina Salomäki,[1,2,3] Antti Saraste,[2,3,4] Päivi Jalava-Karvinen,[1,2] Laura Pirilä,[1,5] and Ulla Hohenthal[1,2]

[1]*Department of infectious Diseases, Division of Medicine, Turku University Hospital, Turku, Finland*
[2]*Faculty of Medicine, Department of Clinical Medicine, University of Turku, Turku, Finland*
[3]*Turku PET Centre, University of Turku and Turku University Hospital, Turku, Finland*
[4]*Heart Center, Turku University Hospital, Turku, Finland*
[5]*Department of Rheumatology, Division of Medicine, Turku University Hospital, Turku, Finland*

Correspondence should be addressed to Ulla Hohenthal; ulla.hohenthal@tyks.fi

Academic Editor: Alfredo E. Rodriguez

Diagnosis of *Candida* spp. infective endocarditis (IE) is challenging, and diagnostic delays are common. We describe two patients with *Candida* spp. prosthetic valve endocarditis (PVE) and ^{18}fluorodeoxyglucose positron emission tomography/computed tomography (^{18}F-FDG-PET/CT) as a part of diagnostic workup. We also refer to 5 other cases we found from the published literature. These cases highlight that ^{18}F-FDG-PET/CT can improve diagnostic accuracy in prosthetic valve *Candida* endocarditis.

1. Background

Candida spp. endocarditis is a rare but devastating disease accounting for <2% of all IE and ~3% of prosthetic valve endocarditis (PVE) [1]. Candida endocarditis is associated with up to 36% in hospital mortality and up to 59% 1-year mortality [2, 3]. Because of the inconsistent and nonspecific presentation, the diagnosis of candida endocarditis is often delayed. Previous studies have shown ^{18}F-FDG PET/CT as a valuable tool in the diagnosis of bacterial PVE but less is known about its role in *Candida* endocarditis [4–7].

We describe 2 cases of prosthetic valve *Candida* endocarditis in which a whole-body or cardiac ^{18}F-FDG-PET/CT scan (Discovery VCT, General Electric Medical Systems, Milwaukee, WI, USA) was used in the diagnostic workup of the disease. Patients were on low-carbohydrate diet for 24 hours before the PET-scan and fasted at least 10 hours before the study.

2. Case Presentations

2.1. Case 1. A 39-year-old man with a history of intravenous drug use (IVDU) and chronic hepatitis C infection presented to our university hospital due to a two-week history of fever, 4-day history of low back pain, and 1-day history of problems in keeping his balance. He had a history of aortic valve replacement with a mechanical prosthesis due to IE 8 years earlier. On admission, the physical examination was remarkable for systolic murmur on auscultation, multiple peripheral emboli of lower limbs, and clumsiness of the right upper limb. His temperature was 37.9°C, oxygen saturation 88%, heart rate 103 beats per minute, and blood pressure 141/81 mmHg. The C-reactive protein (CRP) was 189 mg/L, white blood cells (WBC) 15.8×10^9/L, hemoglobin (Hb) level 106 g/L, and creatinine 89 μmol/L. Transesophageal echocardiography (TEE) confirmed the vegetation of 9×16 mm

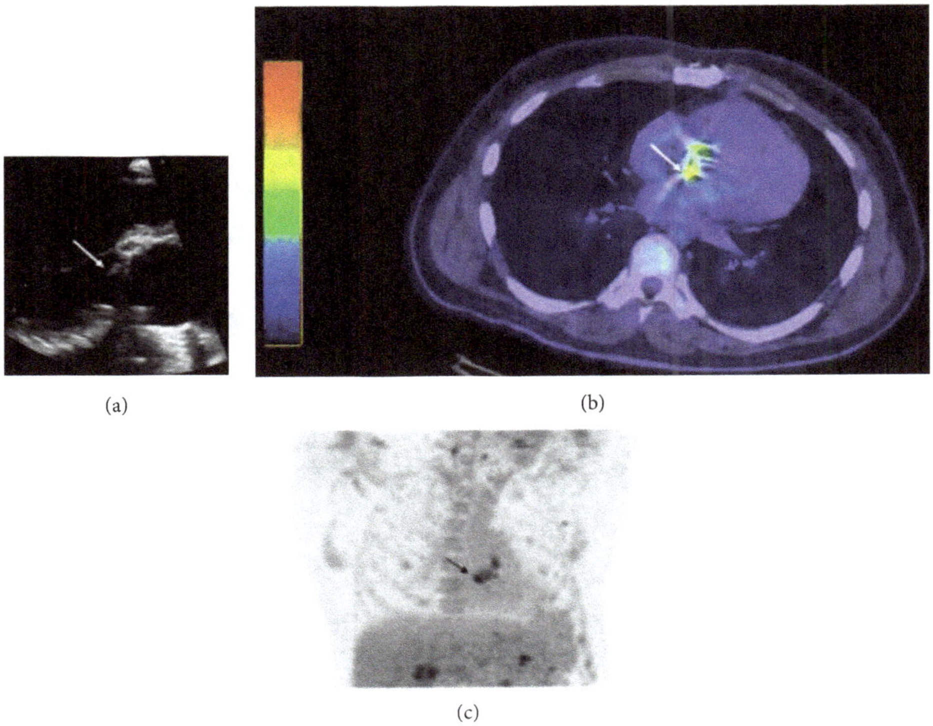

FIGURE 1: Transesophageal echocardiography image of patient 1 (panel (a)); arrow shows vegetation. ^{18}F-FDG-PET/CT images of patient 1 (panels (b) and (c)). Arrows show increased ^{18}F-FDG uptake at the site of aortic valve prosthesis.

(Figure 1) detected at admission with transthoracic echocardiography (TTE). Magnetic resonance imaging (MRI) of the head revealed multiple cerebral hemorrhagic lesions and an abscess in the cerebellum. Embolic infarctions were detected in the spleen and in both kidneys by computed tomography (CT). Blood cultures taken on admission yielded *Candida albicans* on day 4, and therapy with liposomal amphotericin B (LAMB) was started. ^{18}F-FDG-PET/CT of the thoracic region was performed on day 19. Injected dose of ^{18}F-FDG was 392 MBq and 47 minutes later, a whole-body PET acquisition (3 min per bed position) was performed following low-dose CT scan without contrast. High focal uptake was detected at the site of the mechanic aortic valve with a maximal standardized uptake value (SUV_{max}) of 7.4 g/mL (Figure 1). The patient died on day 30 after admission due to massive intracerebral hematoma.

2.2. Case 2. A 31-year-old male with previous IVDU was admitted to our hospital for fever and pain in the left hand and right leg. He had chronic hepatitis C infection and a history of aortic valve replacement with mechanical prosthesis due to IE 4 years earlier. On admission, his temperature was 38.1°C, oxygen saturation 97%, heart rate 94 beats per minute, and blood pressure 140/80 mmHg. On the physical examination, no pulsation was identified in radial or ulnar arteries of the left wrist but the hand was warm. Blood tests showed WBC count of 8.8×10^9/L, Hb 137 g/L, CRP 151 mg/L, and creatinine 82 μmol/L. Blood cultures remained negative. No signs of endocarditis was detected on TTE. However, ^{18}F-FDG-PET/CT (injected dose of ^{18}F-FDG 278 MBq, time from injection to scan 50 min following low-dose CT without contrast) revealed focal uptake consistent with embolic foci in the brachial artery and in arteries of both legs (Figure 2). No accumulation of ^{18}FDG was detected on the prosthetic valve but due to the noncompliance of the patient with the diet before PET/CT, there was physiological uptake in myocardium. CT angiography showed mycotic aneurysm in the brachial artery and thrombosis of the left popliteal artery. The patient was treated with vancomycin, gentamycin, and rifampicin for IE. The patient had intermittently fever, and inflammation values were persistently high, CRP at maximum 322 mg/L and ESR 89 mm/h. Blood cultures were negative until blood culture taken on day 21 after admission yielded *C. albicans*, and treatment with micafungin was commenced. Vegetation on the prosthetic valve was later found on TEE (Figure 2). On day 22. the patient suffered from massive infarct of the right hemisphere followed by hemicraniectomy. The patient remained in poor clinical condition and died 6 months later.

3. Discussion

^{18}FDG-PET/CT has emerged as a valuable diagnostic tool for IE in cases with diagnostic difficulties especially in PVE. There is increasing evidence that besides localizing bacterial infections, ^{18}FDG-PET/CT can also recognize sites of fungal infections [8]. However, less is known about the diagnostic yield of ^{18}F-FDG-PET/CT in fungal PVE. Because of the rarity of the disease, it is challenging to carry out a prospective clinical trial.

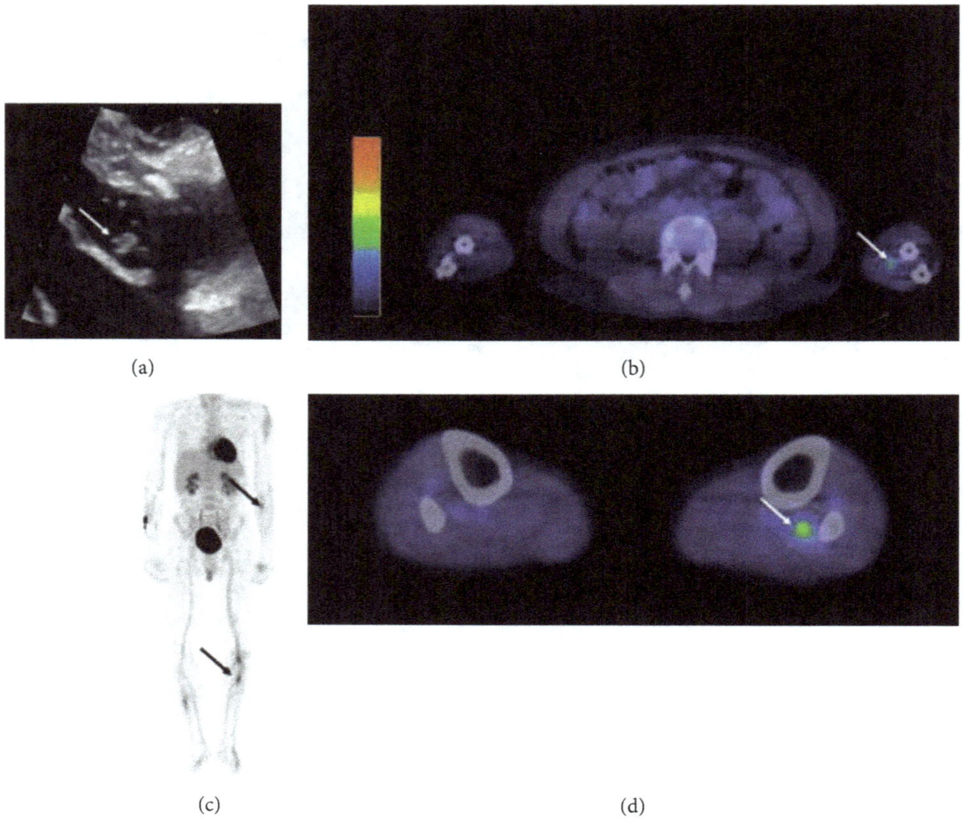

Figure 2: Transesophageal echocardiography images of patient 2 (panel (a)). Arrow shows vegetation. ^{18}F-FDG-PET/CT images of patient 2 (panels (b)–(d)). Arrows show ^{18}F-FDG uptake at the site brachial artery and fibular artery.

Table 1: The characteristics of 7 patients with *Candida* spp. prosthetic valve endocarditis.

Patient [reference number]	*Candida* species	Type and location of prosthetic valve	Transesophageal echocardiography	Visual assessment of valves by FDG-PET/CT	Duke criteria
1 [4]	*C. parapsilosis*	Mechanical AV and MV	Negative[a]	Positive	Definitive
2 [4]	*C. parapsilosis*	Mechanical AV	Fistula[a]	Positive	Definitive
3 [5]	*Candida*[b]	ND[b]	ND	Positive	Definitive
4 [6]	*C. albicans*	AV[c]	Increased wall thickness of the aortic root	Positive	Definitive
5 [9]	*C. albicans*	Mechanical AV	Negative	Positive	Definitive
6 [present case 1]	*C. albicans*	Mechanical AV	Vegetation	Positive	Definitive
7 [present case 2]	*C. albicans*	Mechanical AV	Vegetation	Negative[d]	Definitive

Abbreviations: AV: aortic valve; MV: mitral valve; ND: not done or data not given; [a]Transthoracic echocardiography. [b]Species not given. [c]Type of the prosthetic valve not given. [d] Embolic foci in peripheral arteries detected by ^{18}F-FDG-PET/CT.

To our knowledge, only 5 cases have previously been published in which PET/CT has been used in diagnostic workup of PVE caused by *Candida* sp. [4–6, 9]. As in one of our cases, focal uptake was recognized on the prosthetic valve in all of these 5 previous cases (Table 1). In the other case of ours, no uptake was found on the prosthetic valve. Instead, embolic findings consistent with endocarditis were detected by PET/CT. One explanation for the negative finding of the valve area on PET/CT might be the biofilm formation on prosthesis which is typical for *Candida* species and enables *Candida* to evade the host immune response [10].

One can also question the diagnosis of the etiological agent in our case with the first positive blood culture on day 21 after admission as *C. albicans* might also present secondary infection. However, no other etiological agent was identified, no response was achieved with antibiotic treatment, and course of the illness with multiple emboli was typical for *Candida*. Moreover, the sensitivity of the blood culture to detect *Candida* has been estimated to be only 50-75% [11]. As in our case, the negative blood culture may be one of the reasons for the delayed diagnosis of the disease which is typical for fungal endocarditis.

Embolic complications have been found in up to 46% of the patients with *Candida* endocarditis [3]. As in our case, these can be detected by the whole-body ^{18}FDG-PET/CT which enables detection of several embolic findings with one diagnostic modality and as in our case, these findings on PET/CT may confirm the diagnosis of endocarditis. The multiple arterial findings could have also arisen the suspicion of *Candida* as an etiological agent. Unfortunately, in the other case with multiple emboli, the PET/CT was restricted only to thorax, and we were not able to evaluate the usefulness of PET/CT to detect peripheral embolic foci in this case.

Our 2 cases and one of the previously published cases are case reports. Consequently, findings based on these 7 cases must be interpreted with caution taking into account the possible selection bias of reported cases.

In conclusion, our two cases and the previously published cases indicate that ^{18}F-FDG-PET/CT seems to be a promising and valuable diagnostic tool in *Candida* spp. prosthetic valve endocarditis.

References

[1] P. Muñoz, M. Kestler, A. de Alarcon et al., "Current epidemiology and outcome of infective endocarditis. A multicenter, prospective, cohort study," *Medicine*, vol. 94, no. 43, article e1816, 2015.

[2] C. J. Arnold, M. Johnson, A. S. Bayer et al., "Candida infective endocarditis: an observational cohort study with a focus on therapy," *Antimicrobial Agents and Chemotherapy*, vol. 59, no. 4, pp. 2365–2373, 2015.

[3] C. Rivoisy, A. Vena, L. Schaeffer et al., "Prosthetic valve Candida spp. endocarditis: new insights into long-term prognosis-the ESCAPE study," *Clinical Infectious Diseases*, vol. 66, no. 6, pp. 825–832, 2018.

[4] A. Ricciardi, P. Sordillo, L. Ceccarelli et al., "18-Fluoro-2-deoxyglucose positron emission tomography-computed tomography: an additional tool in the diagnosis of prosthetic valve endocarditis," *International Journal of Infectious Diseases*, vol. 28, pp. 219–224, 2014.

[5] F. Rouzet, R. Chequer, K. Benali et al., "Respective performance of 18F-FDG PET and radiolabeled leukocyte scintigraphy for the diagnosis of prosthetic valve endocarditis," *Journal of Nuclear Medicine*, vol. 55, no. 12, pp. 1980–1985, 2014.

[6] E. Fagman, M. van Essen, J. Fredén Lindqvist, U. Snygg-Martin, and O. Bech-Hanssen, "18F-FDG PET/CT in the diagnosis of prosthetic valve endocarditis," *The International Journal of Cardiovascular Imaging*, vol. 32, no. 4, pp. 679–686, 2016.

[7] S. P. Salomäki, A. Saraste, J. Kemppainen et al., "^{18}F-FDG positron emission tomography/computed tomography in infective endocarditis," *Journal of Nuclear Cardiology*, vol. 24, no. 1, pp. 195–206, 2017.

[8] A. P. Douglas, K. A. Thursky, L. J. Worth et al., "FDG PET/CT imaging in detecting and guiding management of invasive fungal infections: a retrospective comparison to conventional CT imaging," *European Journal of Nuclear Medicine and Molecular Imaging*, vol. 46, no. 1, pp. 166–173, 2019.

[9] M. Bartoletti, F. Tumietto, G. Fasulo et al., "Combined computed tomography and fluorodeoxyglucose positron emission tomography in the diagnosis of prosthetic valve endocarditis: a case series," *BMC Research Notes*, vol. 7, no. 1, p. 32, 2014.

[10] M. B. Lohse, M. Gulati, A. D. Johnson, and C. J. Nobile, "Development and regulation of single- and multi-species Candida albicans biofilms," *Nature Reviews. Microbiology*, vol. 16, no. 1, pp. 19–31, 2018.

[11] M. Cuenca-Estrella, P. E. Verweij, M. C. Arendrup et al., "ESCMID guideline for the diagnosis and management of *Candida* diseases 2012: diagnostic procedures," *Clinical Microbiology and Infection*, vol. 18, suppl 7, pp. 9–18, 2012.

4

Mitral Valve Endocarditis with Perforation from a Urinary Source

Fernando Figueroa Rodriguez, Antonio Faieta Lasarcina, and Francisco Davila Grijalva

Oakland University Beaumont Hospital, West 13 Mile Road, Royal Oak, MI 48073, USA

Correspondence should be addressed to Fernando Figueroa Rodriguez; fernando.figueroarodriguez@beaumont.org

Academic Editor: Ertugrul Ercan

Aerococcus urinae (AU) is a rare pathogen, identified as gram-positive, catalase-negative coccus that grows in pairs and clusters which has been reported to mainly cause urinary tract infections (UTI), especially in elderly males. Treatment for this microorganism is usually with beta-lactams although cultures with antibiotic susceptibility testing are imperative. We present a case of AU endocarditis initially treated with IV antibiotics; nevertheless, the patient required emergent mitral valve replacement due to severe mitral insufficiency and perforation. We also present an analysis with high-yield points summarizing epidemiology, risk factors, microbiology, clinical features, diagnostic workup, and management of AU in general and AU endocarditis. Finally, we post a literature review of relevant cases and the impact of different variables associated with it.

1. Case Presentation

A 55-year-old male with no significant past medical history presented with a one-week history of nonproductive cough, dyspnea at rest, dysuria, and urinary frequency and urgency. He was diagnosed with a urinary tract infection (UTI) and a viral upper respiratory tract infection by his primary care physician two days prior and was prescribed ciprofloxacin. His symptoms did not improve so he decided to go to the emergency department (ED). Upon presentation, his oxygen saturation was noted to be 90%, with tachycardia and a low-grade fever. On exam, he had significant bibasilar crackles as well as a holosystolic apical murmur; additionally, he was found to have 2+ lower extremity edema and several punctuate macular lesions on his feet, highly suspicious for vascular emboli phenomena (Figure 1). His laboratory studies demonstrated leukocytosis with neutrophilia (14.7 bil/L and 11.3 bil/L, respectively) and evidence of acute kidney injury. The urinalysis bacteriuria and leukocytes. A chest X-ray (CXR) was unremarkable. Blood and urine cultures were obtained, and he was empirically started on ceftriaxone. A transthoracic echocardiogram revealed a mobile mass on the posterior leaflet of the mitral valve consistent with a vegetation. Ejection fraction was calculated to be 40% (Figure 2). Preliminary blood cultures reported gram-positive cocci in pairs and clusters. At day 3, AU was identified as the pathogen in both, blood and urine, cultures. The patient was then started on intravenous gentamicin and penicillin G with plans for a 6-week therapy. He was medically treated for acute heart failure with aggressive diuresis. At day 5, the patient received a transesophageal echocardiogram (TEE) which confirmed a "1.4 cm × 2.5 cm" vegetation attached to the posterior leaflet of mitral valve (Figure 3(a)), with severe mitral regurgitation and posterior leaflet perforation (Figure 3(b)). On day 8, the patient was acutely decompensated, and he was endotracheally intubated due to hypoxic respiratory failure and consequently underwent emergent prosthetic mitral valve replacement. He had a prolonged complicated postoperative period requiring mechanical ventilation, vasopressor support, and hemodialysis. Repeat blood cultures showed resolution of AU bacteremia. Finally, after 3 months, the patient was discharged to a subacute rehabilitation unit.

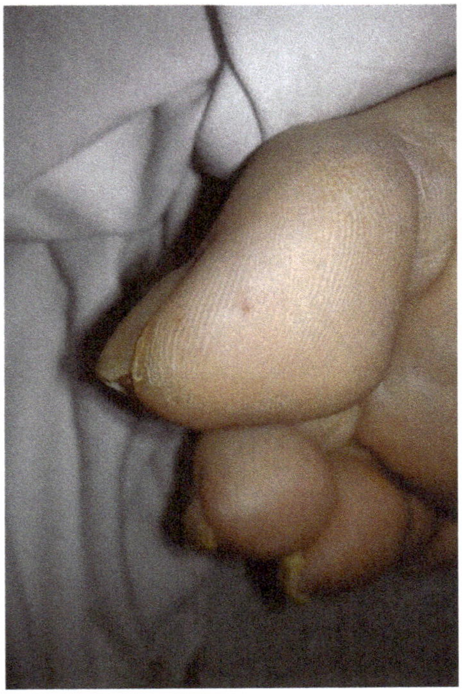

Figure 1: Right first toe with Janeway lesion (vascular emboli phenomena).

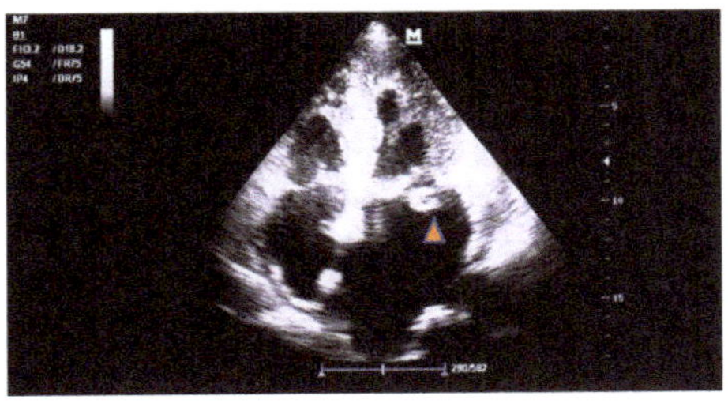

Figure 2: Arrowhead: TTE showing a mobile mass on the posterior leaflet of the mitral valve consistent with a vegetation.

2. Discussion

AU is a rare pathogen, first isolated in 1953 found in lobsters and thought to be of no clinical significance. It was until 1967 when it was first described to cause infection in humans [1]. This organism is a gram-positive, catalase-negative growing coccus in clusters that belongs to a bacterial group referred to as Aerococcus-like organisms (ALO) [2]. It has been associated with UTI mainly, nevertheless there are reports that identify it as the culprit of blood stream infections and endocarditis. Due to difficulties in the biochemical identification, the incidence of infections with this microorganism has likely been underestimated. Currently, it is thought to be the cause of 0.15 to 0.54% of UTIs [1]; additionally, it is responsible for 0.03 to 0.05% of blood stream infections (BSI). There is not enough data regarding the incidence of AU endocarditis as there have been only 45 reports in English literature. Advanced age (>65 years) and underlying urologic conditions are the best-known risk factors for UTI and, potentially, BSI [3] and endocarditis. Both sexes are equally affected [4, 5].

The diagnosis is usually challenging due to the rarity of this pathogen. It is commonly mistaken with Staphylococcus sp. and even Streptococcus viridians; for this reason, molecular diagnostic techniques are often needed to identify it. Testing for leucine aminopeptidase, which is positive only for AU, can be used to differentiate it with Staphylococcus [6]. Secure identification also relies on genetic techniques like 16S ribosomal subunit sequencing or mass spectroscopic methods such as MALDI-TOF [7]. To date, there are no guidelines that recommend starting with any of these modalities, even in the presence of the above risk factors, as they are nonspecific, so the diagnostic algorithms remain the same as for the rest of the pathogens.

Due to the current lack of controlled scientific trials and lack of formalized treatment guidelines, therapy is often empiric and guided by expert opinion. In an effort to standardize a treatment, Yabes et al. in 2018 [8] compiled the reported cases and therapies in literature and found that treatment regimens for AU have largely relied on beta-lactams, with the possible addition of synergistic aminoglycosides for endocarditis. In vitro studies regarding the antibiotic susceptibilities of AU have shown susceptibility to amoxicillin, cefotaxime, ceftriaxone, doxycycline, linezolid, meropenem, penicillin, rifampin, and vancomycin. It had variable resistance to clindamycin, erythromycin, and levofloxacin [9–11]. It is, however, inherently resistant to sulfonamides and fluoroquinolones [10]. The duration of treatment vary from ten days for UTI and phlegmon to 14 to 28 days for BSI and 42 days (6 weeks) for endocarditis [8]. It is important to mention that treatment for the latter very commonly includes surgical intervention as well, but indications are the same as for other etiologies.

Overall mortality of AU infections, including UTI and BSI, has been shown to be equivalent to that of other etiologies. For endocarditis in particular, a higher rate of complications and mortality has been described, with 27% more when compared to other causes. It is thought that this could be associated with an older patient population with multiple other comorbidities, making their surgical profile highly unfavorable, and dependent on medical management only [8].

3. Literature Review

Between 2000 and 2012, the incidence of endocarditis in the United States increased from 11 per 100,000 population to 15 per 100,000 population [12, 13]. Nowadays, the precise incidence is difficult to ascertain because case definitions have varied over time between authors and between clinical centers. In addition, the presence of predisposing conditions such as rheumatic heart disease or injection drug use is variable over time and between regions and in low- and high-income countries [14, 15].

A literature search on PubMed, Web of Science, Cochrane, and Google Scholar databases revealed 45 cases of AU endocarditis in English literature (Table 1). We present a summary with a mathematical analysis and

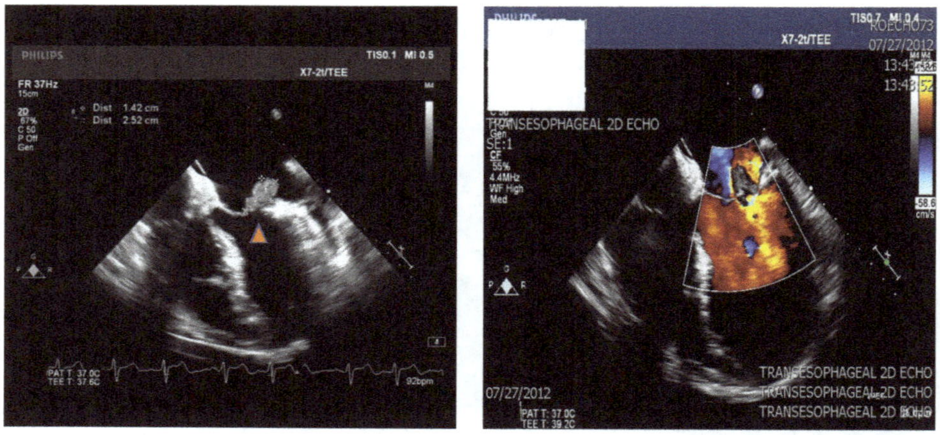

(a) (b)

FIGURE 3: (a) TEE image of vegetation on posterior leaflet of mitral valve, measuring "1.42 cm × 2.52 cm" (arrowhead). (b) TEE image with evidence of blood flow regurgitation with Doppler into the left atrium in the setting of the mitral valve posterior leaflet vegetation.

calculations involving all reports in an effort to identify patterns regarding risk factors, clinical course, treatment modalities, and prognosis.

3.1. General Statistics. The general statistics are as follows:

(i) 85% (39) of the patients were male and only 15% female (7)

(ii) The average age was 72 years, with the youngest patient being 42 years and the oldest 91 years (2)

(iii) Of the forty patients, only three had no reported associated risk factors or comorbidities (6.5%), 93.5% did have risk factors which are as follows:

  (a) 69% of the patients had urologic comorbidities while only four patients (9.5%) had an underlying known cardiac condition (one patient with aortic stenosis, one patient with atrial septal defect, and one patient with pacemaker

  (b) Five patients were also reported to have a non-urologic associated malignancy (11.9%)

  (c) Only two patients (4.6%) had a different risk factor other than the ones mentioned above, a case with untreated hepatitis C and other case with liver failure (2.3% each)

(iv) Regarding urologic risk factors:

  (a) Current or recent presence of indwelling urinary catheter was seen in eight patients (19%), benign prostatic hypertrophy was also seen in eight patients (19%)

  (b) Recurrent UTIs were seen in three patients (6.9%), same goes for urethral strictures (three patients—6.9%)

  (c) History of cystoscopy was found in two patients (4.6%), phimosis was also reported in two patients only (4.6%)

  (d) Transurethral resection of the prostate, ureteral stent, and suprapubic catheter were seen with one patient each (2.3% per patient)

(v) In terms of affected valve: 43.4% (20 patients) had involvement of the mitral valve and the same percentage for aortic valve. One patient, 2.3%, had both valves affected; one patient had aortic and tricuspid valves affected. Finally, one patient (2.3%) had a pacemaker. Affected valves were not reported in 3 patients (6.5%)

(vi) For surgical intervention, in 20 cases, it was not reported whether the patient had surgery or not; for the 26 cases, that it was. Statistics are as follows:

  (a) 14 patients (53.8%) did not have cardiac valve surgery

  (b) 12 patients (46.2%) did have cardiac valve surgery

  (c) 80% of the patients that received surgery survived

(vii) Regarding antibiotic treatment: 98% of the patients received antibiotics. In one patient (2%), treatment was not reported

  (a) In 100% of the cases, a beta-lactam was used

    (1) In 5 patients (11.1%), it was used as a single therapy

    (2) In the rest of the patients (91%), it was used in combination: in 38 patients (83%), it was combined with an aminoglycoside;

Table 1: Summary of clinical characteristics of the forty-five AU endocarditis cases reported in English literature as well as our case.

Case	Age (years)	Gender	Comorbidities or risk factors	Affected valve	Surgery	Antibiotic regimen and duration	Survived?
1 [16]	69	M	Cystoscopy	Aortic	No	Beta-lactam and aminoglycoside for 6 weeks	Yes
2 [17]	54	M	Phimosis	Mitral	Yes	Beta-lactam for 6 weeks	Yes
3 [18]	43	M	Untreated hepatitis C	Aortic	No	Beta-lactam and aminoglycoside for 5 days	No
4 [19]	68	M	Indwelling urinary catheter	Aortic	Yes	Beta-lactam 6 weeks and aminoglycoside for 2 weeks	Yes
5 [20]	80	M	Nonurologic malignancy	Aortic	Yes	Beta-lactam for 2 weeks	Yes
6 [21]	77	M	Benign prostatic hypertrophy	Aortic	No	Beta-lactam and vancomycin; duration not reported	No
7 [22]	68	M	Benign prostatic hypertrophy	Mitral	No	Beta-lactam for 3 weeks; oral aminoglycoside duration not reported	Yes
8 [23]	75	M	Cystoscopy	Aortic	Yes	Beta-lactam and aminoglycoside for 6 weeks	Yes
9 [24]	89	M	Transurethral resection of prostate	Mitral	No	Beta-lactam and aminoglycoside for 7 days	No
10 [25]	81	M	Recurrent UTIs	Aortic	No	Beta-lactam 2 weeks and aminoglycoside for 8 days	No
11 [26]	42	M	None	Aortic	Yes	Beta-lactam and aminoglycoside for 6 weeks	Yes
12 [27]	49	M	Not reported	Aortic	Not reported	Beta-lactam and aminoglycoside; duration not reported	Yes
13 [28]	54	M	Urethral stricture	Tricuspid and aortic	No	Beta-lactam and aminoglycoside; duration not reported	No
14 [29]	69	M	Nonurologic malignancy	Aortic	Yes	Beta-lactam for 12 weeks	Yes
15 [30]	62	M	Benign prostatic hypertrophy	Mitral and aortic	Yes	Beta-lactam and rifampin for 6 weeks and aminoglycoside for 2 weeks	Yes
16 [31]	78	M	Aortic stenosis	Aortic	No	Beta-lactam and aminoglycoside for 10 days	No
17 [32]	74	M	Benign prostatic hypertrophy	Mitral	Yes	Beta-lactam and aminoglycoside for 4 weeks	No
18 [33]	81	M	Benign prostatic hypertrophy	Mitral	No	Beta-lactam and aminoglycoside for 6 weeks	Yes
19 [33]	78	M	Indwelling urinary catheter	Aortic	No	Beta-lactam; duration not reported	No
20 [33]	87	M	Benign prostatic hypertrophy	Mitral	No	Not reported	No
21 [33]	78	F	Ureteral stent	Aortic	No	Beta-lactam and vancomycin for 2 weeks	No
22 [34]	48	M	Atrial septal defect	Mitral	No	Beta-lactam and aminoglycoside; duration not reported	Yes
23 [34]	79	F	Recurrent UTIs	Aortic	No	Beta-lactam and aminoglycoside for 6 weeks	Yes
24 [35]	91	M	Indwelling urinary catheter	Mitral	Not reported	Beta-lactam for 4 weeks and aminoglycoside for 10 days	Yes
25 [35]	91	M	Benign prostatic hypertrophy	Mitral	Not reported	Beta-lactam 4 weeks and aminoglycoside for 10 days	Yes
26 [35]	89	F	Not reported	Mitral	Not reported	Beta-lactam 4 weeks and aminoglycoside for 10 days	Yes
27 [35]	86	M	Urethral stricture	Aortic	Not reported	Beta-lactam 4 weeks and aminoglycoside for 10 days	Yes
28 [35]	83	M	Urethral stricture	Mitral	Not reported	Beta-lactam 4 weeks and aminoglycoside for 10 days	Yes
29 [35]	80	F	Not reported	Mitral	Not reported	Beta-lactam 4 weeks and aminoglycoside for 10 days	Yes
30 [35]	77	M	Not reported	Aortic	Not reported	Beta-lactam for 4 weeks and aminoglycoside for 10 days	Yes
31 [35]	75	M	Benign prostatic hypertrophy	Mitral	Not reported	Beta-lactam for 4 weeks and aminoglycoside for 10 days	Yes
32 [35]	74	M	Suprapubic catheter	Not reported	Not reported	Beta-lactam for 4 weeks and aminoglycoside for 10 days	Yes
33 [35]	65	M	Indwelling urinary catheter	Mitral	Not reported	Beta-lactam for 4 weeks and aminoglycoside for 10 days	Yes
34 [35]	53	M	None	Aortic	Not reported	Beta-lactam 4 weeks and aminoglycoside for 10 days	Yes

Table 1: Continued.

Case	Age (years)	Gender	Comorbidities or risk factors	Affected valve	Surgery	Antibiotic regimen and duration	Survived?
35 [35]	49	F	Intermittent urinary catheter	Aortic	Not reported	Beta-lactam for 4 weeks and aminoglycoside for 10 days	Yes
36 [35]	81	M	Indwelling urinary catheter	Mitral	Not reported	Beta-lactam for 4 weeks and aminoglycoside for 10 days	Yes
37 [35]	74	F	Nonurologic malignancy	Not reported	Not reported	Beta-lactam for 4 weeks and aminoglycoside for 10 days	Yes
38 [36]	87	M	Nonurologic malignancy	Mitral	Not reported	Beta-lactam and aminoglycoside; duration not reported	No
39 [36]	77	M	Liver failure	Aortic	Not reported	Beta-lactam and aminoglycoside; duration not reported	Yes
40 [36]	83	M	Indwelling urinary catheter	Mitral	Not reported	Beta-lactam and aminoglycoside; duration not reported	Yes
41 [36]	73	M	Suprapubic catheter	Not reported	Not reported	Beta-lactam and aminoglycoside; duration not reported	No
42 [36]	88	F	Aortic stenosis	Aortic	Not reported	Beta-lactam and aminoglycoside; duration not reported	Yes
43 [8]	43	M	Indwelling urinary catheter	Mitral	Yes	Beta-lactam and aminoglycoside for 6 weeks	Yes
44 [37]	49	M	Phimosis and recurrent UTIs	Mitral	Yes	Beta-lactam and aminoglycoside for 5 days	No
45 [38]	84	M	Pacemaker and nonurologic malignancy	Pacemaker	Yes	Beta-lactam for 6 weeks	Yes
Present case	55	M	None	Mitral	Yes	Beta-lactam and aminoglycoside for 6 weeks	Yes

in 2 patients (4.5%), it was used along vancomycin; and in 1 patient (2.2%), it was used in combination with aminoglycoside and rifampin

(b) In patients that survived, the duration of beta-lactam ranged from 2 to 12 weeks; meanwhile, aminoglycoside ranged from 1 to 6 weeks. Vancomycin was used for 2 weeks in 1 patient (in the other one duration was not reported), and finally rifampin was used for 6 weeks

3.2. Mortality Statistics. The mortality statistics are as follows:

(i) Overall mortality was 28.2% (13 patients)

 (a) 92.3% (12) were male and only 1 female

 (b) 84.6% (11) were over 50 years old (average age: 71 years)

(ii) In terms of risk factors:

 (a) 69.2% (9) had an underlying urologic condition

 (b) 1 patient (7.6%) had underlying aortic stenosis, and 1 patient (7.6%) had nonurologic malignancy

 (c) In 2 patients, the underlying comorbidities were not reported

(iii) Most patients that eventually died did not undergo surgical intervention, only 2 patients (15%) had it

(iv) Regarding affected valve:

 (a) 46.8% (6 patients) had aortic valve endocarditis

 (b) 38.4% (5 patients) had mitral valve endocarditis

 (c) 1 patient (7.6%) had both aortic and tricuspid involvement

 (d) In 1 patient (7.6%), the affected valve was not reported

3.3. Analysis. As seen in previous reports, most of the patients were elderly males. The majority had underlying urologic comorbidities; baseline cardiac anomalies like valvular diseases were very seldom seen. Additionally, mitral and aortic valves were equally affected.

All of the patients received treatment with beta-lactam antibiotics. In most of them, aminoglycosides were used in combination; other less commonly used add-on therapies were vancomycin and rifampin. More than half of the patients did not undergo surgery, as they were deemed as poor surgical candidates or did not meet criteria for intervention. Interestingly enough, 100% of the patients that received beta-lactam as monotherapy in combination with surgery survived.

Aerococcus urinae endocarditis is associated with a 28% mortality from our calculations, deeming a high grade of aggressiveness to this microorganism. It is unclear at this time if this high mortality is due to the bacteria itself or the fact that most of the patients were elderly and had other comorbidities. Lack of surgical intervention in most patients possibly plays a role as 80% of the patients that underwent a surgical procedure survived. An underlying urologic condition was commonly seen in the patients that died, although it was recurrently seen in patients that survived as well. The affected valve does not seem to have an impact on mortality.

4. Conclusion

AU is an extremely unusual cause of human disease; it has been described to cause urinary tract infections, blood stream infections, and infective endocarditis. We do believe, however, that its actual incidence is higher than reported. Reliable data regarding clinical presentation, diagnosis, and potential treatments of AU are becoming more available to health-care workers making this a promising era in its management. With this case report and literature review, we aim to add critical data to the current medical literature regarding this rare pathogen. We urge health-care professionals to share related experiences in order to build up literature and treat patients in a more appropriate manner; at this time evidently, randomized studies are univariably defiant as with any rare disorder.

References

[1] A. Higgins and T. Garg, "*Aerococcus urinae*: an emerging cause of urinary tract infection in older adults with multimorbidity and urologic cancer," *Urology Case Reports*, vol. 13, pp. 24-25, 2017.

[2] R. E. O. Williams, A. Hirch, and S. T. Cowan, "*Aerococcus*, a new bacterial genus," *Journal of General Microbiology*, vol. 8, no. 3, pp. 475–480, 1953.

[3] P. M. H. Schuur, M. E. E. . Kasteren, L. Sabbe, M. C. Vos, M. M. P. C. Janssens, and A. G. M. Buiting, "Urinary tract infections with *Aerococcus urinae* in the south of the Netherlands," *European Journal of Clinical Microbiology and Infectious Diseases*, vol. 16, no. 12, pp. 871–875, 1997.

[4] E. Senneby, A. C. Petersson, and M. Rasmussen, "Clinical and microbiological features of bacteraemia with *Aerococcus urinae*," *Clinical Microbiology and Infection*, vol. 18, no. 6, pp. 546–550, 2012.

[5] T. J. Cahill and B. D. Prendergast, "Infective endocarditis," *The Lancet*, vol. 387, no. 10021, pp. 882–893, 2016.

[6] K. L. Ruoff, "Miscellaneous catalase-negative, gram-positive cocci: emerging opportunists," *Journal of Clinical Microbiology*, vol. 40, no. 4, pp. 1129–1133, 2002.

[7] M. Rasmussen, "Aerococci and aerococcal infections," *Journal of Infection*, vol. 66, no. 6, pp. 467–474, 2013.

[8] J. M. Yabes, S. Perdikis, D. B. Graham, and A. Markelz, "A rare case of Aerococcus urinae infective endocarditis in an atypically young male: case report and review of the literature," *BMC Infectious Diseases*, vol. 18, no. 1, p. 522, 2018.

[9] C. Hirzel, L. Hirzberger, H. Furrer, and A. Endimiani, "Bactericidal activity of penicillin, ceftriaxone, gentamicin and daptomycin alone and in combination against *Aerococcus urinae*," *International Journal of Antimicrobial Agents*, vol. 48, no. 3, pp. 271–276, 2016.

[10] Clinical and Laboratory Standards Institute, *Performance Standards for Antimicrobial Susceptibility Testing*, CLSI Supplement M100S, 26th edition, 2016.

[11] R. M. Humphries and J. A. Hindler, "*In vitro* antimicrobial susceptibility of *Aerococcus urinae*," *Journal of Clinical Microbiology*, vol. 52, no. 6, pp. 2177–2180, 2014.

[12] S. Pant, N. J. Patel, A. Deshmukh et al., "Trends in infective endocarditis incidence, microbiology, and valve replacement in the United States from 2000 to 2011," *Journal of the American College of Cardiology*, vol. 65, no. 19, pp. 2070–2076, 2015.

[13] N. Toyoda, J. Chikwe, S. Itagaki, A. C. Gelijns, D. H. Adams, and N. N. Egorova, "Trends in infective endocarditis in California and New York State, 1998-2013," *JAMA*, vol. 317, no. 16, pp. 1652–1660, 2017.

[14] I. M. Tleyjeh, A. Abdel-Latif, H. Rahbi et al., "A systematic review of population-based studies of infective endocarditis," *Chest*, vol. 132, pp. 1025–1035, 2007.

[15] J. Ambrosioni, M. Hernandez-Meneses, A. Téllez et al., "The changing epidemiology of infective endocarditis in the twenty-first century," *Current Infectious Disease Reports*, vol. 19, no. 5, p. 21, 2017.

[16] H. Tathireddy, S. Settypalli, and J. J. Farrell, "A rare case of Aerococcus urinae infective endocarditis," *Journal of Community Hospital Internal Medicine Perspectives*, vol. 7, no. 2, pp. 126–129, 2017.

[17] K. D. Kotkar, S. M. Said, H. Michelena, B. Wanta, M. D. Fritock, and L. M. Baddour, "Right coronary artery septic embolization secondary to *Aerococcus urinae* native mitral valve endocarditis," *The Annals of Thoracic Surgery*, vol. 102, no. 4, pp. e295–e297, 2016.

[18] W. Gritsch, M. Nagl, J. Hausdorfer, A. Gschwendtner, C. Pechlaner, and C. J. Wiedermann, "Septicaemia and endomyocarditis caused by Aerococcus urinae," *Wiener Klinische Wochenschrift*, vol. 111, no. 11, pp. 446-447, 1999.

[19] A. Alozie, C. Yerebakan, B. Westphal, G. Steinhoff, and A. Podbielski, "Culture-negative infective endocarditis of the aortic valve due to *Aerococcus urinae*: a rare aetiology," *Heart, Lung & Circulation*, vol. 21, no. 4, pp. 231–233, 2012.

[20] E. Ho, J. Coveliers, B. J. Amsel et al., "A case of endocarditis due to Aerococcus urinae," *The Journal of Heart Valve Disease*, vol. 19, no. 2, pp. 264–266, 2010.

[21] M. Kass, B. Toye, and J. P. Veinot, "Fatal infective endocarditis due to *Aerococcus urinae*—case report and review of literature," *Cardiovascular Pathology*, vol. 17, no. 6, pp. 410–412, 2008.

[22] A. Tekin, G. Tekin, T. Turunç, Z. Demiroğlu, and O. Kızılkılıç, "Infective endocarditis and spondylodiscitis in a patient due to *Aerococcus urinae*: first report," *International Journal of Cardiology*, vol. 115, no. 3, pp. 402-403, 2007.

[23] C. Ebnother, M. Altwegg, J. Gottschalk, J. D. Seebach, and A. Kronenberg, "*Aerococcus urinae* endocarditis: case report and review of the literature," *Infection*, vol. 30, no. 5, pp. 310–313, 2002.

[24] P. M. H. Schuur, L. Sabbe, A. J. van der Wouw, G. J. Montagne, and A. G. M. Buiting, "Three cases of serious infection caused by *Aerococcus urinae*," *European Journal of Clinical Microbiology and Infectious Diseases*, vol. 18, no. 5, pp. 368–371, 1999.

[25] R. L. Skov, M. Klarlund, and S. Thorsen, "Fatal endocarditis due to *Aerococcus urinae*," *Diagnostic Microbiology and Infectious Disease*, vol. 21, no. 4, pp. 219–221, 1995.

[26] M. Gompelman, W. Rozemeijer, and W. Kortmann, "A life-threatening complication of an ordinary urinary tract infection?," *The Netherlands Journal of Medicine*, vol. 72, no. 9, 2014.

[27] K. Westmoreland, D. C. Halstead, and P. V. DuBose, "Infectious endocarditis in 49-year-old man and discussion of phenotypic characteristics of *Aerococcus urinae* and Viridans streptococci," *Laboratory Medicine*, vol. 45, no. 3, pp. e101–e103, 2014.

[28] B. Siddiqui, B. Chaucer, M. Chevenon, D. Fernandes, M. Rana, and J. Nfonoyim, "*Aerococcus urinae* associated aortic and tricuspid valve infective endocarditis," *IDCases*, vol. 4, pp. 30-31, 2016.

[29] M. Slany, T. Freiberger, P. Pavlik, and J. Cerny, "Culture-negative infective endocarditis caused by Aerococcus urinae," *The Journal of Heart Valve Disease*, vol. 16, no. 2, pp. 203–205, 2007.

[30] D. Bruegger, A. Beiras-Fernandez, F. Weis, M. Weis, and F. Kur, "Extracorporeal support in a patient with cardiogenic shock due to Aerococcus urinae endocarditis," *The Journal of Heart Valve Disease*, vol. 18, no. 4, pp. 418–420, 2009.

[31] B. Kristensen and G. Nielsen, "Endocarditis caused by *Aerococcus urinae*, a newly recognized pathogen," *European Journal of Clinical Microbiology and Infectious Diseases*, vol. 14, no. 1, pp. 49–51, 1995.

[32] S. Melnick, S. Nazir, R. Hingorani, and P. Wexler, "*Aerococcus urinae*, a rare cause of infective endocarditis," *BML Case Reports*, vol. 2016, 2016.

[33] M. F. C. de Jong, R. Soetekouw, R. W. ten Kate, and D. Veenendaal, "*Aerococcus urinae*: severe and fatal bloodstream infections and endocarditis," *Journal of Clinical Microbiology*, vol. 48, no. 9, pp. 3445–3447, 2010.

[34] R. Zbinden, P. Santanam, L. Hunziker, B. Leuzinger, and A. von Graevenitz, "Endocarditis due to *Aerococcus urinae*: diagnostic tests, fatty acid composition and killing kinetics," *Infection*, vol. 27, no. 2, pp. 122–124, 1999.

[35] T. Sunnerhagen, B. Nilson, L. Olaison, and M. Rasmussen, "Clinical and microbiological features of infective endocarditis caused by aerococci," *Infection*, vol. 44, no. 2, pp. 167–173, 2016.

[36] E. Senneby, L. Goransson, S. Weiber, and M. Rasmussen, "A population-based study of aerococcal bacteraemia in the MALDI-TOF MS-era," *European Journal of Clinical Microbiology & Infectious Diseases*, vol. 35, no. 5, pp. 755–762, 2016.

[37] D. Adomavicius, M. Bock, C.-F. Vahl, and E. Siegel, "Aerococcus *urinae* mitral valve endocarditis-related stroke: a case report and literature review," *Journal of Investigative Medicine High Impact Case Reports*, vol. 6, 2018.

[38] S. Samuelsson, C. Kennergren, and M. Rasmussen, "A case of pacemaker endocarditis caused by *Aerococcus urinae*," *Case Reports in Infectious Diseases*, vol. 2018, Article ID 9128560, 3 pages, 2018.

5

Rothia dentocariosa Endocarditis in an Unsuspecting Host: A Case Report

Stacy Willner, Zaid Imam, and Ismail Hader

Beaumont, 3601 W 13 Mile Road, Royal Oak, MI 48073, USA

Correspondence should be addressed to Stacy Willner; stacy.willner@beaumont.org

Academic Editor: Tayfun Sahin

Rothia dentocariosa, a gram-positive coccobacillus, is a commensal bacterium that is part of the oropharynx and respiratory tract. In the past, it was known to be a cause for periodontal disease, but in recent years, *Rothia dentocariosa* has been found to be the cause of several other infectious entities, of which endocarditis is the most predominant. We present the case of a healthy 62-year-old female who, after undergoing routine dental cleaning two months prior, developed subacute bacterial endocarditis of the mitral valve, with subsequent cerebral septic emboli causing an occipital hemorrhagic cerebrovascular accident, all secondary to *Rothia dentocariosa*.

1. Introduction

Endocarditis is defined as inflammation of the endocardium, which consists of the inner lining of the heart and heart valves. Bacterial infection remains the most common etiology and is most commonly caused by staphylococcus, streptococcus, and enterococcus species. While a *Rothia dentocariosa* infection predominantly causes endocarditis, having endocarditis secondary to *Rothia dentocariosa* remains a rare entity, with few cases documented in medical literature. To this day, there remains no clear consensus on an optimal therapeutic regimen.

2. Case Report

A 62-year-old female with no significant past medical history presented to the emergency department in November of 2017 with complaints of arthralgias, most notably in her right knee, left shoulder, and bilateral thighs that made it difficult for her to ambulate. She was also admitted due to a headache that was triggered primarily by coughing. Vital signs on admission were as follows: a blood pressure of 202/90 mmHg, a heart rate of 137 bpm, a respiratory rate of 20, and a temperature of 36.6 Celsius. Physical exam revealed Janeway lesions. She was found to have a neutrophilic leukocytosis, with white blood cell count at 20.4 cells/mm^3 and neutrophils at 17.4 bil/L. Troponin was elevated at 1.85; this was deemed to be noncardiac in nature as the patient's pain was relieved with ibuprofen and her EKG showed no acute findings. ESR and CRP were elevated at 95 mm/hr and 24.8 mg/dL, respectively. A computed tomography of the brain showed a high-density mass in the right occipital lobe, with surrounding vasogenic edema. The patient continued to deny any visual changes or symptoms other than what was discussed above. An ophthalmologist was consulted to perform a dilated fundus exam, which was positive for small intraretinal hemorrhages that were deemed to be secondary to the patient's hypertension and less likely positive for Roth's spots. There was no evidence of disc edema. A brain MRI with and without gadolinium showed multiple small punctate bilateral areas of acute or subacute infarctions indicative of embolic phenomenon. The hemorrhagic area in the right occipital lobe was again identified, with subtle surrounding enhancement; the differential diagnosis consisted of neoplasm, vascular malformation, or embolic infarction with hemorrhagic conversion. A transthoracic 2D echo was without vegetation, so a transesophageal echo was ordered, and vegetation was shown on the posterior leaflet of the mitral valve. Two blood cultures from admission then came back positive for *Rothia dentocariosa*. Infectious disease was confirmed, and the patient's current antibiotics, which consisted of vancomycin and ceftriaxone, were switched to penicillin G on a continuous pump. The patient remained largely asymptomatic during her admission and was deemed to be stable for discharge from the hospital after a nine-day stay with penicillin G via a continuous pump for a total of six weeks and was planned for a follow-up MRI in three weeks. The repeat MRI came back showing new subacute strokes. The patient was reported, again, to be asymptomatic but was directed to come straight to the emergency department. A repeat transesophageal echo was done and showed the known vegetation on the mitral valve with new vegetation seen on the PICC line and an abscess between the mitral and aortic valves extending into the ascending aorta. The patient then requested transfer to another institution for further evaluation. A repeat transesophageal echo was completed at this outside institution which showed small anterior and posterior mitral leaflet vegetation with no significant destruction and no abscess. A cardiac MRI was then performed which showed a focal delayed enhancement in the apical inferior and lateral wall, likely secondary to coronary arterial embolization. The patient went on to complete the full six weeks of penicillin therapy, remained asymptomatic, and refused a mitral valve replacement. Her follow-up was continued in the cardiology clinic.

3. Discussion

Georg and Brown first created the genus "*Rothia*" in 1967; it was to include members of the family Actinomycetaceae, which resemble both *Nocardia* and *Actinomyces* but differ in the physiology and cell wall constituents. The first reported case of endocarditis secondary to *Rothia dentocariosa* was reported in 1978. Prior to that, *Rothia dentocariosa* had a well-established role in the oral flora, with only two more well known cases of infectivity: the first being the case of a periappendiceal abscess in a 19-year-old female in 1975 and the second being the case of a pilonidal cyst in a 17-year-old female in early 1978 [1].

To this day, *Rothia dentocariosa* is mostly recognized as a normal oral pathogen, with low pathogenicity. Infective endocarditis remains the most common manifestation of a *Rothia dentocariosa* infection. In 2002, Boudewijns et al. performed a review of all 20 cases of infective endocarditis secondary to *Rothia dentocariosa*. Of the 20 total cases, 18 had cardiac abnormalities, which predisposed them to endocarditis. The 2 cases without cardiac abnormalities had poor dental hygiene and/or extensive dental procedures, predisposing them to *Rothia dentocariosa* infections. 16 of the 20 patients were cured, with only 6 patients without any reported complications [2].

In 2011, another literature review, along with a case report, was published by Shakoor et al. It cited only two new cases of endocarditis due to *Rothia dentocariosa* since the first literature review in 2002, along with five cases of bacteremia without endocarditis and two cases of sepsis. One of the newly published endocarditis cases was written in Spanish and therefore unavailable, while the other case was about a 55-year-old male with baseline mitral valve prolapse and regurgitation who had undergone a dental extraction prior to the onset of his endocarditis. The high rate of complications reported in the first literature review was mentioned, even though the mortality rate for *Rothia dentocariosa* endocarditis had since remained low [3].

Since the abovementioned literature review in 2007, four new cases of infections due to *Rothia* spp. are found on a routine search in PubMed: one case of *Rothia dentocariosa*-associated peritonitis [4] and three cases of endocarditis, in which two were secondary to *Rothia dentocariosa* [5, 6] and one was secondary to *Rothia aeria* [7]. Of the two cases of endocarditis secondary to *Rothia dentocariosa*, one involved a 34-year-old male, an IV methamphetamine abuser [5], and the other a 58-year-old relatively healthy male [6]. In the case of the IV drug abuser, he originally presented with altered mental status, fever, tachycardia, hypertension, a new diastolic murmur, and new left-sided hemiparesis. On computed tomography of the brain, the patient was found to have new ischemic changes in the right middle cerebral artery territory. A transesophageal echo was then performed, in which large vegetation was seen on the aortic valve. Valve tissue was sent out for culture and came back positive for *Rothia dentocariosa*. The patient was treated for two weeks with ceftriaxone after valve replacement and had complete neurologic resolution [5]. The second case involves a patient who was diagnosed with presumptive endocarditis secondary to a new murmur and nonspecific prodromal symptoms by his PCP. Transesophageal echo revealed moderate-to-severe mitral regurgitation with a thickened and myxomatous mitral valve and a posterior flail leaflet, with no vegetation. The presence of *Rothia dentocariosa* in blood cultures was then confirmed, and the patient was sent home with penicillin G via a continuous pump. Two weeks after discharge, the patient woke up with complete loss of vision in his right eye. After evaluation, he was diagnosed with endogenous endophthalmitis, also secondary to *Rothia dentocariosa*. After full treatment, the patient returned to baseline with no residual deficits [6].

Complications secondary to *Rothia dentocariosa* are common and include, but are not limited to, cerebellar hemorrhages [8], cerebral embolism [9], intracranial hemorrhages [10], vertebral osteomyelitis [11], aortic root abscess [12], abdominal aneurysm [13], perivalvular abscess [14], and brain abscess [15].

The current treatment for *Rothia dentocariosa* endocarditis consists of a 4-6-week regimen of penicillin, with or without gentamicin, or monotherapy with ceftriaxone [5]. In 2014, Ramanan et al. published "Rothia Bacteremia: a 10-Year Experience at Mayo Clinic, Rochester, Minnesota." 67 patients from 2002 to 2012 with blood cultures positive for *Rothia* spp. were studied and analyzed. Antimicrobial susceptibility was performed on 21% of the isolates; all were susceptible to vancomycin and most were susceptible to beta-lactams; however, 4 were resistant to oxacillin. In the end, it was determined that more data is needed to develop a standard of care for treating *Rothia* spp. [16].

In conclusion, the presented case was a healthy 62-year-old female, who, despite any known risk factors, developed endocarditis secondary to *Rothia dentocariosa*.

She sustained numerous subacute strokes secondary to cerebral embolization, while remaining largely asymptomatic. She was successfully treated with penicillin G via a continuous pump for a total of weeks, with subsequent imaging showing almost complete recovery of the mitral valve. This case further proves that *Rothia dentocariosa* can cause endocarditis and should always be a consideration, even in the most unlikely hosts.

References

[1] J. Pape, C. Singer, T. E. Kiehn, B. J. Lee, and D. Armstrong, "Infective endocarditis caused by *Rothia dentocariosa*," *Annals of Internal Medicine*, vol. 91, no. 5, pp. 746-747, 1979.

[2] M. Boudewijns, K. Magerman, J. Verhaegen et al., "*Rothia dentocariosa*, endocarditis and mycotic aneurysms: case report and review of the literature," *Clinical Microbiology and Infection*, vol. 9, no. 3, pp. 222–229, 2003.

[3] S. Shakoor, N. Fasih, K. Jabeen, and B. Jamil, "*Rothia dentocariosa* endocarditis with mitral valve prolapse: case report and brief review," *Infection*, vol. 39, no. 2, pp. 177–179, 2011.

[4] T. C. Keng, K. P. Ng, L. P. Tan, Y. B. Chong, C. M. Wong, and S. K. Lim, "*Rothia dentocariosa* repeat and relapsing peritoneal dialysis-related peritonitis: a case report and literature review," *Renal Failure*, vol. 34, no. 6, pp. 804–806, 2012.

[5] M. Chowdhary, B. Farooqi, and R. Ponce-terashima, "*Rothia dentocariosa*: a rare cause of left-sided endocarditis in an intravenous drug user," *The American Journal of the Medical Sciences*, vol. 350, no. 3, pp. 239-240, 2015.

[6] D. Fridman, A. Chaudhry, J. Makaryus, K. Black, and A. N. Makaryus, "*Rothia dentocariosa* endocarditis: an especially rare case in a previously healthy man," *Texas Heart Institute Journal*, vol. 43, no. 3, pp. 255–257, 2016.

[7] R. Collarino, U. Vergeylen, C. Emeraud et al., "Mitral endocarditis due to *Rothia aeria* with cerebral haemorrhage and femoral mycotic aneurysms, first French description," *New Microbes and New Infections*, vol. 13, pp. 40–42, 2016.

[8] A. Sadhu, R. Loewenstein, and S. A. Klotz, "*Rothia dentocariosa* endocarditis complicated by multiple cerebellar hemorrhages," *Diagnostic Microbiology and Infectious Disease*, vol. 53, no. 3, pp. 239-240, 2005.

[9] M. N. Almuzara, A. L. Mariñansky, V. C. Valenzuela, and C. A. Vay, "Endocarditis due to *Rothia dentocariosa* complicated by septic cerebral embolism," *Enfermedades Infecciosas y Microbiología Clínica*, vol. 22, no. 4, pp. 255-256, 2004.

[10] J. C. Ricaurte, O. Klein, V. Labombardi, V. Martinez, A. Serpe, and M. Joy, "*Rothia dentocariosa* endocarditis complicated by multiple intracranial hemorrhages," *Southern Medical Journal*, vol. 94, no. 4, pp. 438–440, 2001.

[11] F. Llopis and J. Carratalà, "Vertebral osteomyelitis complicating *Rothia dentocariosa* endocarditis," *European Journal of Clinical Microbiology & Infectious Diseases*, vol. 19, no. 7, pp. 562-563, 2000.

[12] V. Ferraz, K. Mccarthy, D. Smith, and H. J. Koornhof, "*Rothia dentocariosa* endocarditis and aortic root abscess," *The Journal of Infection*, vol. 37, no. 3, pp. 292–295, 1998.

[13] A. J. L. Weersink, M. Rozenberg-Arska, P. W. Westerhof, and J. Verhoef, "Rothia dentocariosa endocarditis complicated by an abdominal aneurysm," *Clinical Infectious Diseases*, vol. 18, no. 3, pp. 489-490, 1994.

[14] E. J. Sudduth, J. D. Rozich, and W. E. Farrar, "Rothia dentocariosa endocarditis complicated by perivalvular abscess," *Clinical Infectious Diseases*, vol. 17, no. 4, pp. 772–775, 1993.

[15] J. H. Isaacson and R. T. Grenko, "*Rothia dentocariosa* endocarditis complicated by brain abscess," *The American Journal of Medicine*, vol. 84, no. 2, pp. 352–354, 1988.

[16] P. Ramanan, J. N. Barreto, D. R. Osmon, and P. K. Tosh, "*Rothia* bacteremia: a 10-year experience at Mayo Clinic, Rochester, Minnesota," *Journal of Clinical Microbiology*, vol. 52, no. 9, pp. 3184–3189, 2014.

6

Native Aortic and Tricuspid Valve Endocarditis Complicated by Embolic ST Elevation Myocardial Infarction

Mumtaz Zaman,[1] Richard Loynd,[2] and Anthony Donato[1]

[1]*Sidney Kimmel Medical College at Thomas Jefferson University, USA*
[2]*Tower Health System, USA*

Correspondence should be addressed to Richard Loynd; Richard.loynd@towerhealth.org

Academic Editor: Adam Torbicki

Acute myocardial infarction due to a coronary embolic event can occur as a complication of infective endocarditis in up to 2.9% of cases and can frequently be the presenting symptom. A 35-year-old female presented with 4 hours of typical chest pain and was found to have ST elevations in inferior leads as well as an elevated serum Troponin I of 8.29 ng/ml (normal: <0.06 ng/ml). Urgent cardiac catheterization revealed total occlusion of the right coronary artery without other coronary disease or collaterals. Following a failed attempt at thrombus extraction, a 3.0×38 mm bioabsorbable drug-eluting stent was placed. Echocardiography then revealed large mobile aortic valve vegetations with the largest measuring 1.4×1.7 cm, severe tricuspid regurgitation with a 1.1×0.5 cm mobile vegetation on the anterior leaflet along with a patent foramen ovale with right-to-left shunting. Blood cultures identified *Enterococcus faecalis* in 4 of 4 vials. The patient underwent urgent replacement of tricuspid and aortic valves as well as 6 weeks of IV antibiotics followed by chronic antibiotic suppression.

1. Introduction

Endocarditis continues to be the fourth most common life-threatening infection, accounting for 1.58 million disability life-years lost globally [1]. While symptoms of bacteremia, peripheral embolization, and vascular phenomena are the classic symptoms of endocarditis, cardiac embolic disease has been reported in up to 60% of patients in autopsy studies [2] and may present antemortem as acute myocardial infarction (AMI) in up to 2.9% [3]. Recognition of AMI secondary to embolic disease is critical, as it affects decisions on both pharmacologic and mechanical interventions.

2. Case

A 35-year-old female with a past medical history of type 1 diabetes mellitus, hypertension, and hyperlipidemia presented to emergency care with 4 hours of continuous sharp midsternal chest pain. At the time of admission, she admitted to intermittent issues with hyperglycemia over the last several weeks as well as night sweats and malaise but denied fever, weight loss, cough, nausea, vomiting, abdominal pain, dysuria, or vaginal discharge. There was no history of recent travel, cardiac abnormalities, dental procedures, or exposure to tobacco, alcohol, or illicit drugs. Surgical history was pertinent for a Cesarean section performed 3 months prior to admission complicated by postpartum hemorrhage from placental abruption. On exam, she was awake and alert with no respiratory distress. Her vital signs were BP 116/72 mmHg, pulse 97 bpm, temperature 99.7°F, and respiratory rate 24 breaths/minute on room air. The physical examination was normal except for a systolic ejection murmur at the left lower sternal border and a well-healed low transverse Cesarean section incision. Her lab data showed a WBC count of 10,500 c/mm^3 (normal: 4,800–10,800 c/mm^3), hemoglobin of 7.6 g/dl (normal: 12.0–16.0 g/dl), MCV 84.5 fl (normal: 80.0–9.0 fl), creatinine of 1.58 mg/dl (normal: 0.60–1.30 mg/dl), and Troponin I of 8.29 ng/ml (normal: <0.03 ng/ml). EKG demonstrated ST elevations in leads II, III, and aVF consistent with inferior acute myocardial infarction (Figure 1). She was taken emergently to the cardiac catheterization lab where she was noted to have a completely

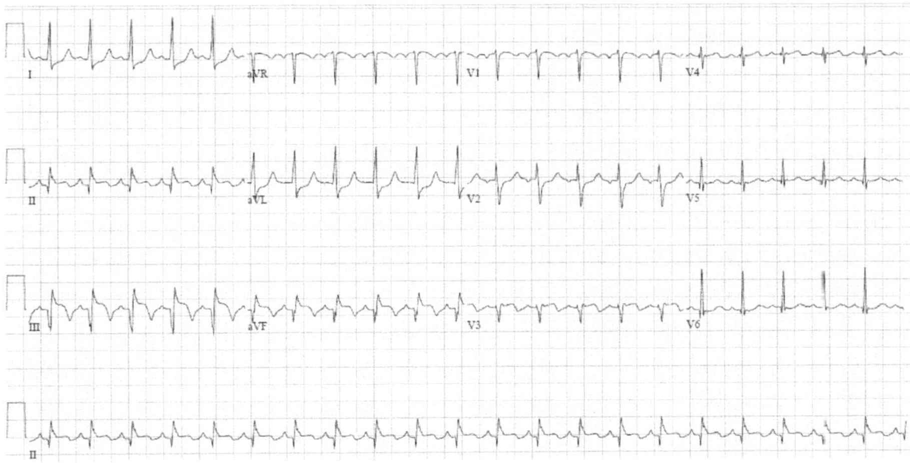

Figure 1: Electrocardiogram on admission showed inferior wall ST elevation myocardial infarction. ST elevations in leads II, III, and aVF.

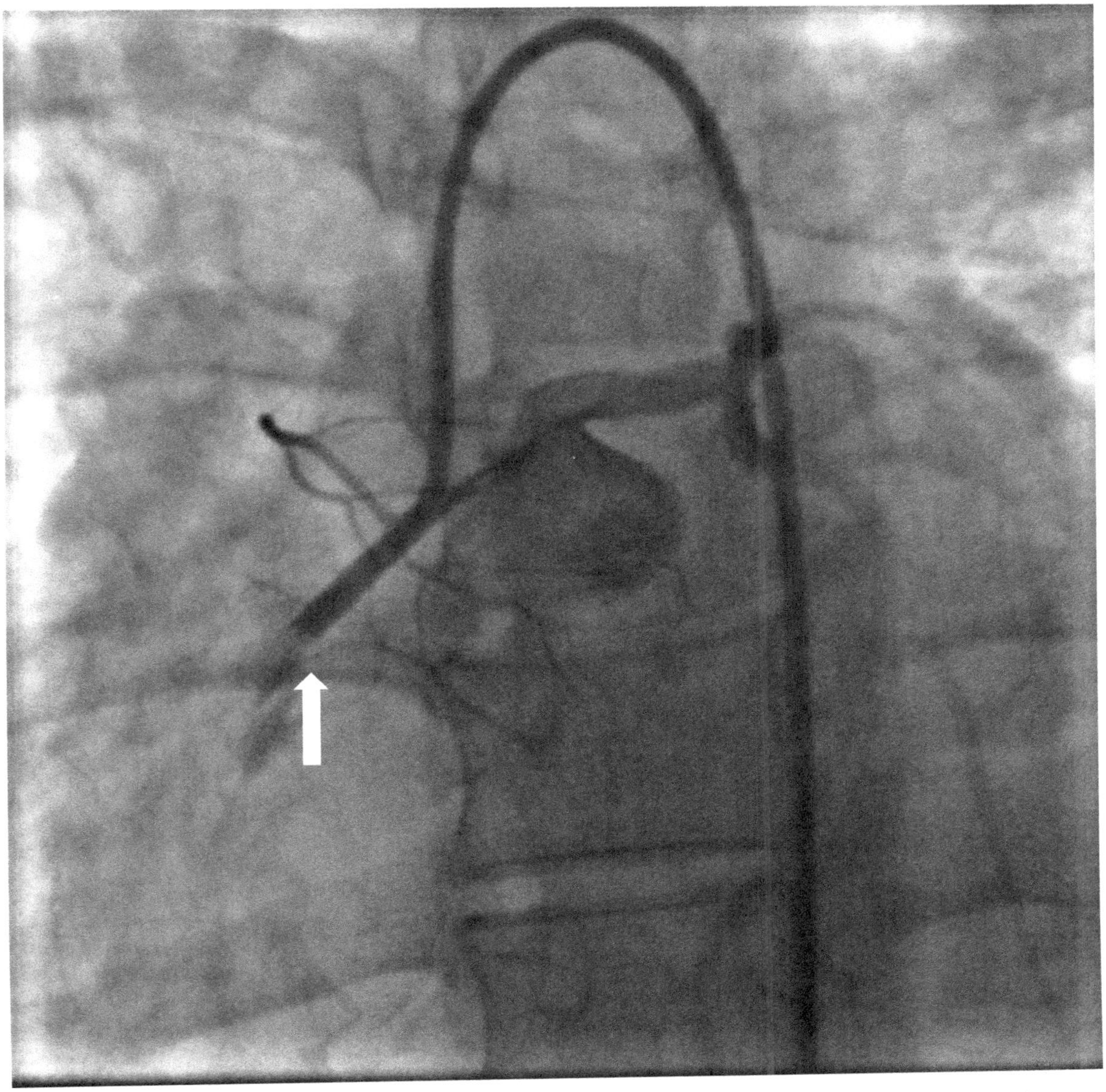

Figure 2: Coronary angiography with 100% occlusion (arrow) at the midsegment of the right coronary artery from infective endocarditis embolus.

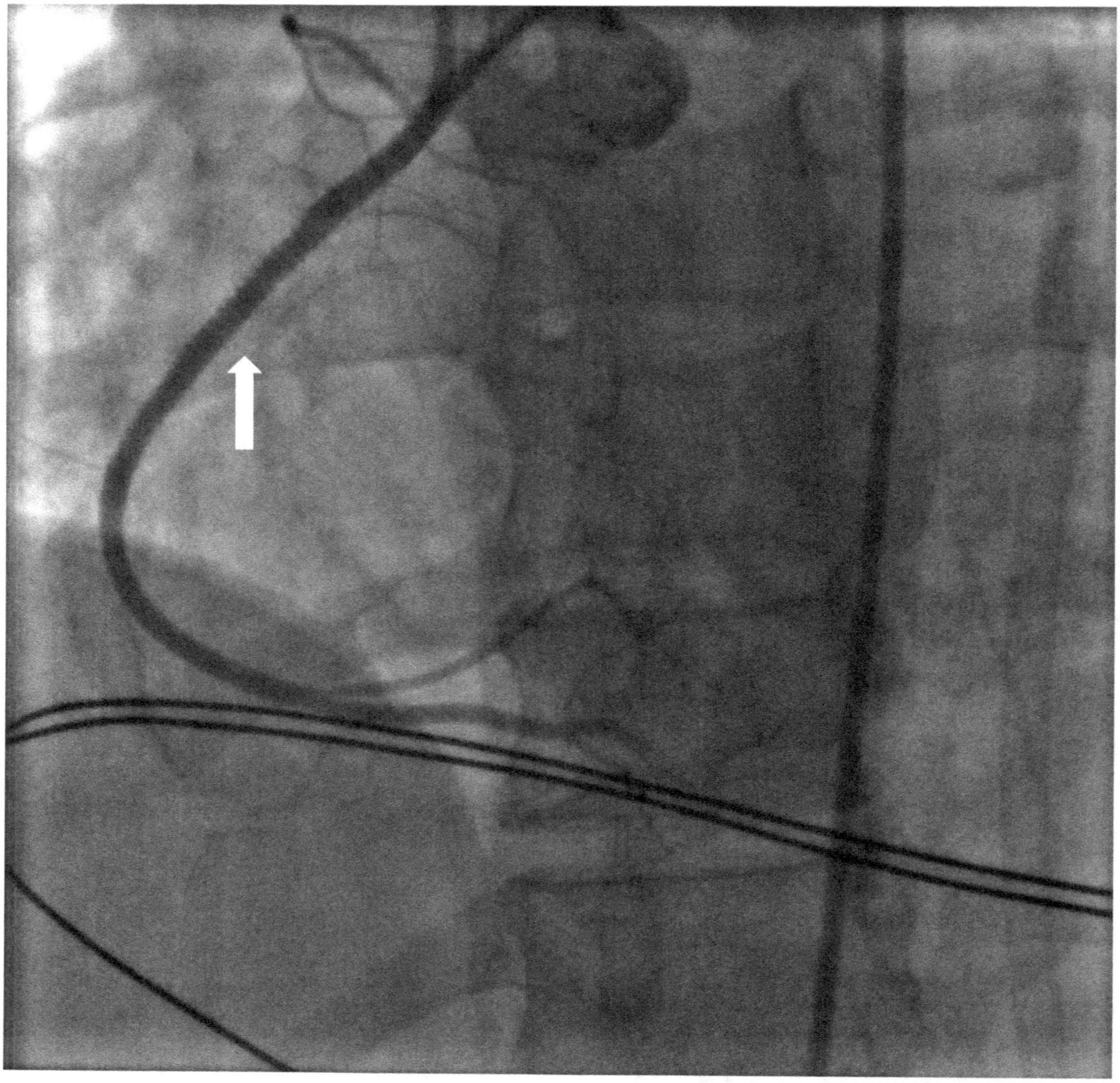

FIGURE 3: Coronary angiography after synergy 3.0 × 38 mm drug-eluting stent (arrow) placed in RCA with return of TIMI 3 flow.

occluded right coronary artery (RCA) (Figure 2). Consistency of the occlusion and absence of calcium suggested acute thrombus or embolus. An aspiration was attempted but was unsuccessful, so a 3.0 × 38 mm bioabsorbable drug-eluting stent was placed into the RCA along with balloon dilation of the proximal aspects of the posterior descending artery and distal RCA (Figure 3). Left-sided coronaries were angiographically normal (Figure 4). A postcatheterization transthoracic echocardiogram then revealed large mobile aortic valve vegetations on all 3 leaflets with the largest measuring 1.4 × 1.7 cm, moderate aortic insufficiency, severe tricuspid regurgitation with a 1.1 × 0.5 cm mobile vegetation on the anterior leaflet of tricuspid valve, and moderate mitral regurgitation without lesions. Ejection fraction was estimated at 50% with inferior and inferolateral wall hypo/akinesis. These findings were later confirmed with transesophageal echocardiogram, which also identified a patent foramen ovale with continuous right-to-left shunt (Figures 5 and 6). Chest CT imaging noted no embolic disease.

Blood cultures grew *Enterococcus faecalis* in 4 of 4 vials. Vancomycin and ceftriaxone were initiated and the patient was transferred to an outside facility where she underwent urgent cardiac surgery with the placement of bioprosthetic aortic and tricuspid valves, as well as PFO closure. Bioprosthetic valves were used as per patient preference. Cultures of removed cardiac tissue were positive for *Enterococcus faecalis*. No evidence of aortic root abscess was noted during the surgery. CT of the chest, abdomen, and pelvis was unrevealing for sepsis source. Endocarditis was ultimately attributed to prior placental abruption.

After valve replacement, she was continued on IV antibiotics. Blood cultures cleared, and on hospital day 15, she was discharged on IV ampicillin and ceftriaxone for synergy. Three weeks after discharge, a repeat ECHO revealed an ejection fraction of 47% and severe hypokinesis of the basal to mid inferior wall with normal function of both aortic and tricuspid bioprosthetic valves. After completing 6 weeks of IV antibiotic therapy, she was transitioned to chronic

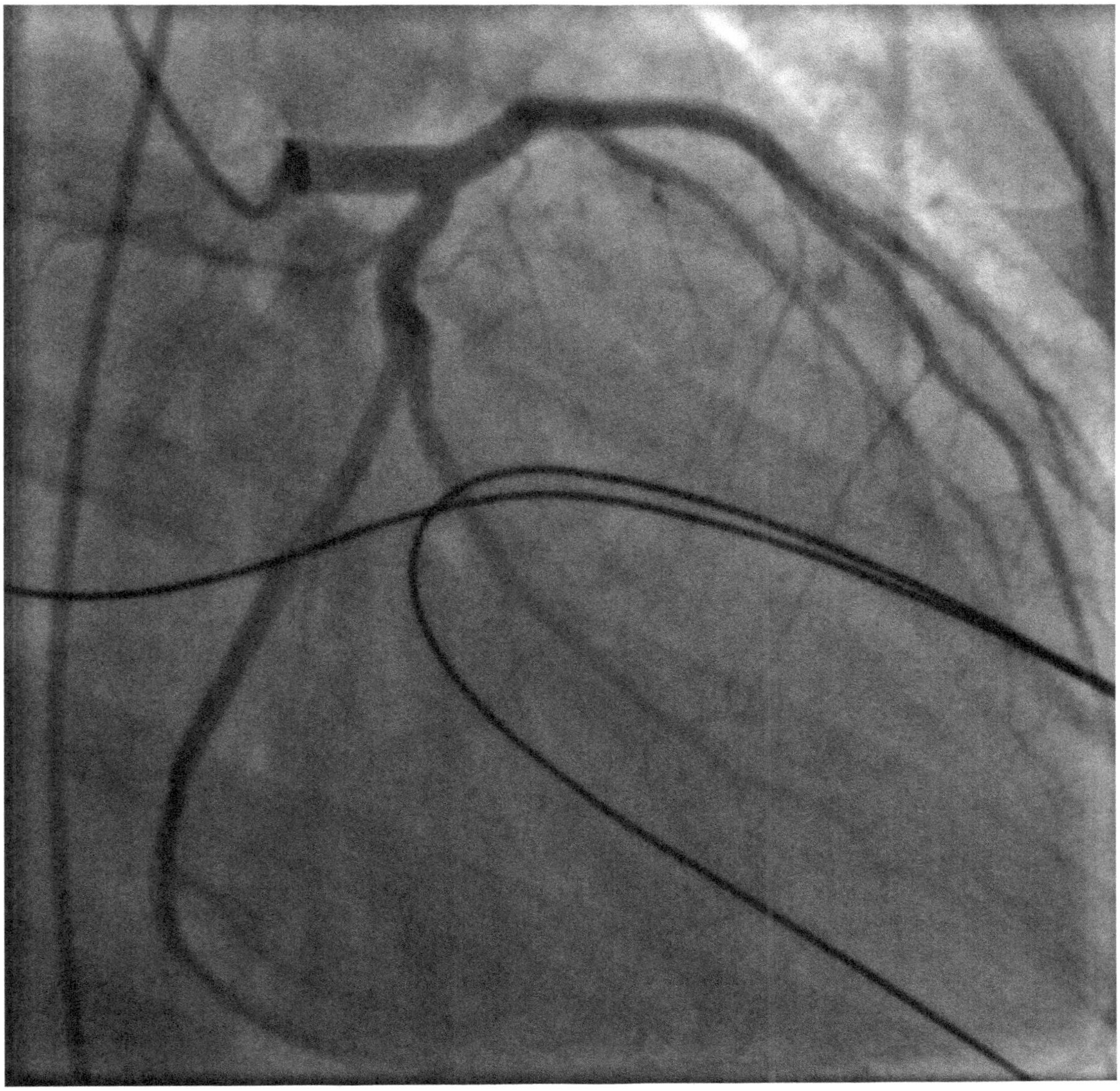

FIGURE 4: Coronary angiography showing widely patent left main, LAD, and circumflex, without evidence of chronic atherosclerosis.

oral suppression with amoxicillin/clavulanic acid. At phone follow-up 6 months later, the patient reported tolerating oral suppressive antibiotic with no clinical signs or symptoms of recurrent infection or complications.

3. Discussion

While most acute myocardial infarctions are secondary to atherosclerotic heart disease, the differential also includes less common nonatherosclerotic causes. These include vasculitis, congenital coronary artery abnormalities, vasospasm, coronary embolism, and coronary artery extrinsic compression by either abscess or pseudoaneurysm [2, 4]. Since the initial description of coronary emboli by Dr. Virchow in 1856 [5], embolic infarction due to infective endocarditis (IE) has remained an underrecognized entity. Sudden onset embolic infarctions are believed to occur in 2.9% of all cases of infective endocarditis [3] and are associated with very high rates of subsequent heart failure (73%) [4] and death (64%) [3].

Presentation with embolic AMI typically occurs within 2 weeks of a known diagnosis of endocarditis [6] but can be the initial presenting symptom in up to 54% of cases [4]. Identified risks for AMI in IE include larger (>1 cm) vegetations, mobile vegetations, and the presence of a valve ring aortic abscess [3, 7]. However, both aortic and mitral valves are associated with AMI. Our case was unusual in that we identified a tricuspid valve vegetation and a PFO with right-to-left shunting without pulmonary infarction or emboli. This suggests that the tricuspid valve was likely infected first, then bypassing the pulmonary circulation through the PFO, led to the infection of the aortic valve, which has only been suspected once before [8].

Clinical findings at cardiac catheterization that suggest embolic disease include abrupt and complete occlusion in a single coronary artery, especially in the absence of

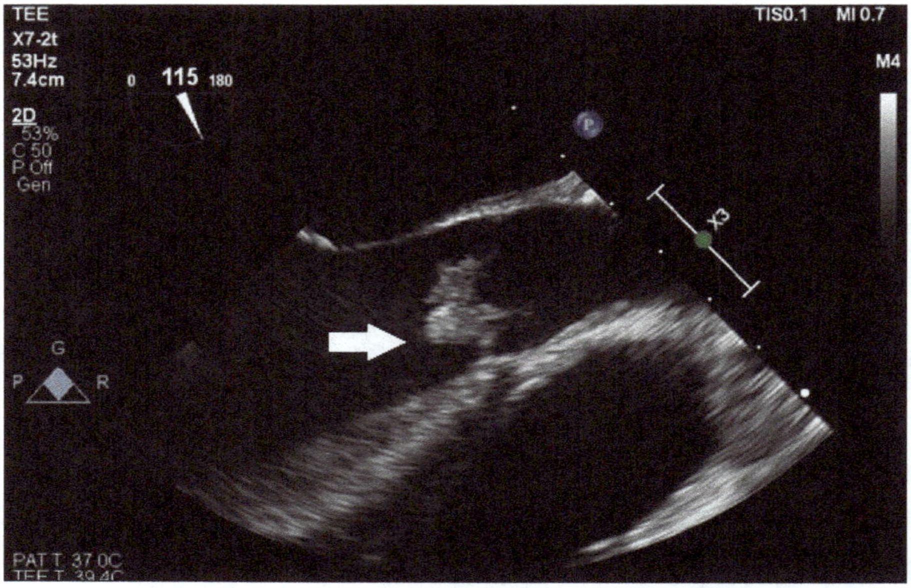

FIGURE 5: Transesophageal echocardiography revealing large aortic vegetation in longitudinal view (arrow).

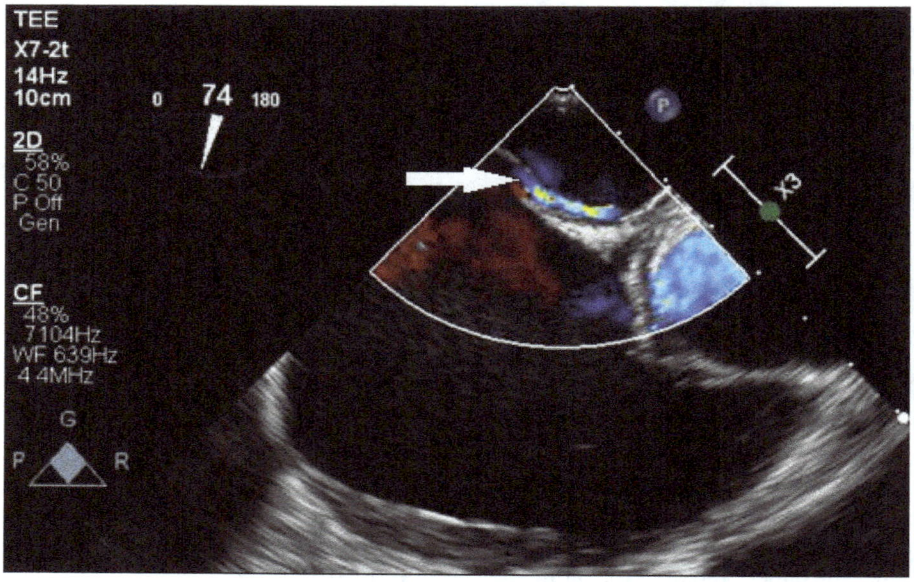

FIGURE 6: Transesophageal echo showing patent foramen ovale (arrow).

other coronary plaques and the absence of collateral blood flow. The management of these infected emboli remains unclear. Thrombolytics seem to release previously walled-off vegetations on valves, resulting in cerebral embolic showers followed by serious intracranial bleeds and the worsening of infection in both animal models [9] and in human case reports [10] and are therefore not recommended. Catheter-based therapies such as angioplasty, PCI, and embolectomy have also been used. Angioplasty is often immediately unsuccessful due to the lack of plaque to expand the vessel lumen, leading to rapid reocclusion [11]. PCI has been shown to be more effective immediately; however, it carries the risk of stent infection and, along with angioplasty, the risk of mycotic aneurysm with ultimate concern for coronary artery rupture and sudden death [12]. Per ACC guidelines, valve replacement is recommended in patients with recurrent emboli (Class IIa recommendation) or heart failure (Class I indication) [13].

While the diagnosis of AMI due to embolic IE remains rare, it is important to consider as treatment and clinical course vary significantly from atherosclerotic AMI. When presented with a young patient without typical risk factors for coronary heart disease, with early fevers, or history of endocarditis, physicians should consider an urgent TEE for evaluation of IE [3], which has a sensitivity of 93% for detecting valvular vegetations [14]. Once diagnosed, we endorse a multidisciplinary approach [4] and propose systemic antibiotics with or without emergent PCI as a bridge to possible surgical valve replacement. Further studies are recommended to help guide future therapy options.

References

[1] L. M. Baddour, W. R. Wilson, A. S. Bayer et al., "Infective endocarditis in adults: diagnosis, antimicrobial therapy, and management of complications: a scientific statement for healthcare professionals from the American Heart Association," *Circulation*, vol. 132, no. 15, pp. 1435–1486, 2015.

[2] C. J. Roxas and A. J. Weekes, "Acute myocardial infarction caused by coronary embolism from infective endocarditis," *The Journal of Emergency Medicine*, vol. 40, no. 5, pp. 509–514, 2011.

[3] M. C. Manzano, I. Vilacosta, J. A. San Román et al., "Acute coronary syndrome in infective endocarditis," *Revista Española de Cardiología*, vol. 60, no. 1, pp. 24–31, 2007.

[4] V. Roux, E. Salaun, C. Tribouilloy et al., "Coronary events complicating infective endocarditis," *Heart*, vol. 103, no. 23, pp. 1906–1910, 2017.

[5] J. G. Brunson, "Coronary embolism in bacterial endocarditis," *The American journal of pathology*, vol. 29, no. 4, pp. 689–701, 1953.

[6] S. Calero-Núñez, V. Ferrer Bleda, M. Corbí-Pascual et al., "Myocardial infarction associated with infective endocarditis: a case series," *European Heart Journal-Case Reports*, vol. 2, no. 1, pp. 1–7, 2018.

[7] A. J. Sanfilippo, M. H. Picard, J. B. Newell et al., "Echocardiographic assessment of patients with infectious endocarditis: prediction of risk for complications," *Journal of the American College of Cardiology*, vol. 18, no. 5, pp. 1191–1199, 1991.

[8] A. M. Johri, K. A. Kovacs, and H. Kafka, "An unusual case of infective endocarditis: extension of a tricuspid valve vegetation into the left atrium through a patent foramen ovale," *Canadian Journal of Cardiology*, vol. 25, no. 7, pp. 429–431, 2009.

[9] C. E. Johnson, H. A. Dewar, and W. A. Aherne, "Fibrinolytic therapy in subacute bacterial endocarditis: an experimental study," *Cardiovascular Research*, vol. 14, no. 8, pp. 482–489, 1980.

[10] T. G. di Salvo, S. B. Tatter, P. T. O'Gara, G. P. Nielsen, and R. W. Desanctis, "Fatal intracerebral hemorrhage following thrombolytic therapy of embolic myocardial infarction in unsuspected infective endocarditis," *Clinical Cardiology*, vol. 17, no. 6, pp. 340–344, 1994.

[11] J. J. Glazier, J. G. McGinnity, and J. R. Spears, "Coronary embolism complicating aortic valve endocarditis: treatment with placement of an intracoronary stent," *Clinical Cardiology*, vol. 20, no. 10, pp. 885–888, 1997.

[12] L. Overend and E. Rose, "Uncertainties in managing myocardial infarction associated with infective endocarditis," *Experimental & Clinical Cardiology*, vol. 17, no. 3, pp. 144-145, 2012.

[13] R. A. Nishimura, B. A. Carabello, D. P. Faxon et al., "ACC/AHA 2008 Guideline update on valvular heart disease: focused update on infective endocarditis: a report of the American College of Cardiology/American Heart Association Task Force on Practice Guidelines endorsed by the Society of Cardiovascular Anesthesiologists, Society for Cardiovascular Angiography and Interventions, and Society of Thoracic Surgeons," *Journal of the American College of Cardiology*, vol. 52, no. 8, pp. 676–685, 2008.

[14] R. L. Popp, "Echocardiography," *New England Journal of Medicine*, vol. 323, no. 3, pp. 165–172, 1990.

7

Acute Myopericarditis after the Second Dose of mRNA COVID-19 Vaccine Mimicking Acute Coronary Syndrome

Chris Pantsios, Zacharias-Alexandros Anyfantakis, Andrew Xanthopoulos, Ioannis Leventis, Spyridon Skoularigkis, Apostolos Dimos, Angeliki Bourazana, Michail Papamichalis, Grigorios Giamouzis, Filippos Triposkiadis, and John Skoularigis

Department of Cardiology, General University Hospital of Larissa, Larissa, Greece

Correspondence should be addressed to Chris Pantsios; chrpantsios@hotmail.com

Academic Editor: Mihaela Mocan

Myocarditis is a rare adverse event of vaccination. Recently, mRNA vaccines for COVID-19 have been reported to correlate with myocarditis, specifically in adolescents and young men. We report a rare case of a 50-year-old man who presented with symptoms of myocardial infarction 3 days after the second dose of vaccination for COVID-19. Cardiac magnetic resonance (CMR) imaging revealed acute myopericarditis. Clinicians should be aware of that rare side effect of mRNA vaccines for COVID-19 that can affect not only younger recipients but also middle-aged patients presenting with symptoms mimicking acute coronary syndrome.

1. Background

Myocarditis is an inflammatory cardiac disease induced by viruses, bacteria, protozoa, and fungi [1]. Severe acute respiratory syndrome coronavirus (SARS-CoV) and SARS-CoV-2 can trigger myocarditis either by direct cardiac injury or indirectly, due to host's immune response [2]. At the same time, myocarditis can be induced by a wide variety of toxic substances, drugs, and vaccines [3]. Postimmunization myocarditis is a known but rare adverse event following some vaccinations, particularly for smallpox [4] but also for influenza, tetanus, and hepatitis B [5]. Although there is a growing literature associating myocarditis with mRNA COVID-19 vaccines, reports are rather rare [6–8].

The clinical manifestations of myocarditis are highly variable and sometimes can mimic acute myocardial infarction, making diagnosis challenging [9].

We present a 50-year-old patient diagnosed with myopericarditis, the term for diagnosis of both myocardial and pericardial inflammation, 3 days after vaccination for COVID-19 with BNT 162b2 vaccine, presenting with symptoms of acute coronary syndrome.

2. Case

A 50-year-old man presented at the emergency department (ED) complaining for retrosternal, constrictive chest pain that awakened him up 2 hours before his arrival to our hospital. Three days before he received the second dose of vaccination for COVID-19 with BNT 162b2 vaccine and the same day, he reported low fever (37.5°C) and diarrhea.

The patient was tested negative at nasopharyngeal swab testing for SARS-CoV-2 PCR, as required prior to hospital admission. His chest pain resolved spontaneously within 6 h of his admission, lasting 8 hours in total.

Our patient did not report past medical history, neither risk factors for CAD, with the exception of a positive family history for premature CAD (his father suffered an acute myocardial infarction at the age of 45 years). He denied any symptom of infectious disease prior to the second dose of vaccination.

Clinical examination was normal. The patient was afebrile, with HR of 75 bpm and normal blood pressure (130/80 mmHg). Oxygen saturation was 99% on room air. Auscultation of the heart and lungs was normal. Electrocardiogram

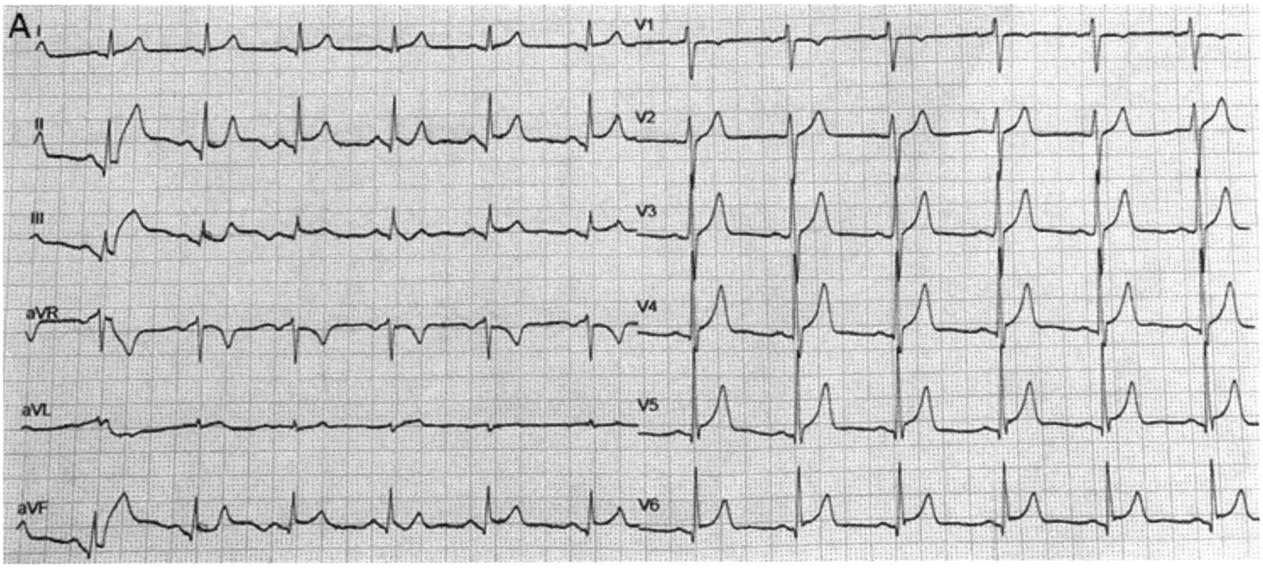

(a)

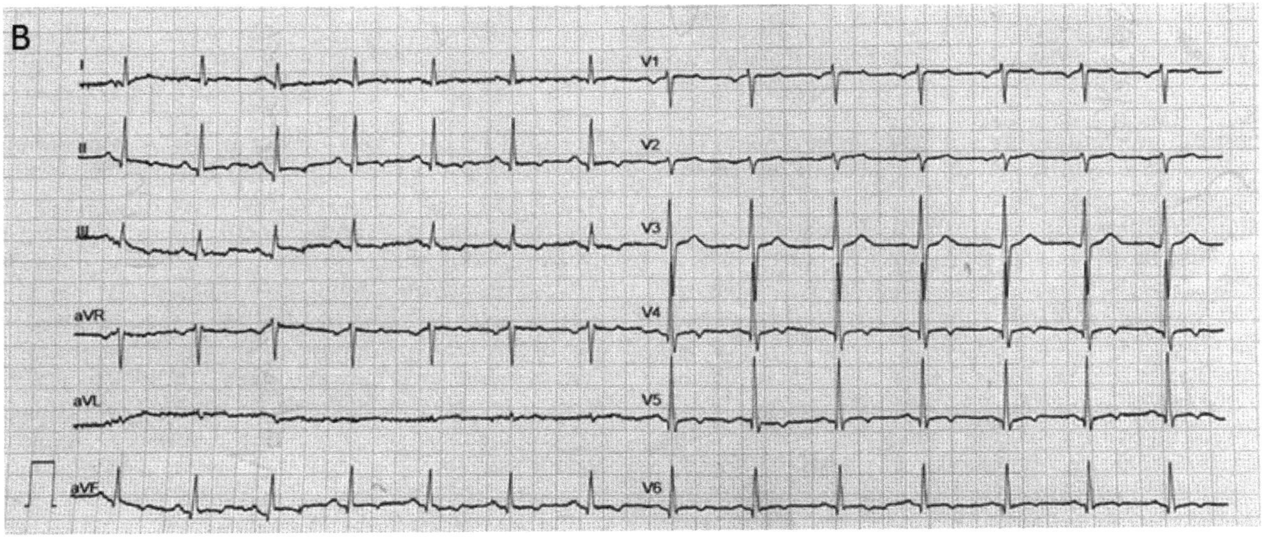

(b)

FIGURE 1: ECG at presentation (a) and at day 4 after admission (b). (a) ST elevation in inferior and lateral leads with concave up and PR segment depression can be noticed. (b) ST resolution and T wave inversion in inferior and lateral leads.

(ECG) in the ED showed ST segment elevation in inferior and lateral leads, pointing inferolateral wall involvement, with concave up and PR segment depression in the same leads (Figure 1(a)).

Troponin T was elevated at admission (0.088 μg/L) and peaked at 0.71 μg/L the next day (normal value < 0.017 μg/L). Creatine kinase was also elevated (345 U/L, normal value < 198 U/L).

Clinical presentation, electrocardiographic changes, and elevated cardiac markers led the patient to the catheterization lab. Thirty minutes after the patient's arrival at the emergency department, an emergent coronary angiography was performed to rule out acute coronary syndrome revealing normal epicardial arteries (Figure 2). As myocarditis emerged as the most likely diagnosis, antithrombotic and antiplatelet therapy was discontinued and the patient remained in the coronary care unit (CCU) for monitoring. During his first day of hospitalization, he reported two episodes of mild chest pain, of 30 min duration each, with no ECG changes and spontaneous resolution.

The echocardiogram was normal with neither regional wall motion abnormalities nor pericardial effusion. CMR was performed 6 days after the admission (SIEMENS AVANTO 1.5 T). It demonstrated normal left ventricular size and ejection fraction (60%), postgadolinium diffuse subepicardial enhancement in the inferior and inferolateral LV wall, and increase in T1 (1159 s) and T2 (57ms) time in comparison with the rest myocardium, confirming the

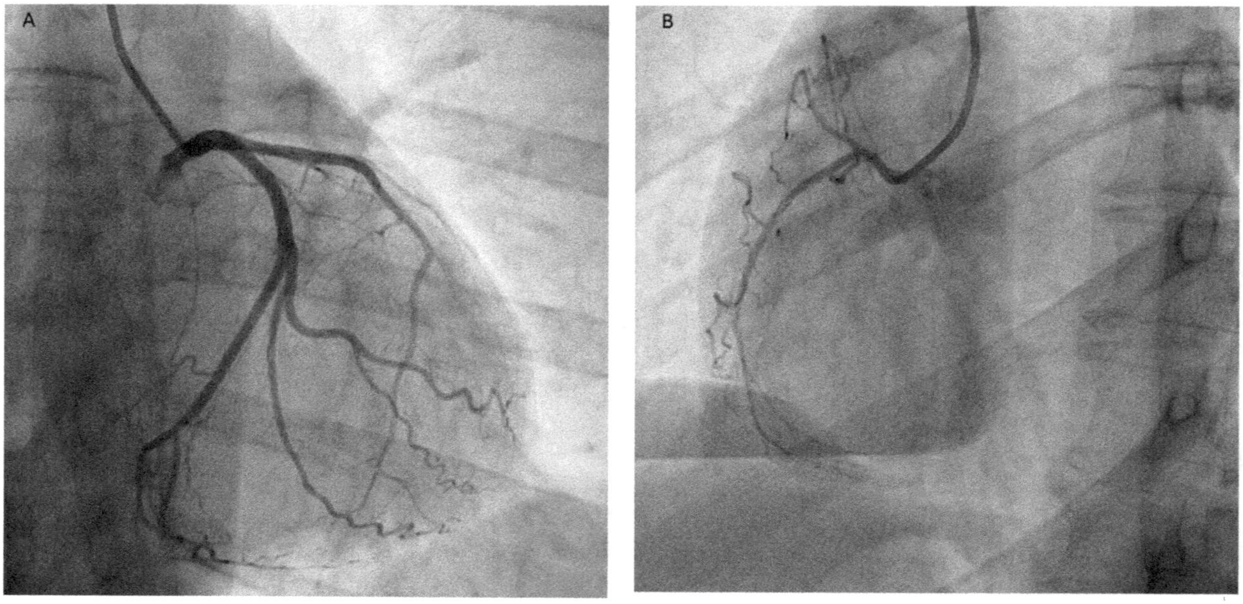

(a) (b)

Figure 2: Coronary angiogram ((a) left coronary artery and (b) right coronary artery) demonstrating normal coronary arteries.

diagnosis of myocarditis (revised Lake Louise criteria) [10]. Thickening and enhancement of the adjacent pericardium were also shown (Figure 3).

Due to mild in-hospital symptomatology and absence of heart failure, the patient did not receive specific treatment for myocarditis or pericarditis. During his six-day hospitalization, he remained well appearing, hemodynamically stable, and in sinus rhythm. Viral studies for related to myocarditis viruses were performed and did not reveal IgM antibodies nor fourfold increase in IgG antibodies. The workup concerned Epstein-Barr virus, cytomegalovirus, adenovirus, enterovirus (coxsackie A, coxsackie B1), hepatitis B and C viruses, and human herpes 1 and 2 viruses.

Cardiac troponin T and creatine kinase progressively decreased, and ECG showed ST segment resolution with T wave inversion (Figure 1(b)). The patient was discharged home with the recommendation to avoid intense physical activity for three to six months.

Six months after his admission, CMR was repeated and revealed normal left ventricular size and function and mild postgadolinium subepicardial enhancement in the inferior and inferolateral LV wall, compatible with healed myocarditis (Figure 4). T1 time was decreased to 1036 ms (from 1159 ms) showing inflammation remission. The patient remains well appearing and asymptomatic.

A written informed consent was provided by the patient for the publication.

3. Discussion

Our patient meets the criteria for confirmed acute myocarditis (clinical symptoms and pathologic troponin levels and CMR findings consistent with myocarditis and no other identifiable cause of the symptoms and findings) [11, 12]. He also meets criteria for acute pericarditis (acute chest pain and compatible ECG changes). This case is rare as until 11th of June 2021, only 50 cases of people over 50 years have been reported to the US Vaccine Adverse Events Reporting System (VAERS) after over 34 million doses of mRNA COVID-19 vaccines administered [11].

One potential cause of COVID-19 vaccine myocarditis may be the pathologic immune response to vaccine's mRNA. Certain predisposed individuals detect mRNA molecules of vaccine as antigens and activate immunologic pathways and proinflammatory cascades that may play a role in myocarditis [13]. Another potential mechanism may be the molecular mimicry between the spike protein of SARS-CoV-2 and self-antigens. Antibodies against SARS-CoV-2 spike glycoproteins have been shown to cross-react with structurally similar human peptide proteins, including α-myosin [14].

The incidence of myocarditis after vaccination is very low. The estimated incidence of at least one dose of the BNT162b2 mRNA vaccine was reported to be 2.13 cases per 100,000 vaccinated persons in the first 42 days after receipt [15]. The CDC COVID-19 Vaccine Task Force has reported until 11th of June 2021 a rate of myopericarditis ranging from 18.1/1.000.000 doses in adolescents of 12-17 y. to 1.7/1.000.000 doses in people older than 50 years [11].

On the contrary, nearly 2.3% of highly fit athletes with mild COVID-19 infection have evidence of myocarditis on CMR [16] and recently, in a second study, 0.6% of professional athletes have demonstrated detectable inflammatory heart disease on CMR [17]. While the actual prevalence of myocarditis in COVID-19 patients remains unknown, it is estimated that cardiac injury after COVID-19 infection is as high as 19-28% and may reach 60% in seriously ill patients [18]. It is obvious that there is a significantly higher

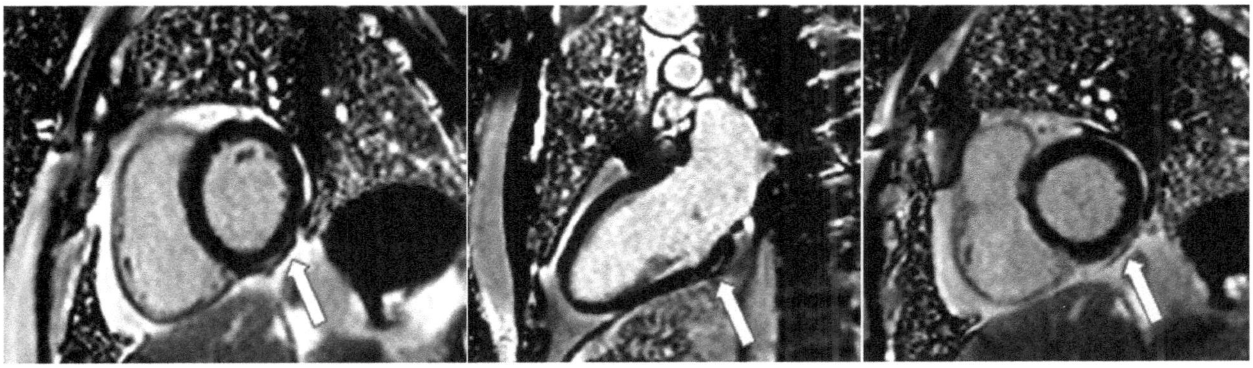

FIGURE 3: Postcontrast images of cardiac magnetic resonance (6 days after the patient's admission) in short and long views showing subepicardial enhancement in the basal and midinferior and inferolateral wall of the left ventricle (white arrows).

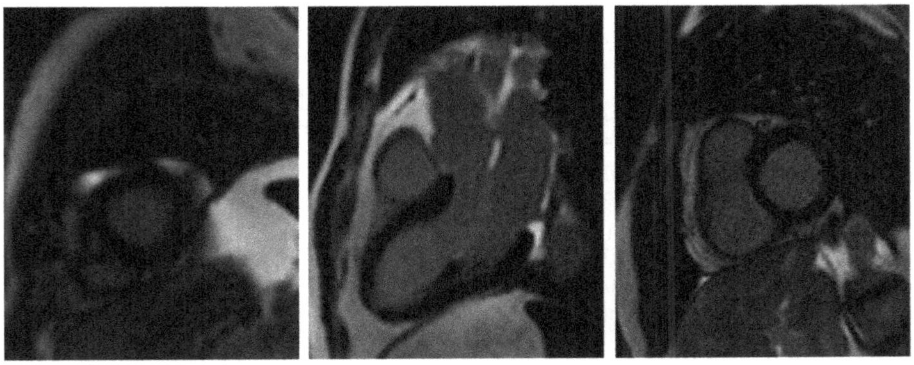

FIGURE 4: Postcontrast images of cardiac magnetic resonance (at 6 months) in short and long views showing minimal subepicardial enhancement in the basal inferior and inferolateral wall of the left ventricle.

risk of cardiac involvement from COVID-19 infection compared to COVID-19 vaccination.

Given that the majority of cases have a mild clinical course, COVID-19 vaccination should remain the cornerstone for population immunity. It is important to note that a causal relation between the mRNA-COVID-19 vaccine and myocardial inflammation has not been proven yet.

The retrosternal, constrictive chest pain which made our patient seek medical care subsided a few minutes after his arrival to the ED. His symptoms thereafter—during his hospitalization—were mild. Patients with myocarditis mimicking AMI have a favorable long-term prognosis [19]. It is noteworthy that after six months, our patient remains asymptomatic.

Recognition of vaccine-associated myocarditis is important, as diagnosis impacts management, recommendations for exercise, and surveillance. Whether vaccination schedule needs to be modified for patients who have a history of myocarditis, how should these cases be managed, and what type of cardiac follow-up would be appropriate remain to be answered.

Clinicians should be aware that myopericarditis after COVID-19 vaccination may not exclusively affect younger individuals but it should be also considered in middle-aged patients presenting with acute coronary syndrome symptoms.

4. Conclusion

Myocarditis is a rare adverse event of mRNA vaccines for COVID-19. Clinicians should be aware that myopericarditis can affect not only younger vaccine recipients but also middle-aged patients presenting with symptoms mimicking acute coronary syndrome. Given that there is a significantly higher risk of cardiac involvement from COVID-19 infection compared to mRNA vaccines, vaccination should remain the cornerstone for population immunity.

References

[1] C. Tschope, E. Ammirati, B. Bozkurt et al., "Myocarditis and inflammatory cardiomyopathy: current evidence and future directions," *Nature Reviews. Cardiology*, vol. 18, no. 3, pp. 169–193, 2021.

[2] S. Van Linthout, K. Klingel, and C. Tschope, "SARS-CoV-2-related myocarditis-like syndromes Shakespeare's question: what's in a name?," *European Journal of Heart Failure*, vol. 22, no. 6, pp. 922–925, 2020.

[3] J. R. Hu, R. Florido, E. J. Lipson et al., "Cardiovascular toxicities associated with immune checkpoint inhibitors," *Cardiovascular Research*, vol. 115, no. 5, pp. 854–868, 2019.

[4] J. S. Halsell, J. R. Riddle, J. E. Atwood et al., "Myopericarditis following smallpox vaccination among vaccinia-naive US military personnel," *JAMA*, vol. 289, no. 24, pp. 3283–3289, 2003.

[5] R. Mei, E. Raschi, E. Forcesi, I. Diemberger, F. De Ponti, and E. Poluzzi, "Myocarditis and pericarditis after immunization: gaining insights through the Vaccine Adverse Event Reporting System," *International Journal of Cardiology*, vol. 273, pp. 183–186, 2018.

[6] S. Abu Mouch, A. Roguin, E. Hellou et al., "Myocarditis following COVID-19 mRNA vaccination," *Vaccine*, vol. 39, no. 29, pp. 3790–3793, 2021.

[7] E. Albert, G. Aurigemma, J. Saucedo, and D. S. Gerson, "Myocarditis following COVID-19 vaccination," *Radiology Case Reports*, vol. 16, no. 8, pp. 2142–2145, 2021.

[8] J. Montgomery, M. Ryan, R. Engler et al., "Myocarditis following immunization with mRNA COVID-19 vaccines in members of the US military," *JAMA Cardiology*, vol. 6, no. 10, pp. 1202–1206, 2021.

[9] J. W. Magnani and G. W. Dec, "Myocarditis," *Circulation*, vol. 113, no. 6, pp. 876–890, 2006.

[10] V. M. Ferreira, J. Schulz-Menger, G. Holmvang et al., "Cardiovascular magnetic resonance in nonischemic myocardial inflammation: expert recommendations," *Journal of the American College of Cardiology*, vol. 72, no. 24, pp. 3158–3176, 2018.

[11] T. Shimabukuro, "Covid-19 vaccine safety updates," *Advisory Committee on Immunization Practices (ACIP)*August 2021, https://www.cdc.gov/vaccines/acip/meetings/downloads/slides-2021-06/03-COVID-Shimabukuro-508.pdf.

[12] A. L. Caforio, S. Pankuweit, E. Arbustini et al., "Current state of knowledge on aetiology, diagnosis, management, and therapy of myocarditis: a position statement of the European Society of Cardiology Working Group on Myocardial and Pericardial Diseases," *European Heart Journal*, vol. 34, no. 2636-48, pp. 2648a–2648d, 2013.

[13] F. Caso, L. Costa, P. Ruscitti et al., "Could Sars-coronavirus-2 trigger autoimmune and/or autoinflammatory mechanisms in genetically predisposed subjects?," *Autoimmunity Reviews*, vol. 19, no. 5, article 102524, 2020.

[14] A. Vojdani and D. Kharrazian, "Potential antigenic cross-reactivity between SARS-CoV-2 and human tissue with a possible link to an increase in autoimmune diseases," *Clinical Immunology*, vol. 217, article 108480, 2020.

[15] G. Witberg, N. Barda, S. Hoss et al., "Myocarditis after Covid-19 vaccination in a large health care organization," *The New England Journal of Medicine*, vol. 385, no. 23, pp. 2132–2139, 2021.

[16] C. J. Daniels, S. Rajpal, J. T. Greenshields et al., "Prevalence of clinical and subclinical myocarditis in competitive athletes with recent SARS-CoV-2 infection: results from the big ten COVID-19 cardiac registry," *JAMA Cardiology*, vol. 6, no. 9, pp. 1078–1087, 2021.

[17] M. W. Martinez, A. M. Tucker, O. J. Bloom et al., "Prevalence of inflammatory heart disease among professional athletes with prior COVID-19 infection who received systematic return-to-play cardiac screening," *JAMA Cardiology*, vol. 6, no. 7, pp. 745–752, 2021.

[18] R. O. Bonow, G. C. Fonarow, P. T. O'Gara, and C. W. Yancy, "Association of coronavirus disease 2019 (COVID-19) with myocardial injury and mortality," *JAMA Cardiology*, vol. 5, no. 7, pp. 751–753, 2020.

[19] M. Anzini, M. Merlo, G. Sabbadini et al., "Long-term evolution and prognostic stratification of biopsy-proven active myocarditis," *Circulation*, vol. 128, no. 22, pp. 2384–2394, 2013.

Right Ventricular Myocardial Infarction Complicated by Cardiac Arrest: Utilization of Extracorporeal Membrane Oxygenation

Alisha Alabre-Bonsu, Saurav Uppal, Ernest L. Mazzaferri Jr., and Konstantinos Dean Boudoulas

Division of Cardiovascular Medicine, The Ohio State University, Columbus, Ohio, USA

Correspondence should be addressed to Konstantinos Dean Boudoulas; konstantinos.boudoulas@osumc.edu

Academic Editor: Manabu Shirotani

A 44-year-old male with an out-of-hospital cardiac arrest due to an acute left ventricular (LV) inferoposterior wall myocardial infarction (MI) involving the right ventricle (RV) is presented. This case highlights the challenges in the management of patients with cardiac arrest, indications for use of ventricular assist devices, potential effects of LV assist devices on the RV in the setting of RV MI, and culprit versus complete coronary artery revascularization in these patients.

1. Introduction

Combined left ventricular (LV) and right ventricular (RV) myocardial infarction (MI) is associated with greater morbidity and mortality as compared to an isolated LV MI. RV dilatation and marked decrease in RV stroke volume may occur in RV MI leading to systemic hypotension, tissue hypoperfusion, and cardiogenic shock. Further, cardiac arrest is not uncommon during the acute phase of MI leading to a poor prognosis [1]. While LV assist devices have been shown to be effective in the management of LV failure due to an acute MI, in cases of combined RV and LV MI, these devices may increase RV work due to increased volume return to the RV resulting in deterioration of its function [2]. A 44-year-old male with an out-of-hospital cardiac arrest due to an acute LV inferoposterior wall MI associated with a RV MI is presented, and current management of cardiac arrest in these patients is briefly discussed.

2. Case Presentation

A 44-year-old man without a significant past medical history developed chest pain for approximately one hour while at his office prior to being found unconscious by one of his colleagues. Bystander cardiopulmonary resuscitation (CPR) was not performed at that time. Emergency medical services (EMS) arrived within 5 minutes and initiated advanced cardiovascular life support (ACLS). The patient was intubated and underwent multiple unsuccessful defibrillation attempts for ventricular fibrillation. Since return of spontaneous circulation (ROSC) could not be obtained, an automated CPR device (LUCAS chest compression system, Stryker Medical, Portage, Michigan) was placed and initiated at 100 beats per minute. The patient was emergently transported directly to the cardiac catheterization laboratory (CCL) at The Ohio State University as part of an extracorporeal cardiopulmonary resuscitation (ECPR) program that utilizes venoarterial extracorporeal membrane oxygenation (ECMO) as an adjunct to CPR for out-of-hospital cardiac arrest due to refractory ventricular tachycardia/fibrillation despite three defibrillation attempts [3]. Upon arrival to CCL, the patient was found to be in persistent ventricular fibrillation; thus, he was defibrillated once again; this time, ROSC was achieved.

Coronary arteriography demonstrated complete thrombotic occlusion in the proximal right coronary artery (RCA; Figure 1(a)) and 90% stenosis in the proximal and 95% stenosis in the mid left anterior descending (LAD) coronary artery (Figure 1(b)). Percutaneous coronary intervention (PCI) with the placement of drug eluting stents in the RCA (culprit lesion) was performed restoring coronary

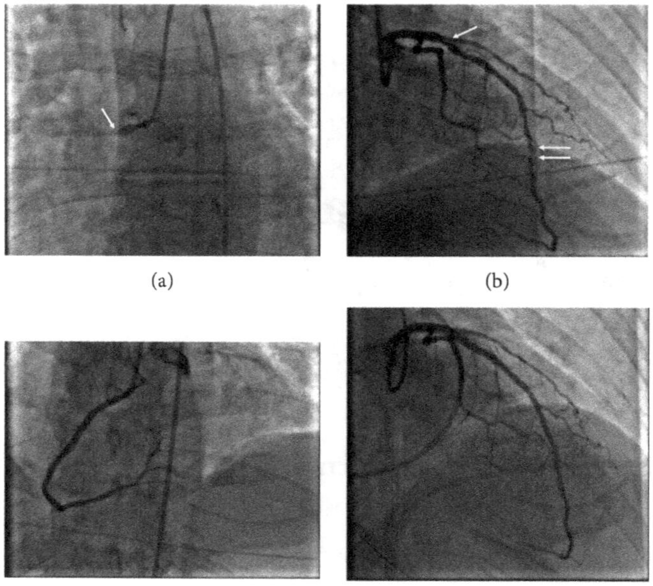

(a) (b) (c) (d)

FIGURE 1: (a) Diagnostic arteriogram demonstrating acute complete thrombotic occlusion in the proximal right coronary artery (arrow) representing the culprit lesion and (b) 90% stenosis in the proximal left anterior descending (LAD) coronary artery (arrow) and 95% stenosis in the mid LAD (double arrow). (c) Coronary arteriogram post-percutaneous coronary intervention (PCI) of the RCA with placement of drug eluting stents with restoration of coronary blood flow. (d) Coronary arteriogram post-PCI of the proximal and mid LAD with placement of drug eluting stents.

blood flow (Figure 1(c)). PCI was not performed in the LAD stenoses. After PCI and despite an epinephrine infusion, the patient remained in cardiogenic shock with a systemic arterial pressure of 75/47 mmHg. At that time, a left and right heart catheterization demonstrated LV end diastolic pressure (LVEDP) 18 mmHg, right atrial pressure (RAP) 14 mmHg (mean), pulmonary artery pressure 28/16 mmHg, pulmonary capillary wedge pressure (PCWP) 16 mmHg (mean), and cardiac index (CI) 1.1 L/min/m^2. The pulmonary artery pulsatility index (PAPi) (pulmonary artery pulse pressure over RAP) when <1.0 is considered an index of RV failure in acute MI [2]. A ratio of RAP to PCWP >0.86 is also considered an index of RV failure in acute MI [2]. The PAPi in this case was 0.9, and RAP/PCWP was 0.87; both of these indices were borderline for RV failure. Since the patient was in cardiogenic shock with an elevated LVEDP and low CI with borderline values for RV failure, the decision at that time was to support the LV with an Impella CP percutaneous LV assist device (Abiomed, Inc., Danvers, Massachusetts) that was placed via the femoral artery (Figure 2(a)). Impella was chosen due to its ease and quickness of implantation compared to ECMO, which can be more cumbersome to set-up, implant, and initiate. The patient was then admitted to the cardiovascular intensive care unit (CVICU) for further management.

Upon arrival to the CVICU, an electrocardiogram (ECG) was obtained that demonstrated supraventricular tachycardia (ectopic atrial versus junctional tachycardia), early R-wave transition in the precordial leads, diffuse ST and T wave changes, and QT prolongation most likely secondary to myocardial injury/ischemia and metabolic abnormalities due to cardiac arrest (Figure 3). Shortly after his arrival to the CVICU, the patient had a recurrent ventricular fibrillation in which he underwent ACLS and one defibrillation achieving ROSC. At that time, the lactate (14 mmol/L), serum creatinine (2.1 mg/dL), alanine aminotransferase (183 U/L), and aspartate aminotransferase (348 U/L) were elevated. A transthoracic echocardiogram (TTE) demonstrated severe LV systolic dysfunction (ejection fraction approximately 20%), RV enlargement with moderately severe RV systolic dysfunction, and septal flattening suggestive of RV volume/pressure overload (Figures 2(b) and 2(c)). Due to recurrent ventricular fibrillation and persistent cardiogenic shock despite intravenous pressor and Impella support, the decision was made to take the patient back to the CCL for placement of ECMO for escalated hemodynamic support and PCI of the LAD. Successful PCI of the proximal and mid LAD stenoses with placement of drug eluting stents was performed (Figure 1(d)). In addition, the Impella was removed, and the patient was placed on venoarterial ECMO through cannulas placed in the femoral artery and vein.

The patient had a prolonged hospital stay that was further complicated by persistent acute kidney injury requiring hemodialysis. Support with dobutamine infusion was required. Eventually, ECMO support was slowly weaned over several days, and on hospital day 5, the ECMO cannulas were successfully removed in the operative room. Following removal of ECMO, the patient did require additional inotropic support; thus, a milrinone infusion was initiated along with the preexisting dobutamine infusion. Milrinone was able to be weaned off after 48 hours. The dobutamine infusion was slowly weaned off after a total therapy of 13 days.

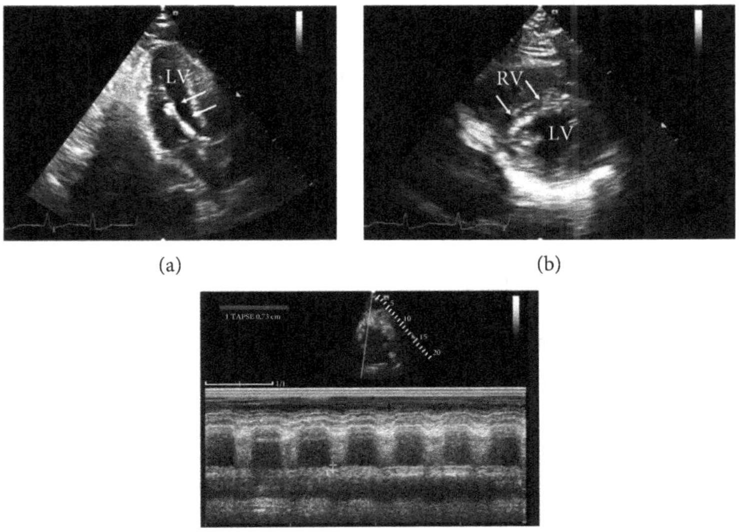

FIGURE 2: (a) Transthoracic echocardiogram (TTE) 3-chamber showing the Impella CP percutaneous left ventricular assist device (arrows) within the left ventricle (LV). (b) TTE short axis view demonstrating septal flattening (arrows) indicating right ventricular (RV) pressure/volume overload; the RV is dilated as well. (c) TTE M-mode of the tricuspid annulus showing decreased (dashed line) tricuspid annular plane systolic excursion (TAPSE) of 0.73 cm suggesting RV dysfunction.

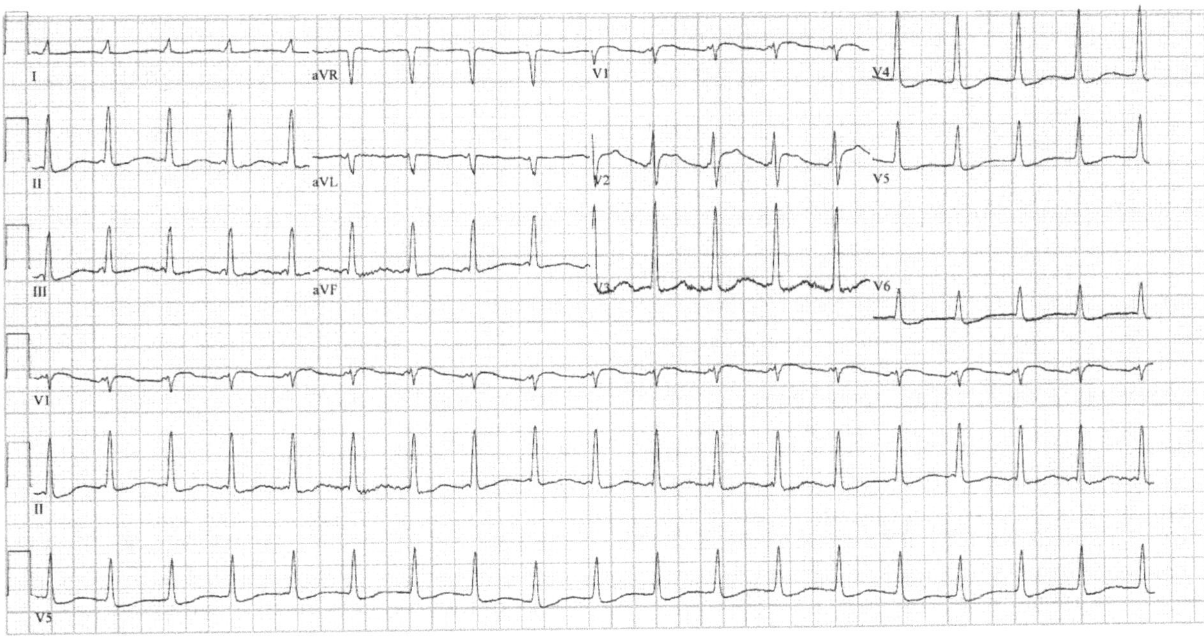

FIGURE 3: Electrocardiogram obtained upon arrival to the cardiovascular intensive care unit demonstrating supraventricular tachycardia (ectopic atrial versus junctional tachycardia), early R-wave transition in the precordial leads, diffuse ST and T wave changes, and QT prolongation most likely secondary to myocardial injury/ischemia and metabolic abnormalities due to cardiac arrest.

A TTE was repeated 2 weeks after his initial presentation that demonstrated almost full recovery of LV (ejection fraction approximately 55%) and RV function. Physical therapy was performed initially at the bedside on day 10 of hospitalization, and by day 16, the patient was ambulating the hospital hallway without difficulty. The patient was evaluated by the electrophysiologist for possible placement of an implantable cardioverter defibrillator (ICD) given presentation of ventricular fibrillation cardiac arrest; however, this was deferred due to successful coronary artery revascularization and recovery of LV systolic function. Optimal guideline directed medical therapy for heart failure was initiated and slowly titrated over the course of patient's hospitalization including carvedilol 25 mg twice daily, hydralazine 50 mg every 8 hours, and isosorbide mononitrate 60 mg daily. Renin angiotensin aldosterone system inhibitor was not initiated due to acute renal failure. In addition, the patient was taking aspirin 81 mg daily and clopidogrel 75 mg daily due to coronary artery stent placement. The patient was discharged to home on day 20 of hospitalization with full neurologic capacity and with outpatient hemodialysis and cardiology follow-up.

The patient was evaluated in cardiology clinic 2 weeks after hospital discharge. He was asymptomatic and was attending cardiac rehabilitation. His acute renal failure had improved (serum creatinine 1.8 mg/dL) and he no longer required hemodialysis. Eighteen months after hospital discharge, the patient remained asymptomatic and was training for a 5-kilometer race.

3. Discussion

Despite recent medical progress, the prognosis in cardiac arrest due to MI remains poor and the management is quite challenging. This case highlights the importance of aggressive and timely therapy in this group of patients [1]. Emergent coronary artery revascularization of the culprit lesion is the mainstay of therapy, and fluid resuscitation may be required in cases of RV MI. The high RV preload, however, needed to maintain a cardiac output may result in an increase in RV work in the setting of an ischemic myocardium [1, 2]. In addition, RV volume overload can lead to leftward shifting of the LV septum resulting in a further decrease in LV stroke volume and cardiac output [4].

The diagnosis and the severity of RV dysfunction that leads to failure can be established by echocardiography and hemodynamic assessment (Figures 2(b) and 2(c)). Echocardiogram will demonstrate a dilated and hypokinetic RV with diminished ejection fraction. Right heart catheterization can be utilized to determine various hemodynamic parameters including PAPi (<1.0) and ratio of RAP to PCWP (>0.86) that suggest RV failure in the setting of an acute MI [2]. Limitations including accuracy of these pressure-related indices, mostly based on recordings using fluid-filled catheters, should be acknowledged [1]. Since the patient was in cardiogenic shock with an elevated LV end diastolic pressure and low CI, and borderline values for RV failure, the decision made at that time was to support the LV with placement of an Impella percutaneous LV assist device. Shortly after his arrival in the CVICU, the patient developed another episode of ventricular fibrillation. If this was partially related to an increase in cardiac output after the placement of the LV assist device that resulted in an increase in RV work due to an increase volume return to the RV cannot be proven or disproven. Likewise, if the last episode of ventricular fibrillation could have been avoided if ECMO was initially placed to provide full cardiac support not only to the LV but also to the RV, cannot be proven after the fact; however, such an approach in patients with LV and RV failure should be considered.

ECMO is effective in providing hemodynamic support for individuals with refractory cardiogenic shock due to LV and/or RV failure [5, 6]. Pulmonary vasodilators may have some utility in supporting acute RV failure [7]. In addition, RV assist devices can be utilized for RV support [2]. However, ECMO was eventually chosen in this particular case due to the need to support both ventricles. While ECMO can provide hemodynamic support in LV failure, it is important to be aware of the LVEDP, as an increase in LVEDP may result in an increase in pulmonary edema, increase in myocardial oxygen demand, and vulnerability to ischemia-mediated necrosis [5, 8]. Interventions that may assist in decreasing an elevated LVEDP while on EMCO include use of inotropes, vasodilators, intra-aortic balloon pump, and percutaneous left ventricular assist devices [6, 9]. Since ECMO is often used as a bridge to recovery in patients with reversible cardiac injury, it is important when initiating ECMO to assess which patients may derive the most benefit and likelihood of recovery; various risk scores are available to assist with this; however, nothing replaces sound clinical judgement and experience [5].

It is important to be aware that after placement of a LV assist device, RV failure has been reported in approximately 13-44% of patients [10]. Reassessing hemodynamic parameters with a right heart catheterization, as described previously, after placement of a LV assist device should be performed when there is concern for RV failure. In addition, several echocardiographic variables such as RV fractional area change, RV/LV diameter ratio, RV free wall longitudinal strain by velocity vector imaging, and tricuspid annular plane systolic excursion (TAPSE; Figure 2(c)) have been found to be useful in predicting RV failure after placement of a LV assist device [10].

Another dilemma in this case was the decision to either only perform PCI of the culprit lesion or pursue complete coronary artery revascularization during the index procedure. There are several studies including the PRAMI, COMPLETE, and DANAMI-3 PRIMULTI trials that demonstrated improved cardiovascular outcomes with complete coronary artery revascularization immediately or staged within the index hospitalization for patients presenting with ST-elevation myocardial infarction (STEMI) without cardiogenic shock [11–13]. Conversely, the CULPRIT SHOCK trial demonstrated that patients with an acute MI and cardiogenic shock had a significantly lower risk of mortality and required less often renal-replacement therapy at 30 days when PCI was only performed on the culprit lesion as compared to immediate multivessel PCI, and there was no significant difference in mortality between the two groups at 1-year follow-up [14]. There is limited data, however, to guide management of patients who present with cardiac arrest and cardiogenic shock who are found to have multivessel coronary artery disease. "Individualization" is essential, as in these cases, one size does not fit all. In our case, the initial revascularization was targeted towards the culprit RCA lesion. It is unclear as to whether or not upfront PCI to the LAD could have prevented further decompensation in this patient. Further, it is unclear if acute renal failure could have been avoided or if the outcome of the patient could have been different if LAD revascularization was deferred for a later time.

4. Conclusion

This case highlights the challenges in the management of a patient with cardiac arrest even after achieving ROSC.

Understanding the pathophysiology of LV and RV infarction and their interrelationship is critical in order to provide optimal care. It is also important to understand the potential effects on the RV in the setting of RV MI when unloading the LV with a LV assist device and the potential benefits of ECMO. In addition, the risk of complete revascularization due to longer procedural times and increase use of contrast material should always be taken into consideration. It is difficult to establish fixed rules for these critically ill and unstable patients in which individualized therapy based on knowledge, clinical experience, and common sense should be applied.

References

[1] D. P. Zipes, P. Libby, R. O. Bonow, D. L. Mann, and G. F. Tomaselli, *Braunwald's Heart Disease: A Textbook of Cardiovascular Medicine*, Elsevier, Philadelphia, 11th edition, 2019.

[2] N. K. Kapur, M. L. Esposito, Y. Bader et al., "Mechanical circulatory support devices for acute right ventricular failure," *Circulation*, vol. 136, no. 3, pp. 314–326, 2017.

[3] K. D. Boudoulas, B. A. Whitson, D. P. Keseg et al., "Extracorporeal cardiopulmonary resuscitation (ECPR) for out-of-hospital cardiac arrest due to pulseless ventricular tachycardia/fibrillation," *Journal of Interventional Cardiology*, vol. 2020, article 6939315, 9 pages, 2020.

[4] R. Naeije and R. Badagliacca, "The overloaded right heart and ventricular interdependence," *Cardiovascular Research*, vol. 113, no. 12, pp. 1474–1485, 2017.

[5] P. Rao, Z. Khalpey, R. Smith, D. Burkhoff, and R. D. Kociol, "Venoarterial extracorporeal membrane oxygenation for cardiogenic shock and cardiac arrest," *Circulation. Heart Failure*, vol. 11, no. 9, article e004905, 2018.

[6] C. Grant Jr., J. B. Richards, M. Frakes, J. Cohen, and S. R. Wilcox, "ECMO and right ventricular failure: review of the literature," *Journal of Intensive Care Medicine*, vol. 36, no. 3, pp. 352–360, 2021.

[7] C. E. Ventetuolo and J. R. Klinger, "Management of acute right ventricular failure in the intensive care unit," *Annals of the American Thoracic Society*, vol. 11, no. 5, pp. 811–822, 2014.

[8] D. Burkhoff, G. Sayer, D. Doshi, and N. Uriel, "Hemodynamics of mechanical circulatory support," *Journal of the American College of Cardiology*, vol. 66, no. 23, pp. 2663–2674, 2015.

[9] S. M. Patel, J. Lipinski, S. G. Al-Kindi et al., "Simultaneous venoarterial extracorporeal membrane oxygenation and percutaneous left ventricular decompression therapy with Impella is associated with improved outcomes in refractory cardiogenic shock," *ASAIO Journal*, vol. 65, no. 1, pp. 21–28, 2019.

[10] S. Hayek, D. B. Sims, D. W. Markham, J. Butler, and A. P. Kalogeropoulos, "Assessment of right ventricular function in left ventricular assist device candidates," *Circulation. Cardiovascular Imaging*, vol. 7, no. 2, pp. 379–389, 2014.

[11] D. S. Wald, J. K. Morris, N. J. Wald et al., "Randomized trial of preventive angioplasty in myocardial infarction," *The New England Journal of Medicine*, vol. 369, no. 12, pp. 1115–1123, 2013.

[12] T. Engstrøm, H. Kelbæk, S. Helqvist et al., "Complete revascularisation versus treatment of the culprit lesion only in patients with ST-segment elevation myocardial infarction and multivessel disease (DANAMI-3–PRIMULTI): an open-label, randomised controlled trial," *Lancet*, vol. 386, no. 9994, pp. 665–671, 2015.

[13] D. A. Wood, J. A. Cairns, J. Wang et al., "Timing of staged nonculprit artery revascularization in patients with ST-segment elevation myocardial infarction: complete trial," *Journal of the American College of Cardiology*, vol. 74, no. 22, pp. 2713–2723, 2019.

[14] H. Thiele, I. Akin, M. Sandri et al., "PCI strategies in patients with acute myocardial infarction and cardiogenic shock," *The New England Journal of Medicine*, vol. 377, no. 25, pp. 2419–2432, 2017.

9

Infective Aortic Valve Endocarditis Causing Embolic Consecutive ST-Elevation Myocardial Infarctions

Kanksha Peddi[1] **Alexander L. Hsu**[2] **and Tomas H. Ayala**[2]

[1]*Saba University School of Medicine, Saba, Dutch Caribbean, Netherlands*
[2]*Department of Medicine, MedStar Harbor Hospital, Baltimore, MD, USA*

Correspondence should be addressed to Alexander L. Hsu; alexhsu3211@gmail.com

Academic Editor: Hajime Kataoka

ST-elevation myocardial infarction (STEMI) is a rare and potentially fatal complication of infective endocarditis. We report the ninth case of embolic native aortic valve infective endocarditis causing STEMI and the first case to describe consecutive embolisms leading to infarctions of separate coronary territories. Through examination of this case in the context of the previous eight similar documented cases in the past, we find that infective endocarditis of the aortic valve can and frequently affect more than a single myocardial territory and can occur consecutively. Further, current treatment modalities for embolic infective endocarditis causing acute myocardial infarction are limited and unproven. This index case illustrates the potential severity of complications and the challenges in developing standardized management for such patients.

1. Introduction

Infective endocarditis as a result of injection drug use is an increasingly prevalent condition in the United States [1]. With the increase in frequency of injection use-associated endocarditis, there is an associated increase in the complications associated with the disease. Symptomatic embolisms are a well-known complication of infective endocarditis (IE). Prior studies have reported embolisms in 13-49% of IE patients [2]. However, embolism to the coronary arteries is much rarer, and of these cases, even fewer describe ST-elevation myocardial infarctions (STEMIs) caused by such emboli [2]. We report a case of a unique nature: two consecutive STEMIs caused by infective endocarditis of the aortic valve. A thorough review of current literature yields only eight other previously reported cases of STEMI caused by embolic infective endocarditis of a native aortic valve [3–10]. Here, we discuss the ninth case of embolic native aortic valve infective endocarditis causing STEMI and the first case to describe consecutive embolisms leading to infarctions of separate coronary territories.

2. History of Presentation

A 31-year-old female with a past medical history of intravenous drug abuse (IVDA) presented with a four-day history of generalized weakness, shortness of breath, and chest pain. She described her chest pain as pleuritic and associated with a nonproductive cough. She also reported fevers with diffuse body and joint pains. The patient injected heroin daily but denied any other substance abuse. On arrival to the emergency department, the patient was afebrile, tachycardic, normotensive, and saturating well on room air. Physical exam was significant for a chronic appearing left lateral forearm wound that was approximately five by five centimeters without drainage or significant erythema. Another chronic appearing wound was found on the left lateral calf that was approximately five by seven centimeters with several foci of purulent drainage with edema and erythema of the surrounding area. Imaging later revealed a five by twelve by ten millimeter abscess in the left lateral calf. She had multiple stigmata of injection drug use along her bilateral upper and lower extremities. On this encounter, the patient was

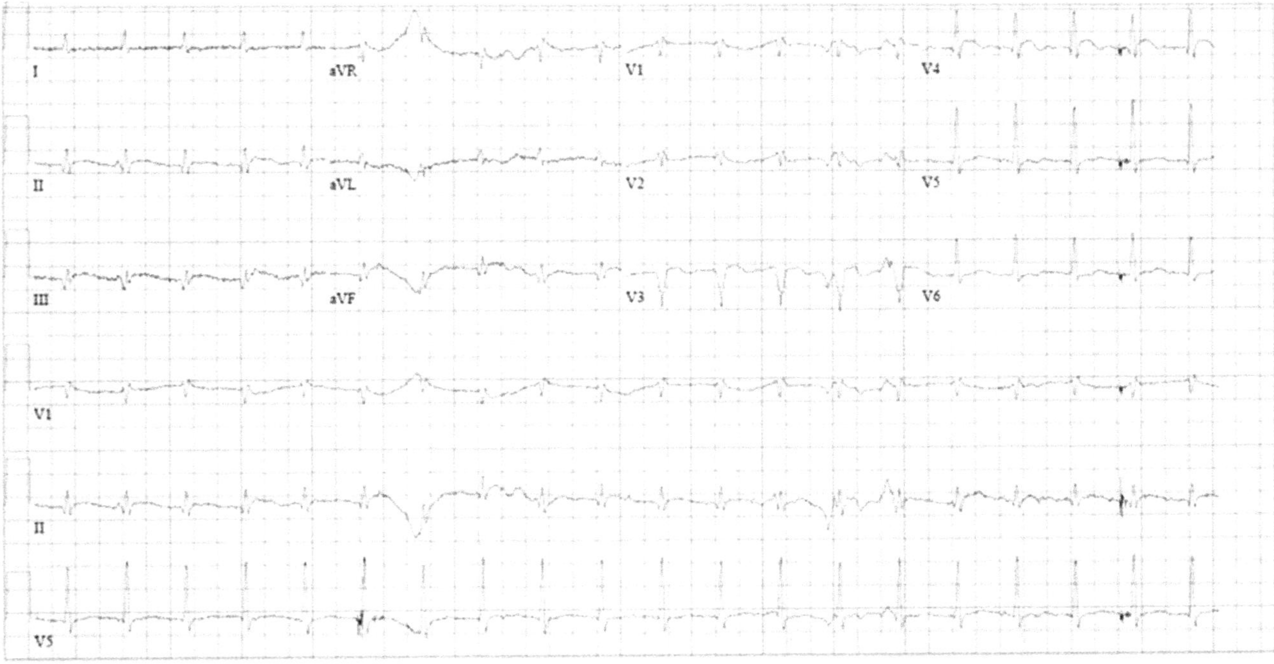

FIGURE 1: Electrocardiogram performed on patient arrival demonstrating ST-elevation in leads V3-V4.

admitted for treatment of sepsis secondary to cellulitis but elected to leave against medical advice from the emergency department and was provided with a course of doxycycline and sulfamethoxazole-trimethoprim. One day following the encounter, blood cultures drawn at the time of the encounter grew methicillin-resistant Staphylococcus aureus (MRSA).

Three days following the initial encounter, the patient again presented to the emergency department. Upon arrival, the patient was confused with nonsensical speech and was unable to provide medical history. She was febrile at 39.4°C. Physical examination was notable for pale conjunctiva, jugular venous distension, tachypnea, tachycardia, a one out of six systolic ejection murmurs at the right upper sternal border, and extensive skin wounds as described prior.

2.1. Past Medical History. The patient is with a past medical history of intravenous drug use.

2.2. Investigations. Initial blood work of the second encounter was significant for a white blood cell count of 33.1 k/μL, hemoglobin of 6.2 g/dL, hematocrit of 18.4%, mean corpuscular volume of 69.2 fL, absolute neutrophil count of 29.3 k/μL, sodium of 132 mmol/L, potassium of 3.4 mmol/L, bicarbonate of 18 mmol/L, blood urea nitrogen of 27 mg/dL, troponin of 30.5 ng/mL, N-terminal pro-B-type natriuretic peptide of 27,028 pg/mL, cocaine-positive urine toxicology, and lactic acid of 3.1 mmol/L.

2.3. Differential Diagnosis

(i) Infective endocarditis

(ii) Cellulitis, abscess

(iii) Opioid overdose

(iv) Drug-induced vasospasm

2.4. Imaging. An electrocardiogram performed on arrival demonstrated an anterolateral STEMI (Figure 1). Echocardiogram revealed anterior wall motion abnormalities and an aortic valve vegetation that filled more than half of the left ventricular outflow tract measuring 1.8 by 1.3 centimeters (Figures 2 and 3).

2.5. Management. The patient was started on vancomycin, piperacillin, tazobactam, and ceftriaxone. Acute cardiac intervention, which would have required transfer to a tertiary care center with cardiothoracic surgery capabilities, was deferred due to the patient's unstable hemodynamic state and comorbid conditions. A repeat electrocardiogram five hours later as the patient became more hypotensive revealed evolution of anterior MI with diffuse Q waves and an inferior lead STEMI (Figure 4). In the following hours, the patient became more hypotensive and hypoxic and required vasopressors and intubation with ventilator support. Subsequently, the patient became pulseless requiring cardiopulmonary resuscitation with return of spontaneous circulation after six minutes of advanced cardiac life support. Approximately twelve hours after presentation, the patient expired from cardiovascular collapse. An autopsy was not performed postmortem.

3. Discussion

There are few documented cases of acute myocardial infarction caused by IE particularly of the aortic valve. In IVDA patients, infective endocarditis most frequently affects tricuspid valves (50%) and aortic (20%) and mitral valves (20%) less frequently [11]. Most emboli stem from mitral valve vegetations and in patients with prior valve replacement. This

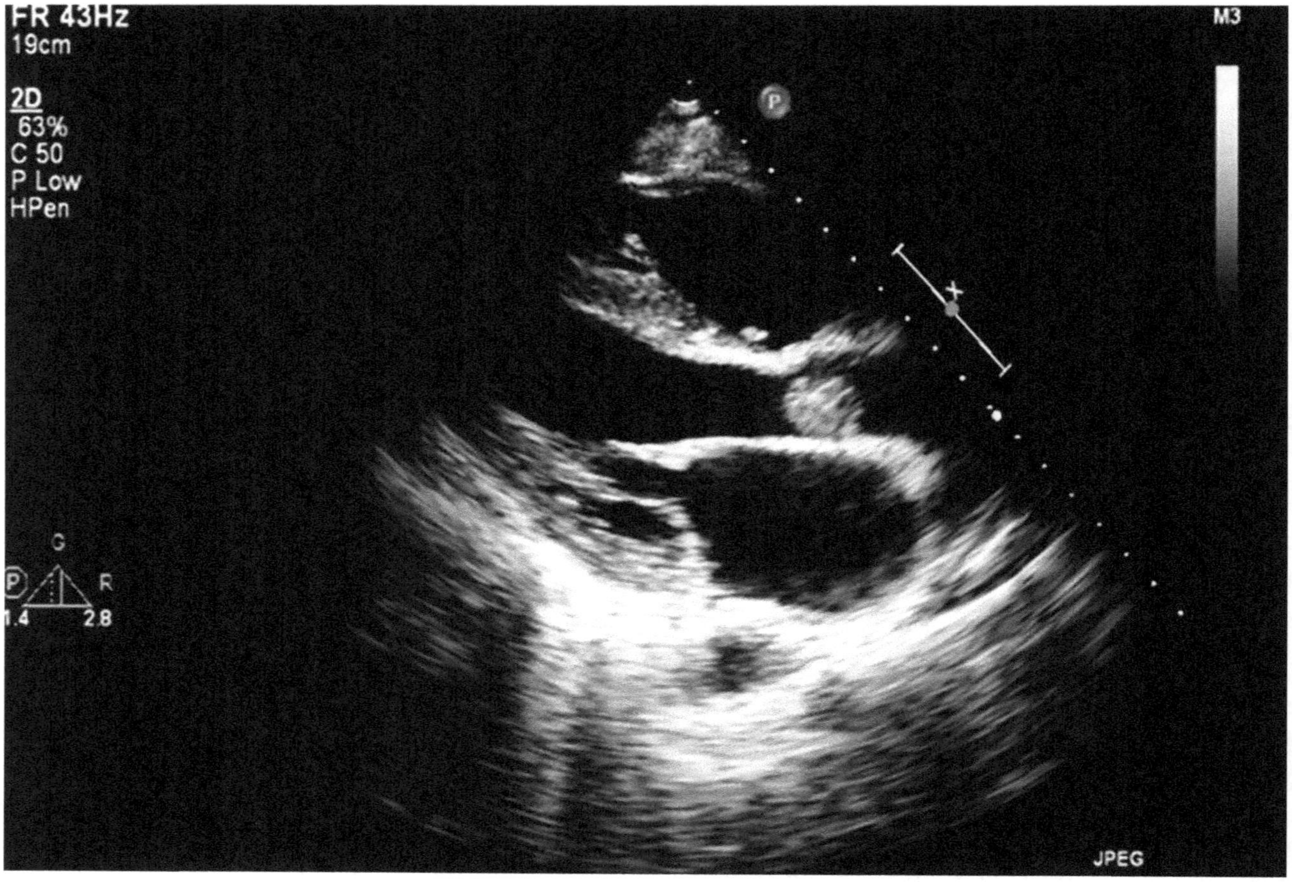

FIGURE 2: Echocardiogram demonstrating a vegetation measuring 1.8 cm × 1.3 cm.

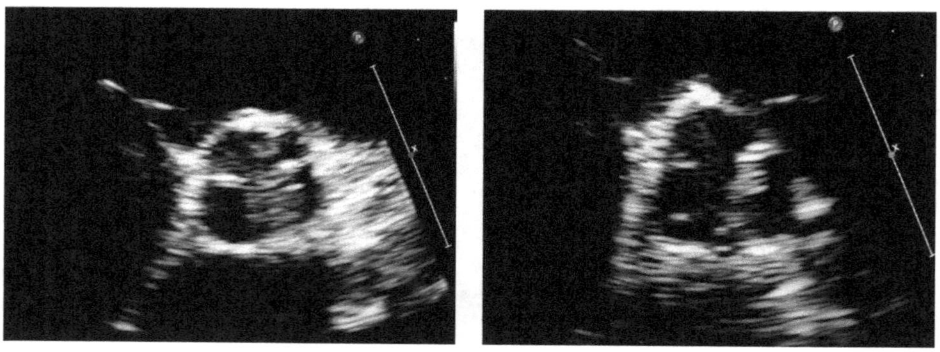

(a) (b)

FIGURE 3: Echocardiogram demonstrating a vegetation proximal to the left aortic cusp (a) and the vegetation mobilizing toward the left coronary artery origination anastomosis upon valve opening (b).

case is unique in that the patient presented with a native aortic valve vegetation that embolized to cause two consecutive acute ST-elevation myocardial infarctions affecting two distinct coronary artery territories. However, it is also necessary to consider two factors that increase the likelihood of embolization unique to this case: vegetation length and microbiology. In 2018, Mahananey et al. suggest that vegetation size of greater than 10 mm may be associated with increased embolization risk [12]. In the case presented, the patient had an 18 mm vegetation [12]. Further, Hubert et al. find that Staphylococcus aureus is also associated with an increased risk of embolization, which conforms to the microbiology found in this case [13].

There are eight previously documented cases of ST-elevation myocardial infarctions caused by embolic native aortic valve endocarditis [3–10]. The cases illustrate a spectrum of embolized coronary vessels and corresponding myocardial territories. Including the case presented here, infarcted myocardial territories are nearly all equally represented with several cases describing multiple affected territories [3–10]. In

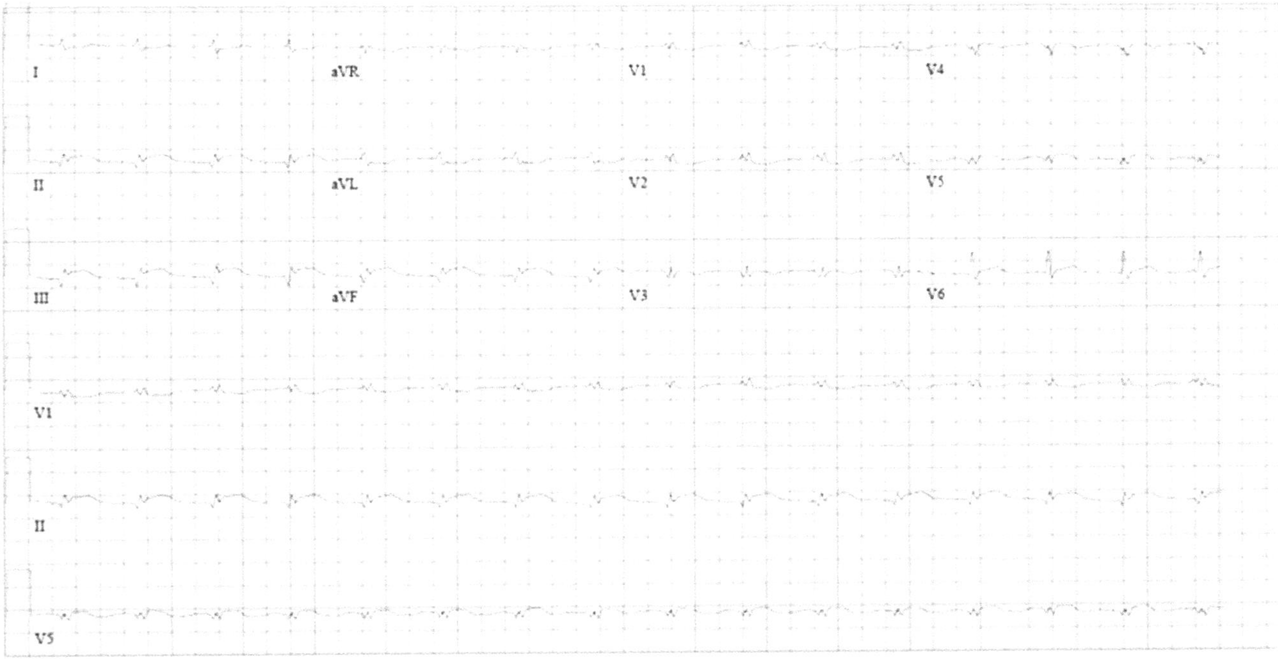

FIGURE 4: Electrocardiogram performed five hours after first electrocardiogram (Figure 1) demonstrating ST-elevation in leads II, III, and AVF.

the documented cases, 3/9 demonstrate anterior myocardial infarctions [4, 5], 2/9 demonstrate anterolateral infarctions [7, 10], 4/9 demonstrate inferior territory infarctions [6, 8, 10], and 1/9 demonstrates lateral territory infarction [9]. While there are other cases that demonstrate multiterritory infarcted myocardium, we present the first case to illustrate two consecutive infarctions. Further, infective endocarditis of the aortic valve can and frequently affect more than a single myocardial territory and can occur consecutively. This case serves as notice for clinicians to remain vigilant of the potential for sequential STEMIs in these patients.

Current treatment modalities for embolic infective endocarditis causing acute myocardial infarction are limited and unproven. Detailed guidelines for managing STEMI and for managing infective endocarditis as separate conditions exist but recommendations for concurrent diagnoses are lacking. The treatment modalities applied in the nine cases of STEMI caused by embolic aortic valve endocarditis varied considerably, as did the affected patient characteristics and associated outcomes. Of the nine cases, three underwent angioplasty; two of the three were reported to survive beyond the immediately observed period [4, 5, 7]. Three patients underwent aortic valve replacement with two surviving beyond the observed period; in one case, the final survival status was not reported [6, 9, 10]. One patient was administered fibrinolytic therapy and survived with complication of a major gastrointestinal bleed [3]. Finally, in two cases, including the one presented here, the patient received neither invasive nor fibrinolytic therapy; one patient reportedly survived beyond the observed period [8]. Given the small treatment group sizes and the infrequency of the condition, it is difficult to draw conclusions regarding treatment superiority. It is essential to evaluate each patient individually, particularly as there are no clear guidelines to direct clinicians in managing patients presenting with myocardial infarction in the setting of infective endocarditis.

Due to the rarity of this case, we consider possible predisposing factors as well as an alternative explanation to this presentation. Rather than two distinct emboli affecting different vessels, it is necessary to consider the possibility that a single embolus propagated through a wrap-around left anterior descending (LAD) artery supplying both the anterior and inferior cardiac territories. Indeed, such a scenario could feasibly present as consecutive STEMI of different coronary myocardial territories. However, while a definitive answer attained through perhaps a coronary angiogram is not available in this case, we believe the presented electrocardiograms and echocardiogram support that there were indeed two distinct emboli. First, in the initial electrocardiogram (Figure 1), the absence of inferior ischemic findings with an upstream blockage lends support that the inferior myocardial territory is not supplied by a wrap-around LAD but likely rather supplied by the right coronary artery (RCA). This is further reinforced by an echocardiogram acquired during the first insult that revealed only anterior wall motion abnormality without evidence of apical or inferior wall motion abnormality. Finally, there would likely be preferential embolization to the RCA following injury to the flow of the anterior territory.

4. Conclusion

Among the reported cases of infective aortic valve endocarditis causing embolic acute myocardial infarction, we present the first case with consecutive infarctions involving separate myocardial territories. This index case illustrates the potential severity of complications and the challenges in developing standardized management for such patients. Through this case, we hope to expand the fund of knowledge and judicious approach for similar future patients.

References

[1] S. E. Rudasill, Y. Sanaiha, A. L. Mardock et al., "Clinical outcomes of infective endocarditis in injection drug users," *Journal of the American College of Cardiology*, vol. 73, no. 5, pp. 559–570, 2019.

[2] E. Mylonakis and S. B. Calderwood, "Infective endocarditis in adults," *New England Journal of Medicine*, vol. 345, no. 18, pp. 1318–1330, 2001.

[3] D. L. Connolly, P. S. Dardas, J. J. Crowley, A. Kenny, and M. C. Petch, "Acute coronary embolism complicating aortic valve endocarditis treated with streptokinase and aspirin. A case report.," *The Journal of Heart Valve Disease*, vol. 3, no. 3, pp. 245-246, 1994.

[4] E. Ural, U. Bildirici, G. Kahraman, and B. Komsuoğlu, "Coronary embolism complicating aortic valve endocarditis: treatment with successful coronary angioplasty," *International Journal of Cardiology*, vol. 119, no. 3, pp. 377–379, 2007.

[5] B. Hibbert, M. Kazmi, J. P. Veinot, E. R. O'Brien, and C. Glover, "Infective endocarditis presenting as ST-elevation myocardial infarction: an angiographic diagnosis," *Canadian Journal of Cardiology*, vol. 28, no. 4, pp. 515.e15–515.e17, 2012.

[6] M. Singh, A. Mishra, and E. Kaluski, "Acute ST-elevation myocardial infarction due to septic embolism: a case report and review of management options," *Catheterization and Cardiovascular Interventions*, vol. 85, no. 6, pp. E166–E171, 2015.

[7] G. Murtaza, Z. U. Rahman, P. Sitwala et al., "Case of acute ST segment elevation myocardial infarction in infective endocarditismanagement with intra coronary stenting," *Clinics and Practice*, vol. 7, no. 3, 2017.

[8] J. Jose, K. Narayanan, S. T. Chacko, and O. K. George, "Infective endocarditis presenting with ST segment elevation," *Journal of Heart Valve Disease*, vol. 20, no. 4, pp. 468–470, 2011.

[9] C. J. Roxas and A. J. Weekes, "Acute myocardial infarction caused by coronary embolism from infective endocarditis," *The Journal of Emergency Medicine*, vol. 40, no. 5, pp. 509–514, 2011.

[10] F. Casazza, F. Faorista, F. Donatelli, and A. Grossi, "Acute myocardial infarction in bacterial endocarditis," *Giornale Italiano di Cardiologia*, vol. 26, no. 2, pp. 207–211, 1996.

[11] E. A. Ashley and J. Niebauer, *Cardiology Explained*, Remedica, London, 2004, Chapter 10, Infective endocarditis.

[12] S. Hubert, F. Thuny, N. Resseguier et al., "Prediction of symptomatic embolism in infective endocarditis: construction and validation of a risk calculator in a multicenter cohort," *Journal of the American College of Cardiology*, vol. 62, no. 15, pp. 1384–1392, 2013.

[13] D. Mohananey, A. Mohadjer, G. Pettersson et al., "Association of vegetation size with embolic risk in patients with infective endocarditis: a systematic review and meta-analysis," *JAMA Internal Medicine*, vol. 178, no. 4, pp. 502–510, 2011.

Simultaneous Multi-Vessel Very Late Stent Thrombosis in Acute ST-Segment Elevation Myocardial Infarction

Yuefeng Chen, Michael Amponsah, and Cyril Nathaniel

Department of Cardiology, Conemaugh Memorial Medical Center, Johnstown, Pennsylvania 15905, USA

Correspondence should be addressed to Yuefeng Chen; cyf.usa@gmail.com

Academic Editor: Dirk Bandorski

Simultaneous multi-vessel very later stent thrombosis (VLST) is a very rare complication of percutaneous coronary intervention (PCI). We present a case of simultaneous multi-vessel VLST as the cause of acute ST-segment elevation myocardial infarction (STEMI). PCI of the culprit vessel was performed at acute presentation. Resolution of in-stent thrombosis in non-culprit vessels was noted on coronary angiography 2 days later. Our case suggests that PCI for culprit lesion in acute setting may be a reasonable option for simultaneous multi-vessel VLST.

1. Introductions

VLST is defined as stent thrombosis that occurs after first year after the initial implantation [1]. It is a very rare complication of stent implantation with an incidence of less than 1% during a 4-year follow-up [2]. Simultaneous multi-vessel thrombosis in the setting of acute STEMI has been reported [3], but simultaneous multi-vessel VLST in acute STEMI is extremely rare. Here we report a case of acute STEMI with simultaneous multi-vessel VLST with the last stent implantation of 5 years prior.

2. Case Presentation

The patient is a 71-year-old male with history of coronary artery disease (CAD) was brought to emergency room for left-sided chest pain for 45 minutes, associated with shortness of breath, diaphoresis and nausea. He has history of PCI of proximal to mid left anterior descending artery (LAD) and proximal left circumflex artery (LCX) with drug-eluting stents (DES) in March, 2012, repeated PCI of mid LAD with DES in March, 2015, and PCI of mid and distal right coronary artery (RCA) in January, 2016. He also has history of hypertension, type II diabetes mellitus and morbid obesity. He was taking Aspirin 325 mg daily, Prasugrel 10 mg daily, Quinapril 40 mg daily, Atorvastatin 80 mg daily. Physical exam revealed body mass index 43.1 kg/m^2, blood pressure 157/122 mmHg, heart rate 131 beats/minute, respiration rate 24/minute, oxygen saturation 97%, he was in acute respiratory distress, with diaphoresis, tachycardia, tachypnea and bilateral lungs decreased breath sounds, but no wheezing or crackles. Laboratory studies showed SARS-CoV-2 negative, hemoglobin A1C 6.9%, eGFR 60 ml/min, White blood cell 10.8x10^3/ul, platelet 316x10^3/ul, B-type natriuretic peptide 340 pg/ml, Troponin I 0.01 ng/ml, Total cholesterol 199 mg/dl, Low-density lipoproteins 140 mg/dl. Initial electrocardiography showed anterior ST segment elevation. He was intubated due to respiratory distress and unable to lie flat. Emergency cardiac catheterization revealed 100% occlusion of proximal to mid LAD with instent thrombosis, and 90% stenosis in proximal LCX and mid RCA stents (Figure 1(a)–1(c)). PCI of proximal to mid LAD was performed and TIMI-3 flow to distal LAD was restored, a Synergy 3.0 x 24 mm DES was then placed and post dilated with a 3.5 mm non-compliant balloon (Figure 1(d)). The patient was hemodynamically stable and brought back to catheterization laboratory 2 days later for staged PCI of LCX and RCA lesions. However, angiography showed that previously found severe stenosis in the above vessels was no longer visualized (Figure 1(e) and 1(f)), it turned out that previously noted instent stenosis was actually caused by thrombus at the time of acute STEMI and had dissolved

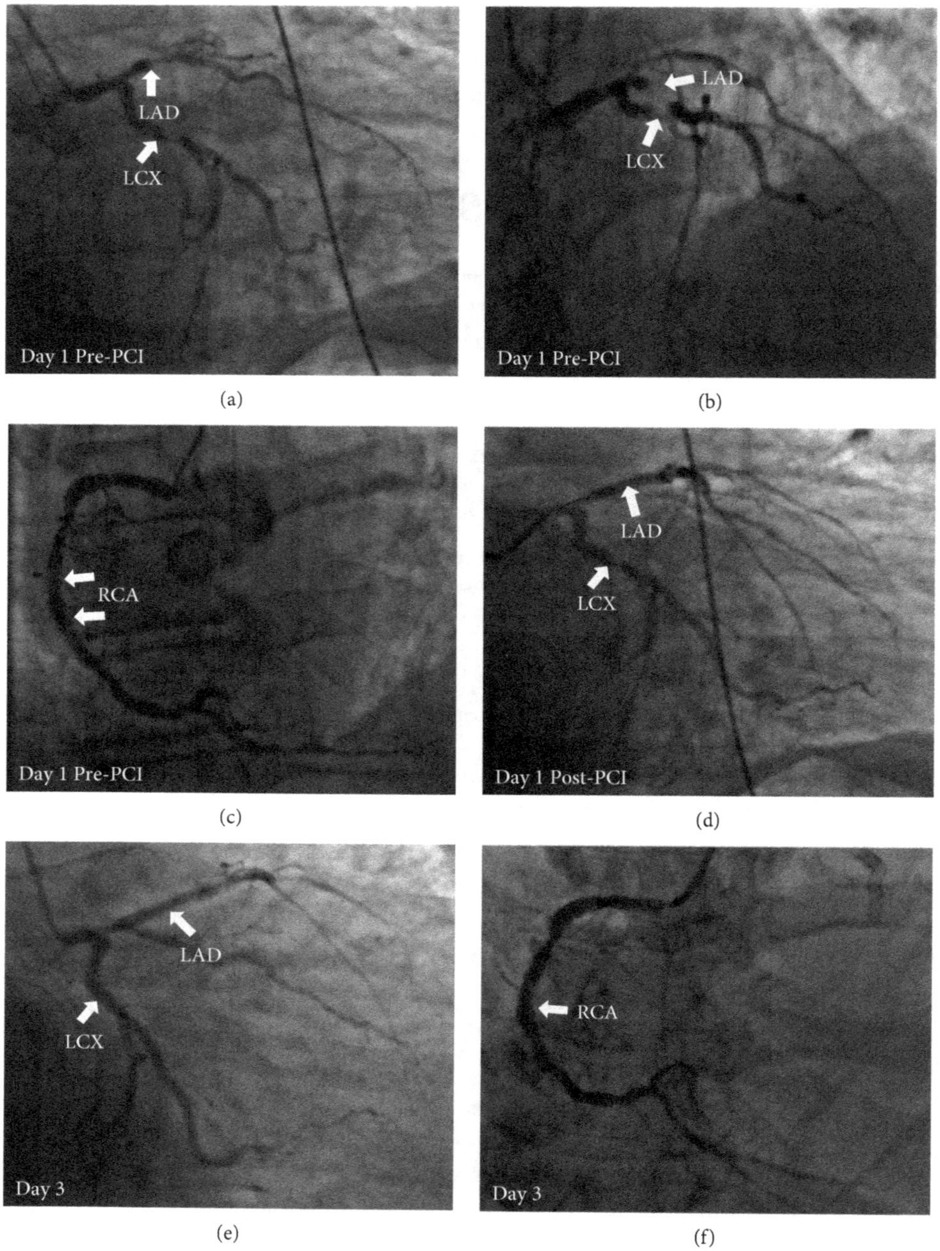

Figure 1: Coronary angiography and LAD primary PCI. Thrombotic occlusion at the site of the proximal LAD stent with TIMI 0 flow (A, B, arrow) and evidence of thrombus at the site of the proximal LCX stent (A, B, arrow) and the mid RCA stent (C, arrows). Following PCI and restoration of TIMI 3 flow in the LAD, there was evidence of remaining thrombus at the site of proximal LCX stent (D, arrow). Resolution of thrombus at the site of the proximal LCX stent (E, arrow) and the mid RCA stent (F, arrow) on day 3 of admission. LAD: left anterior descending artery; LCX: left circumflex artery; RCA: right coronary artery; PCI: percutaneous coronary intervention.

spontaneously over time. No PCI of mid LCX and RCA was performed. Patient recovered well and was discharged later.

3. Discussions

VLST is an uncommon complication of stent implantation, the incidence is generally less than 1% in newer generation DES [4], and is especially rare after 5 years of initial stenting. In our case, the last stent in the culprit vessel (LAD) was placed 6 years ago, and the stents in LCX and RCA were placed 9 years and 5 years ago, respectively. VLST has been reported to be more often associated with DES than with BMS [5]. It usually presents as acute STEMI, but compared to patients with early and late ST, patients with VLST had better prognosis with lower incidence of major adverse cardiac events and mortality [6–8]. The mechanism of VLST is not fully understood, but is thought to be related to delayed incomplete stent strut endothelialization [9, 10], stent strut malapposition secondary to positive remodeling [10, 11], stent fracture [12], hypersensitivity reaction to polymers [13, 14], chronic inflammation [9, 15], rupture of lipid-laden-like neointima within the DES [10], and discontinuation of antiplatelet therapy [16]. In our case, we did not notice anything from his medical history that known to contribute to VLST, and there was no delay in patient transfer or patient care. Simultaneous triple vessel VLST is extremely rare, only a few cases have been reported [17, 18]. Treatment for multi-vessel ST can be challenging, whether PCI should be performed on all lesions at initial presentation is not certain. In our case, VLST caused 100% occlusion of LAD, while LCX and RCA remained TIMI 3 flow during the procedure, only culprit lesion was treated with PCI initially, the thrombus in the other two vessels dissolved spontaneously in 2 days, suggesting that as long as blood flow is not comprised in non-culprit vessels, culprit lesion only management at presentation may be reasonable. VLST is a multifactorial event and prevention can be difficult, some patients may need oral anticoagulation or long term DAPT therapy. More research needs to be done to identify those who are at high risk for VLST, especially in current era of trending toward short DAPT treatment duration.

4. Conclusions

Simultaneous triple vessel VLST is a very rare complication following stent implantation. When blood flow in non-culprit vessels is not comprised, PCI for culprit lesion only at initial presentation may be a reasonable option.

References

[1] D. E. Cutlip, S. Windecker, R. Mehran et al., "Clinical end points in coronary stent Trials," *Circulation*, vol. 115, no. 17, pp. 2344–2351, 2007.

[2] L. Mauri, W. H. Hsieh, J. M. Massaro, K. K. Ho, R. Agostino, and D. E. Cutlip, "Stent thrombosis in randomized clinical trials of drug-eluting stents," *The New England Journal of Medicine*, vol. 356, no. 10, pp. 1020–1029, 2007.

[3] A. Mahmoud, M. Saad, and I. Y. Elgendy, "Simultaneous multi-vessel coronary thrombosis in patients with ST-elevation myocardial infarction: a systematic review," *Cardiovascular Revascularization Medicine*, vol. 16, no. 3, pp. 163–166, 2015.

[4] L. Räber, M. Magro, G. G. Stefanini et al., "Very late coronary stent thrombosis of a newer-generation everolimus-eluting stent compared with early-generation drug-eluting stents: a prospective cohort study," *Circulation*, vol. 125, no. 9, pp. 1110–1121, 2012.

[5] B. Brodie, Y. Pokharel, N. Fleishman et al., "Very late stent thrombosis after primary percutaneous coronary intervention with bare-metal and drug-eluting stents for ST-segment elevation myocardial infarction: a 15-year single-center experience," *JACC. Cardiovascular Interventions*, vol. 4, no. 1, pp. 30–38, 2011.

[6] T. Kimura, T. Morimoto, K. Kozuma et al., "Comparisons of baseline demographics, clinical presentation, and long-term outcome among patients with early, late, and very late stent thrombosis of sirolimus-eluting stents: observations from the registry of stent thrombosis for review and reevaluation (RESTART)," *Circulation*, vol. 122, no. 1, pp. 52–61, 2010.

[7] S. Kubo, K. Kadota, T. Ichinohe et al., "Comparison of long-term outcome after percutaneous coronary intervention for stent thrombosis between early, late, and very late stent thrombosis," *Circulation Journal*, vol. 78, no. 1, pp. 101–109, 2014.

[8] E. J. Armstrong, D. N. Feldman, T. Y. Wang et al., "Clinical presentation, management, and outcomes of angiographically documented early, late, and very late stent thrombosis," *JACC. Cardiovascular Interventions*, vol. 5, no. 2, pp. 131–140, 2012.

[9] M. Joner, A. V. Finn, A. Farb et al., "Pathology of drug-eluting stents in humans: delayed healing and late thrombotic risk," *Journal of the American College of Cardiology*, vol. 48, no. 1, pp. 193–202, 2006.

[10] S. Miyazaki, Y. Hiasa, T. Takahashi et al., "In vivo optical coherence tomography of very late drug-eluting stent thrombosis compared with late in-stent restenosis," *Circulation Journal*, vol. 76, no. 2, pp. 390–398, 2012.

[11] S. Cook, P. Wenaweser, M. Togni et al., "Incomplete stent apposition and very late stent thrombosis after drug-eluting stent implantation," *Circulation*, vol. 115, no. 18, pp. 2426–2434, 2007.

[12] Z. Y. Huang, J. Y. Qian, and J. B. Ge, "Very late stent thrombosis due to multiple stent fracture and stent malapposition," *Chinese Medical Journal*, vol. 126, no. 1, pp. 186–189, 2013.

[13] R. Virmani, G. Guagliumi, A. Farb et al., "Localized hypersensitivity and late coronary thrombosis secondary to a sirolimus-eluting stent: should we be cautious?," *Circulation*, vol. 109, no. 6, pp. 701–705, 2004.

[14] R. Rayoo, M. Rayoo, G. Ferrante, and P. Barlis, "Histological confirmation of hypersensitivity as a contributor to very-late coronary stent thrombosis," *International Journal of Cardiology*, vol. 157, no. 2, pp. e29–e30, 2012.

[15] S. Cook, E. Ladich, G. Nakazawa et al., "Correlation of intravascular ultrasound findings with histopathological analysis of thrombus aspirates in patients with very late drug-eluting stent thrombosis," *Circulation*, vol. 120, no. 5, pp. 391–399, 2009.

[16] K. N. Huang, S. M. Grandi, K. B. Filion, and M. J. Eisenberg, "Late and very late stent thrombosis in patients with second-generation drug-eluting stents," *The Canadian Journal of Cardiology*, vol. 29, no. 11, pp. 1488–1494, 2013.

[17] S. Narasimhan, N. R. Krim, G. Silverman, and E. S. Monrad, "Simultaneous very late stent thrombosis in multiple coronary arteries," *Texas Heart Institute Journal*, vol. 39, no. 5, pp. 630–634, 2012.

[18] M. S. Vieira, A. Luz, D. Anjo et al., "Trombose tripla, simultanea, muito tardia de _stents_ coron arios," *Revista Portuguesa de Cardiologia*, vol. 32, no. 3, pp. 247–252, 2013.

Symptomatic Supraventricular Tachycardia Resistant to Adenosine Therapy in a Patient with Chronic Theophylline Use

Seyedeh Maryam Hosseini,[1] Muhammad Ajmal,[1] and Ranjith Shetty[2]

[1]*University of Arizona College of Medicine, USA*
[2]*Carondelet Medical Group, USA*

Correspondence should be addressed to Seyedeh Maryam Hosseini; shosseini@deptofmed.arizona.edu

Academic Editor: Assad Movahed

Theophylline is a potent adenosine receptor antagonist with indirect adrenergic effects that can lead to arrhythmias and metabolic abnormalities such as hypokalemia. Therapeutic toxicity cases have declined over the years mainly due to decreased recommended therapeutic doses and overall decreased usage of this medication due to newer available COPD treatment options. We present a clinical case of symptomatic supraventricular tachycardia resistant to adenosine therapy in a patient with theophylline use. This case highlights the importance of comprehensive medication review in acute settings to aid in identifying the underlying etiologies and initiating prompt treatments. It also signifies the importance of reviewing chronic medications in each outpatient visits to ensure continued indication for their use and be able to change them to newer agents per guidelines whenever possible.

1. Introduction

Theophylline is well known for its bronchodilation effects. It is used for pulmonary obstructive disease, severe bradycardia, apnea, and asthma in certain premature and pediatric patients. It is also associated with adrenergic effects that can predispose patients to arrhythmias. We present a case of symptomatic supraventricular tachycardia unresponsive to adenosine.

2. Clinical Case Description

A 62-year-old male with a past medical history significant for hypertension, heart failure with persevered ejection fraction (HFpEF), alcohol abuse, chronic obstructive pulmonary disease (COPD) on chronic theophylline presented with epigastric abdominal pain, and vomiting after one day of heavy alcohol drinking. He denied hematemesis, melena, fall, and change in mental status. He was admitted with protocol in place for acute alcohol toxicity and alcohol withdrawal care. His initial presentation was significant for sinus tachycardia that resolved with fluid resuscitation. He had negative troponin values, positive elevated serum alcohol levels, metabolic acidosis, and normal hepatic function enzymes with no signs of acute infection or bleeding.

On the second day of admission, the patient developed shortness of breath and palpitations. EKG showed supraventricular tachycardia, atrioventricular tachycardia nodal reentrant type, with a heart rate of 181 beats per minute (Figure 1). 6 milligram (mg) of adenosine was administered as rapid IV push but did not terminate the arrhythmia, and the next dose of 12 mg of adenosine rapid IV push was administered which was also unsuccessful (Figure 2). Because of the failure of adenosine to terminate arrhythmia and decreasing blood pressure measurements most likely secondary to ongoing SVT, cardioversion for unstable SVT was considered; however, patient regained hemodynamic stability quickly with administration of intravenous bolus of fluids as well as amiodarone 150 mg which was able to terminate the arrhythmia (Figure 3). His blood pressure improved from 85/60 mmHg to 122/74 mmHg after arrhythmia termination. Patient remained responsive, alert, and oriented and only complained of palpitations while having SVT. Serum theophylline level was found to be 4.67ug/mL (Table 1).

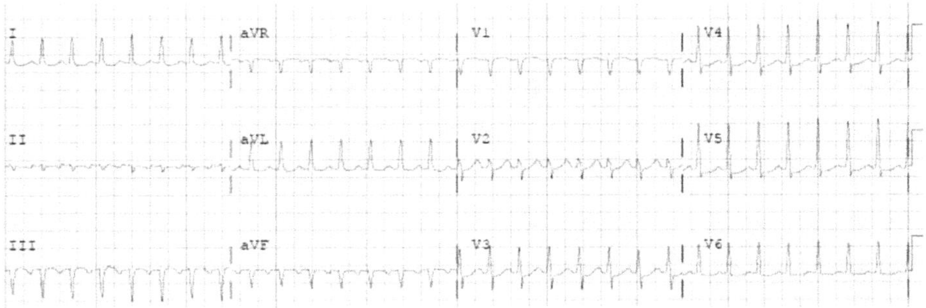

FIGURE 1: Initial EKG showing supraventricular tachycardia with heart rate of 181 beats per minute.

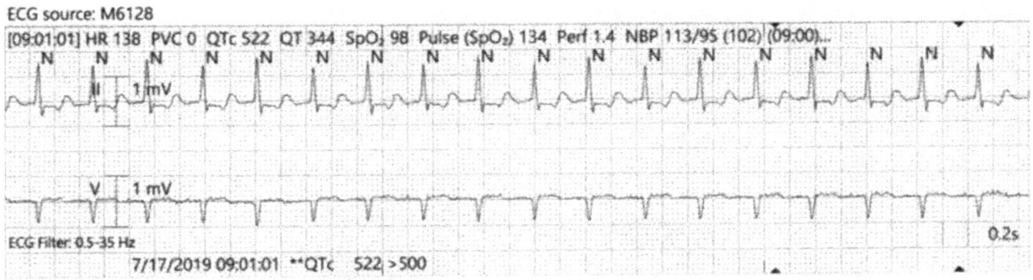

FIGURE 2: Patient's rhythm strip showing no improvement in response to adenosine.

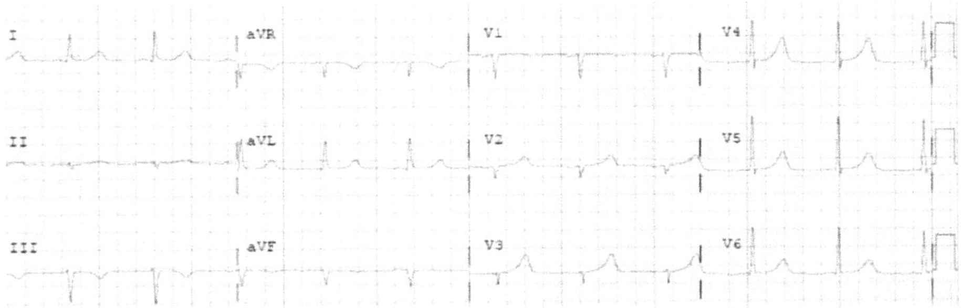

FIGURE 3: Patient's EKG after completion of amiodarone bolus showing resolution of supraventricular tachycardia.

Patient's theophylline was stopped. He was started on tiotropium, an inhaled long-acting muscarinic antagonist as well as rescue inhaler albuterol, short acting beta agonist, for his COPD management. Patient was monitored in Coronary Care Unit for 24 hours and remained symptom free. He was transferred to medicine unit and discharged after two additional days of hospitalization. At discharge patient was recommended to take his new inhaler medications for COPD while stopping theophylline. Patient was discharged in stable condition with no further need or indication of amiodarone or any other antiarrhythmic drug.

3. Discussion

Theophylline metabolism and kinetics have a wide variation as a function of age. It is rapidly absorbed, metabolized by the liver, and excreted by the kidney. Toxic levels are seen mainly in serum concentrations of above 20 μg/mL, but symptoms of toxicity can be seen at even lower end of therapeutic levels in some older patients and in those with chronic theophylline use such as in our case [1]. Theophylline effects are well explained by its mechanism of action. It is a potent adenosine receptor antagonist. In a case series study done in Massachusetts Children's Hospital, theophylline intoxication was shown to be associated with increased catecholamine serum levels in humans [2]. This was also shown on animal studies [3]. Theophylline is an antagonism of all adenosine receptor types, A1, A2A, A2B, and A3 which leads to increased norepinephrine release causing overall indirect adrenergic effects and thus metabolic abnormalities such as hypokalemia, hyperglycemia, and metabolic acidosis. It also predisposes to arrhythmias and can cause hypotension that is likely mediated by not only arrhythmias but also by beta adrenergic vasodilatory mechanism. Theophylline is also a nonselective competitive inhibitor of phosphodiesterases (PDE) 3 and 4 which results in relaxation of smooth muscle cells in the airways, and this in fact is the main mechanism of theophylline bronchodilation effect [2]. In addition, there are studies suggesting theophylline rule in stimulation of calcium release from intracellular stores and also in IL-10 secretion and apoptosis of inflammatory cells [1].

Being an adenosine receptor antagonist, patients on theophylline, as seen in our case, when in tachycardia state, may

Table 1: Complete blood count, comprehensive metabolic panel, troponin, and theophylline blood test results.

Blood test	Result	Normal range
White blood cell count	4.2 K/MM3	4-11 K/MM3
Red blood cell (RBC) count	3.86 M/MM3 L	4.30-6.00 M/MM3 L
Hemoglobin	12.0 g/dL L	13.5-17.00 g/dL L
Hematocrit	36.8% L	40.0-53.0 L
Mean corpuscular volume	95 fL	78-100 fL
Mean corpuscular hemoglobin	31.1 pg	27.0-34.0 pg
Mean corpuscular hemoglobin concentration	32.6 g/dL	31.0-37.0 g/dL
Red cell distribution width—coefficient of variation	15.6% H	11.0-15.0%
Red cell distribution width—standard deviation	54.4 fL H	38.0-49.9 fL
Nucleated RBC, automated	0%	≤0%
Platelet count	173 K/MM3	130-450 K/MM3
Mean platelet volume	10.1 fL	9.0-12.0 fL
Albumin/globulin ration	1.3	1.0-2.0
Albumin	3.9 g/dL	3.4-5.0 g/dL
Alkaline phosphatase	89 IU/L	40-150 IU/L
Alanine aminotransferase	19 IU/L	10-60 IU/L
Anion gap	12	4-16
Aspartate aminotransferase	38 IU/L	10-50 IU/L
Bilirubin total	1.1 mg/dL	0.2-1.3 mg/dL
Blood urea nitrogen (BUN)	4 mg/dL	8-25 mg/dL
BUN/creatinine ratio	4	10-28
Calcium	9.2 mg/dL	8.3-10.4 mg/dL
Chloride	104 mmol/L	96-110 mmol/L
CO2	21 mmol/L	21-31 mmol/L
Creatinine	0.90 mg/dL	0.60-1.50 mg/dL
Estimated glomerular filtration rate (African descent)	105 mL/min/1.73 m^2	≥60 mL/min/1.73 m^2
Glucose	134 mg/dL	65-99 mg/dL
International normalized ratio (INR)	1.0	0.9-1.1
Lipase	24 IU/L	8-78 IU/L
Potassium	3.5 mmol/L	3.5-5.2 mmol/L
Protein, total	7.0 g/dL	6.0-8.0 g/dL
Sodium	137 mmol/L	135-145 mmol/L
Troponin-I, conventional	<0.01 ng/mL	0.00-0.02 ng/mL
Theophylline	4.67 μg/mL	10.00-20.00 μg/mL

be resistant to treatment with adenosine, due to blocked receptors by the theophylline in the serum. Therefore, failure of regular dose treatment with adenosine is not surprising. Adenosine may still be attempted however as there have been case reports of successful SVT treatment with repeated adenosine therapy [4]. It has been known that most common types of arrhythmias associated with theophylline are supraventricular tachycardia (SVT) [5]. This is seen in our patient's case as well. Adenosine, either on initial or repeated dosing, can reverse theophylline induced supraventricular tachycardia [6]. But it should be given with caution in patients with severe pulmonary obstructive disease due to its bronchoconstriction effect. In such cases, selective beta 1 antagonist such as esmolol can safely be used to terminate SVT [7]. Calcium channel blockers such as diltiazem or verapamil can also be used but in caution in patients with hypotension [8]. In our case, given failure of response to initial therapies and patient's hemodynamic instability by hypotension, amiodarone and fluid resuscitation was used with eventual success in stabilizing patient. Amiodarone is an antiarrhythmic medication with known severe potential side effects, and given no prolonged use indication or requirement in our patient, it was not continued beyond the initial bolus administration in our patient.

It is important to recognize the possibility of multifactorial etiology for our patient's presentation. Alcohol and dehydration can also contribute and exacerbate tachycardia. Termination of SVT was therefore most likely multifactorial secondary to spontaneous resolution, fluid resuscitation, and amiodarone therapy. Our patient was recommended to follow-up with cardiology and pulmonary clinics for better guideline-based therapies for his chronic conditions.

4. Conclusion

Theophylline and adenosine interactions are well known and used in laboratory settings for years, but clinical cases are rarely reported in literature. This case is significant in showing clinical manifestation of these interactions. Providers' careful medication review not only can aid in timely diagnosis and understanding the underlying pathophysiology of an acute situation but can also help to prevent adverse effects. It is also important to regularly review chronic medications and substitute for any possible newer options that might have less adverse effects compared to older medications.

References

[1] P. J. Barnes, "Theophylline?," *American Journal of Respiratory and Critical Care Medicine*, vol. 188, no. 8, pp. 901–906, 2013.

[2] M. Shannon, "Hypokalemia, hyperglycemia and plasma catecholamine activity after severe theophylline intoxication," *Journal of Toxicology. Clinical Toxicology*, vol. 32, p. 41, 2008.

[3] M. P. Biberstein, M. G. Ziegler, and D. M. Ward, "Use of beta-blockade and hemoperfusion for acute theophylline poisoning," *The Western Journal of Medicine*, vol. 141, p. 485, 1984.

[4] A. A. Giagounidis, S. Schäfer, R. M. Klein, C. Aul, and B. E. Strauer, "Adenosine is worth trying in patients with paroxysmal supraventricular tachycardia on chronic theophylline medication," *European Journal of Medical Research*, vol. 3, no. 8, pp. 380–382, 1998.

[5] M. Shannon, "Predictors of major toxicity after theophylline overdose," *Annals of Internal Medicine*, vol. 119, no. 12, p. 1161, 1993.

[6] C. B. Cairns and J. T. Niemann, "Intravenous adenosine in the emergency department management of paroxysmal supraventricular tachycardia," *Annals of Emergency Medicine*, vol. 20, no. 7, pp. 717–721, 1991.

[7] R. J. Hoffman, N. E. Flomenbaum, L. R. Goldfrank, and R. S. Hoffman, Eds., "Methylxanthines and selective beta2-adrenergic agonists," in *Goldfrank's Toxicologic Emergencies*, p. 989, McGraw-Hill, New York, 8th edition, 2006.

[8] N. A. Minton and J. A. Henry, "Treatment of theophylline overdose?," *The American Journal of Emergency Medicine*, vol. 14, no. 6, pp. 606–612, 1996.

12

Severe Prinzmetal's Angina Inducing Ventricular Fibrillation Cardiac Arrest

Bashar Khiatah, [1] **David Philips,** [2] **Jonathan Dukes,** [2] **and Amanda Frugoli** [3]

[1] *Department of Internal Medicine, Community Memorial Hospital, 147 N Brent St, Ventura, CA 93003, USA*
[2] *Cardiology Associates Medical Group, Ventura, CA, USA*
[3] *Department of GME Internal Medicine, Community Memorial Hospital, Ventura, CA, USA*

Correspondence should be addressed to Bashar Khiatah; bkhiatah@cmhshealth.org

Academic Editor: Assad Movahed

Prinzmetal's angina is a vascular spasm of the coronary artery that can mimic acute coronary syndrome. It is rarely responsible for ventricular arrhythmias and cardiac arrest; however, survivors with these complications are at increased risk for recurrent ventricular arrhythmias and sudden cardiac death. This is true despite the presence of normal cardiac function and optimal medical therapy. Thus, this select population should be considered for an implantable cardioverter defibrillator (ICD). In this case vignette, we describe a healthy 48-year-old female with ventricular fibrillation arrest, followed by recurrent ventricular tachyarrhythmias caused by Prinzmetal's angina.

1. Introduction

Vasospastic angina (VSA), variant angina (VA), or Prinzmetal's angina is a focal spasm of one or more coronary arteries, without clinically significant atherosclerosis or atherosclerotic plaque. These spasms are responsible for inducing anginal symptoms and temporary ischemia [1, 2]. Research has shown many eliciting factors that increase the sensitivity of the coronary arteries, which in turn cause a hyperconstrictive reaction of the smooth muscles in the coronary arteries [3]. For example, endothelial dysfunction in noncritical plaque can facilitate the vasospasm, which we believe is the electing factor in our case. Rarely, Prinzmetal's angina is responsible for cardiac arrest [4]. Despite optimal medical treatment with calcium channel blockers and nitrates, 5% to 30% of patients continue to have recurrent anginal episodes. Both myocardial infarction and arrhythmia resulting in sudden cardiac death may occur [5]. Thus, treatment choices for this population of patients can be challenging. While vasodilator therapy provides relief of anginal symptoms and ventricular arrhythmia episodes, implantable cardioverter defibrillator (ICD) implantation is the treatment of choice in the case of recurrence, combined with medical therapy [6].

2. Clinical Case

A 48-year-old healthy, athletic Japanese female with a past medical history of right renal agenesis presented to the emergency department after being found unconscious by her husband. This occurred just minutes after she reported having severe 10/10 chest pressure with radiation to her jaw. Her husband called 911, and emergency medical service arrived within 7 min. She was found to be in ventricular fibrillation arrest and CPR was immediately started. No epinephrine was administered, but she was defibrillated twice with return of spontaneous circulation. Subsequently, she was brought to the hospital for further evaluation.

The patient states that she has never had this before and has no prior cardiac history. A detailed review of systems included 2-3 loose stools a day, for several days, which started shortly after completing a 30-mile marathon earlier in the week. She reports being unable to finish the run, due to recurrent anginal symptoms. Otherwise, she denied any significant symptoms. Her family history consists of a mother with breast cancer and a father with no significant medical history. Socially, the patient is married and just moved to the United States from Japan 2 years ago. She quit smoking 15 years ago and previously was smoking 6 cigarettes a day for approximately 10 years. She denied any prior recreational drug use. She reports drinking one beer a day.

Her emergency room labs included a normal troponin, as well as hypokalemia at 2.7. Her ECG showed normal sinus rhythm, no ST segment elevations or depressions, and nonspecific T wave abnormalities (Figure 1). She was started on medical therapy with aspirin 325 mg po daily, 80 mEq of potassium, metoprolol 12.5 mg BID, and a heparin drip. Her follow-up studies demonstrated minimally uptrending troponins after 6 hours, with a peak level of 0.18 ng/ml. A transthoracic echocardiogram was completed and was unremarkable, demonstrating preserved left ventricular systolic function and normal wall motion.

A subsequent cardiac catheterization was performed, which showed no obstructive atherosclerotic disease. She did have mild mid left anterior descending artery stenosis, which did improve with intracoronary nitroglycerin (Figure 2). Otherwise, her coronary arteries were normal.

Her clinical course within the first 24 hours of admission was complicated by recurrent episodes of chest pain, associated with dynamic ST elevation on ECG (Figure 1(b)). She subsequently developed nonsustained ventricular tachycardia (Figures 1(c) and 1(d)). Metoprolol was discontinued, and she was started on amlodipine 5 mg and isosorbide mononitrate 30 mg daily. An external defibrillator LifeVest was ordered.

Additional work-up at this point included a procainamide drug challenge, in order to exclude Brugada syndrome. The patient was given 10 mg/kg of procainamide over 10 min. Her baseline ECG demonstrated normal sinus rhythm, with no notable ST segment abnormalities in the precordial leads V1-V2. No changes in the ST segments or T waves occurred with the procainamide drug challenge. Other possible etiologies for recurrent ventricular arrhythmias were considered but were felt to be less likely the cause in her case: long QT interval (normal QTc on exam and all other ECGs), catecholaminergic polymorphic ventricular tachycardia ((CPVT) VT events were monomorphic and occurred at rest), short QT, and early repolarization (no ECG evidence). Autoimmune etiology was excluded with negative serology including antinuclear antibody, anti-double-stranded deoxyribonucleic acid, and rheumatoid factor. A cardiac magnetic resonance imaging was scheduled to evaluate for infiltrative disease and arrhythmogenic right ventricular cardiomyopathy (ARVC).

Given the presentation of cardiac arrest and her ongoing nonsustained ventricular tachycardia, the tentative plan at this time is to proceed with ICD implantation. After the initiation of the calcium channel blocker and long-acting nitrate, the patient's symptoms and events completely subsided. She was discharged home on these medications and the LifeVest, with a follow-up appointment for ICD placement and magnetic resonance imaging. A couple of weeks after, her MRI was negative for any infiltrative disease and ICD was implanted.

3. Discussion

VSA is a widespread diagnosis that includes documented spontaneous attacks of angina pectoris elicited by coronary epicardial vasospasm (EV) and/or coronary microvascular dysfunction (CMD). The diagnostic criteria for VSA, as proposed by the Coronary Vasomotor Disorders International Study Group (COVADIS) [7], includes nitrate sensitive angina with one of the following: rest angina; marked diurnal variation in exercise tolerance; hyperventilation-induced episode or calcium channel blocker-sensitive angina (7); transient ischemic ECG changes, including 0.1 mV ST elevation or depression or new negative U waves in at least two contiguous leads (7); and total or subtotal coronary artery spasm with angina and ischemic ECG changes, either spontaneously or in response to a provocative stimulus (7). Prinzmetal's angina differs from traditional stable angina pectoris anatomically, as it is not driven by atherosclerotic lumen encroachment within the coronary vasculature [8].

Although VSA may coexist with coronary microvascular disorders and/or structural CAD, it is a clinical entity that involves hyperreactivity of the epicardial arteries to vasoconstrictor stimuli [4]. The significance of diagnosing VSA is tied to the major complications correlated with this disorder, including acute myocardial infarction, arrhythmias, or sudden cardiac death (SCD) [9–11], and, in turn, the potential to prevent these life-threatening events by using nitrates and calcium channel blockers and by avoiding potential vasospasm stimuli (2).

Treatment for these patients consists of smoking cessation, weight loss, and avoiding psychological stress or excessive exercise. Also, cardiac rehabilitation and exercise training with behavioral therapy is a cornerstone in therapy [12]. Medical therapies consist of calcium channel blockers and nitrates, with preference given to calcium channel blockers due to concern that long-acting nitrates may produce nitrate intolerance. However, combination therapy with a calcium channel blocker and a nitrate may have a synergistic effect and provide relief when a patient has VSA refractory to monotherapy. Despite the association of vasospasm with atherosclerotic lesions, data regarding the use of aspirin is currently lacking; however, based on current knowledge, low-dose aspirin (<100 mg daily) appears to be safe and may be effective in preventing acute attacks [13]. High-dose aspirin (≥325 mg daily) and beta blockers should both be avoided, as they may elicit an episode of VSA [14]. Finally, invasive treatment includes stent implantation, implantable cardioverter defibrillator, and partial sympathetic denervation. These options are case by case dependent. For example, in a patient with consistent vasospasm due to arterial injury, stenting is a reasonable option. ICD implantation, on the other hand, may be considered for secondary prevention in patients who have had a cardiac arrest secondary to VSA [15]. A recent publication in the *Journal of Arrhythmia*, by Akiko et al., suggested that combined medical treatment using CCB with an ICD may be effective for reducing recurrent ventricular dysrhythmias for some patients with coronary vasospasm who have been successfully resuscitated from ventricular fibrillation or ventricular tachycardia arrest [16]. Additionally, a retrospective review over 18 years by Ahn et al. evaluated a small number of patients with aborted sudden cardiac death (ASCD) and ICD and found there was a nonsignificant trend of cardiac deaths in patients with ICDs compared to those without [17].

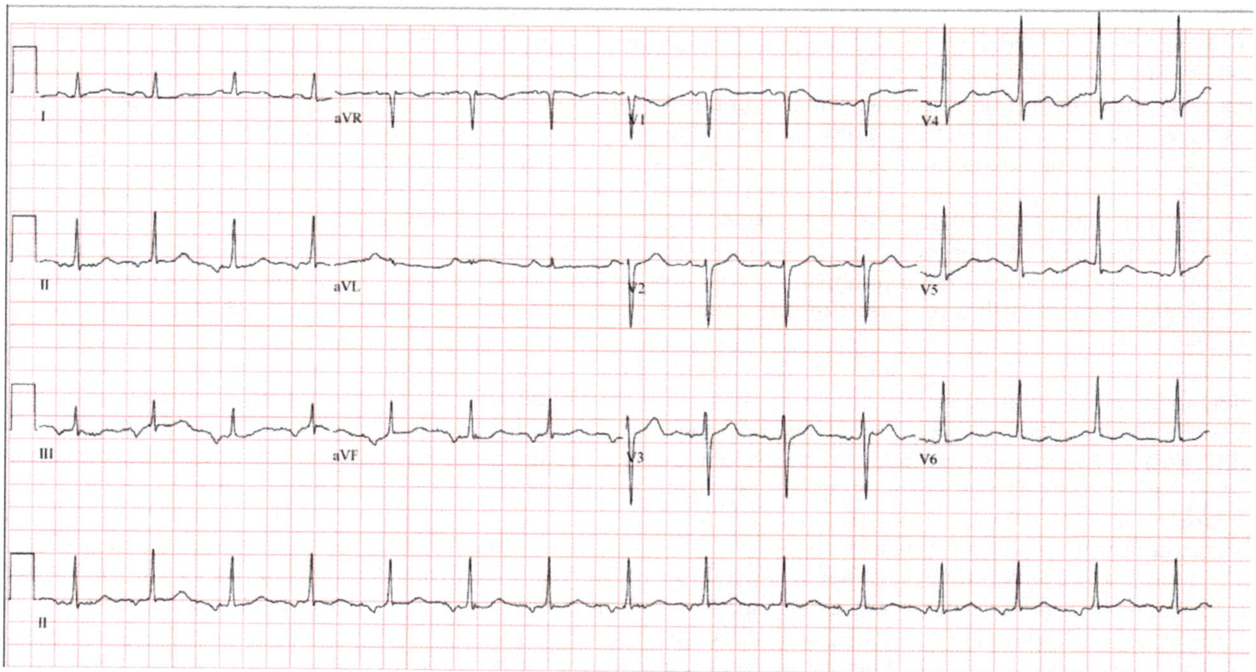

(a)

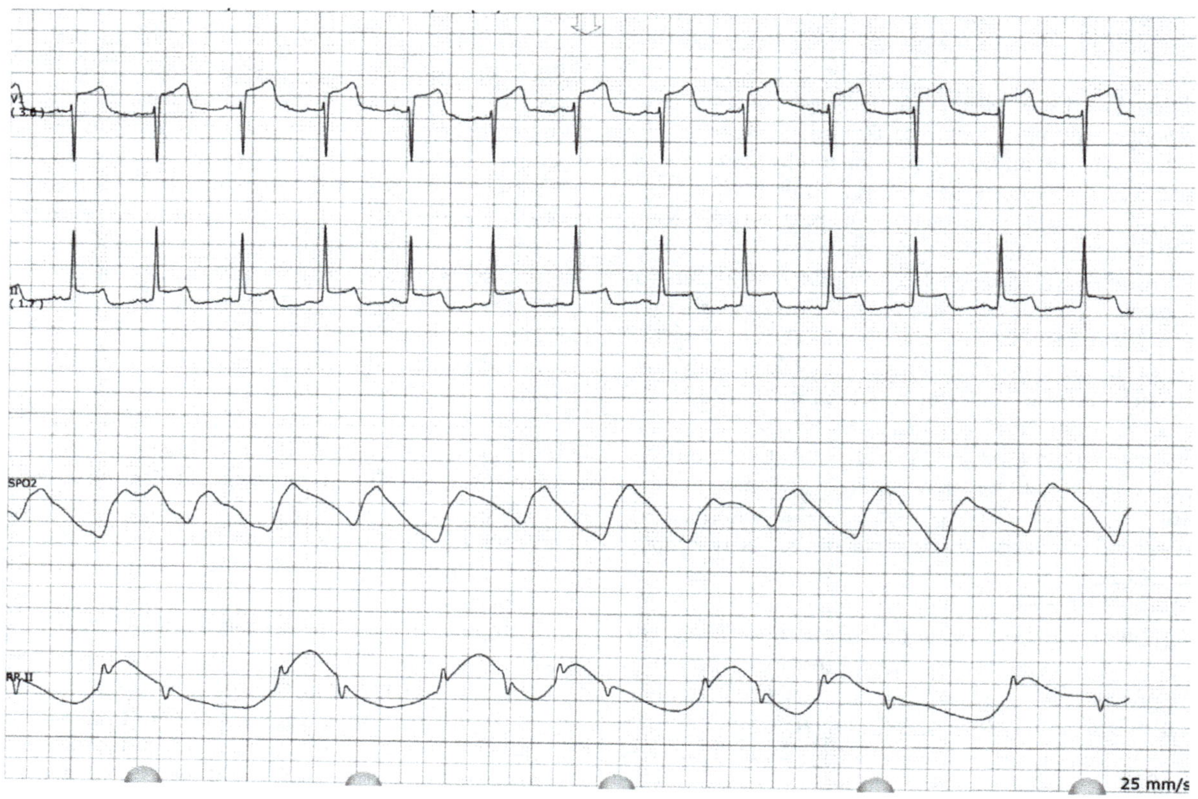

(b)

FIGURE 1: Continued.

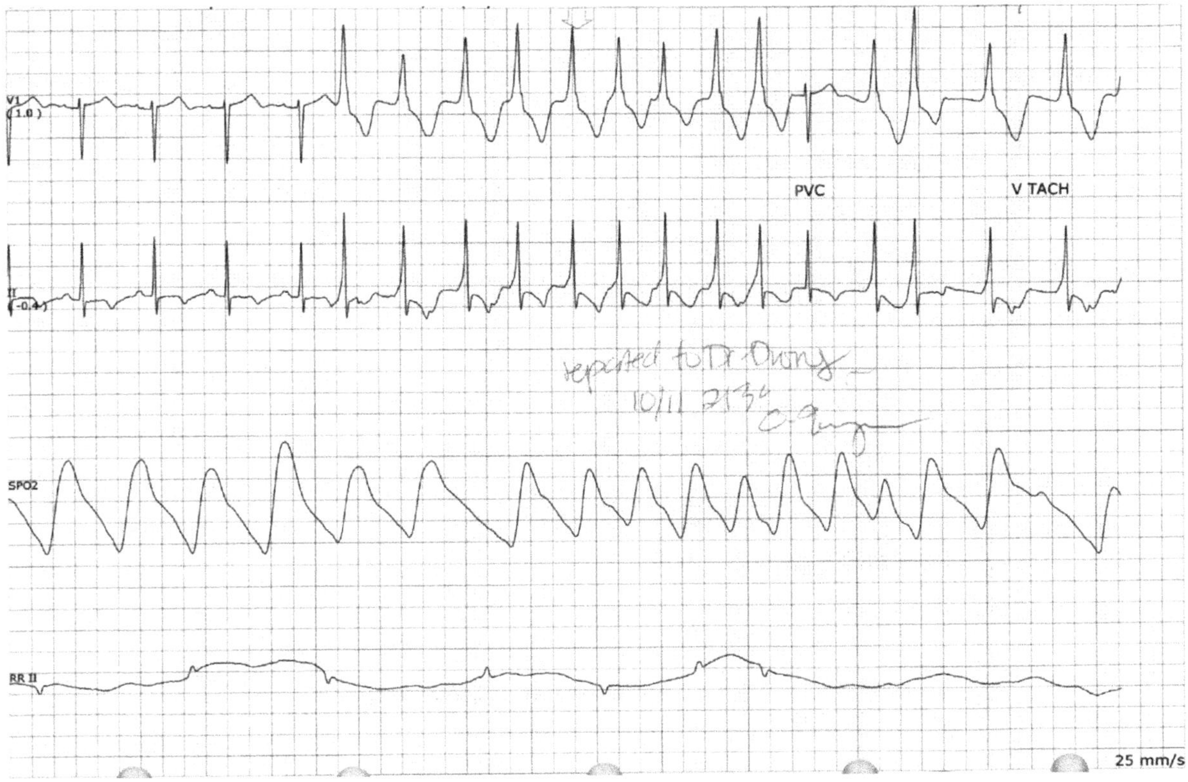

(c)

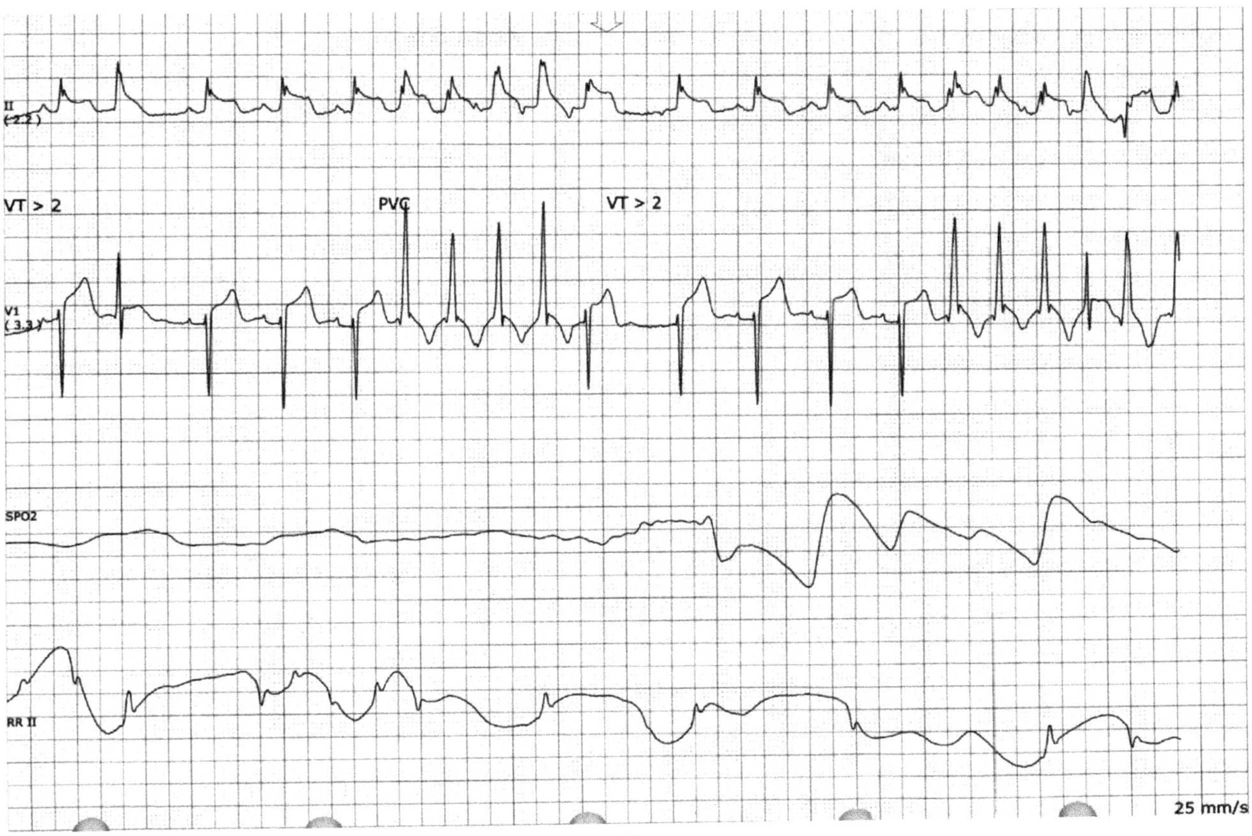

(d)

FIGURE 1: (a) Normal sinus rhythm, no ST segment elevations or depressions, and nonspecific T wave abnormalities. (b) Dynamic ST elevation on ECG. (c, d) Nonsustained ventricular tachycardia.

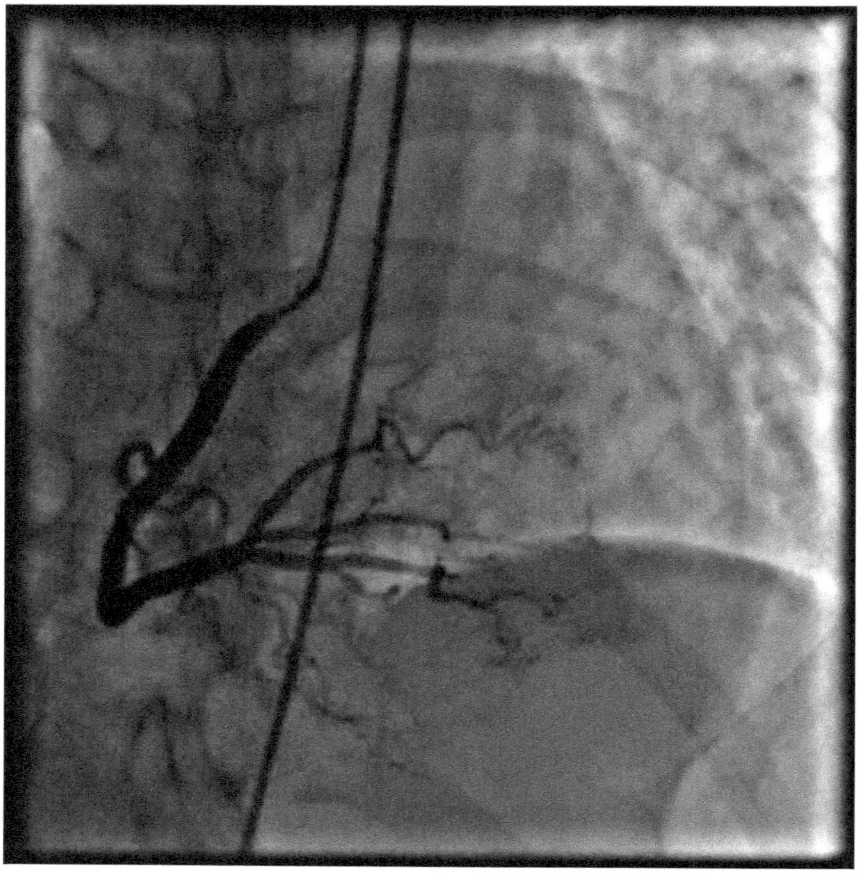

(a)

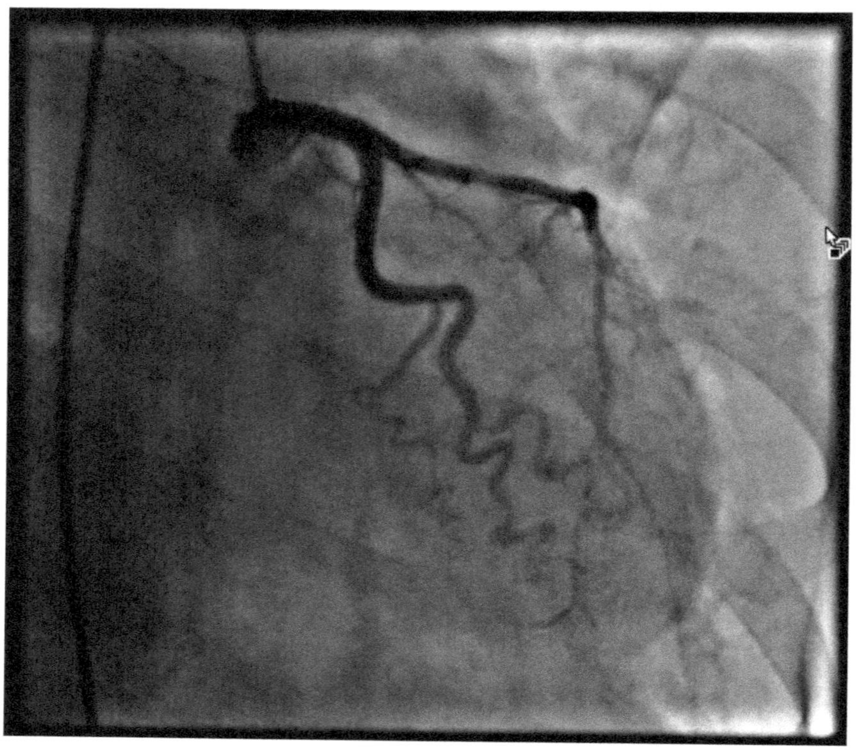

(b)

Figure 2: Continued.

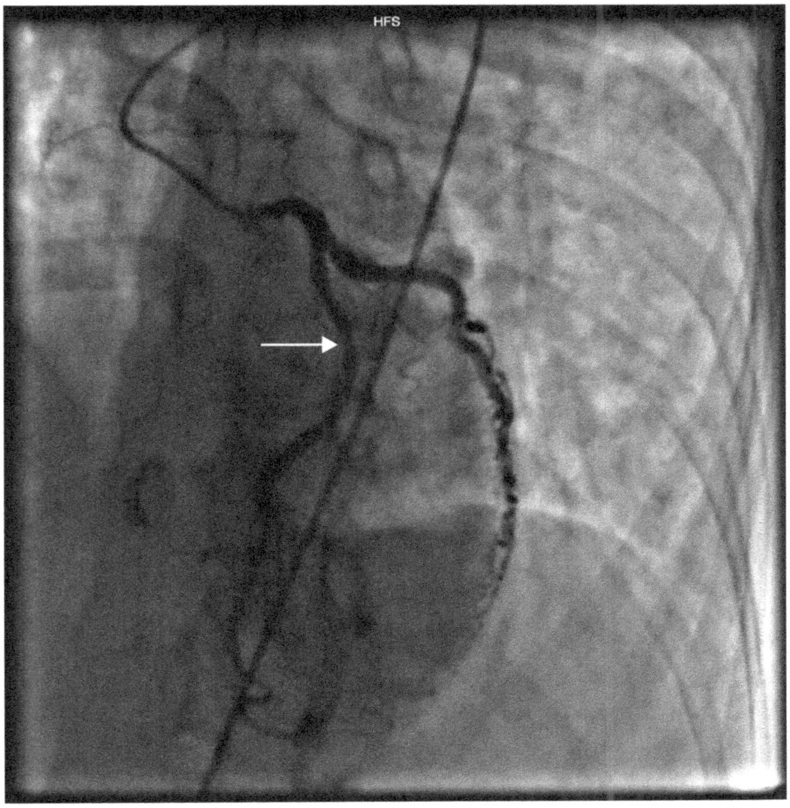

(c)

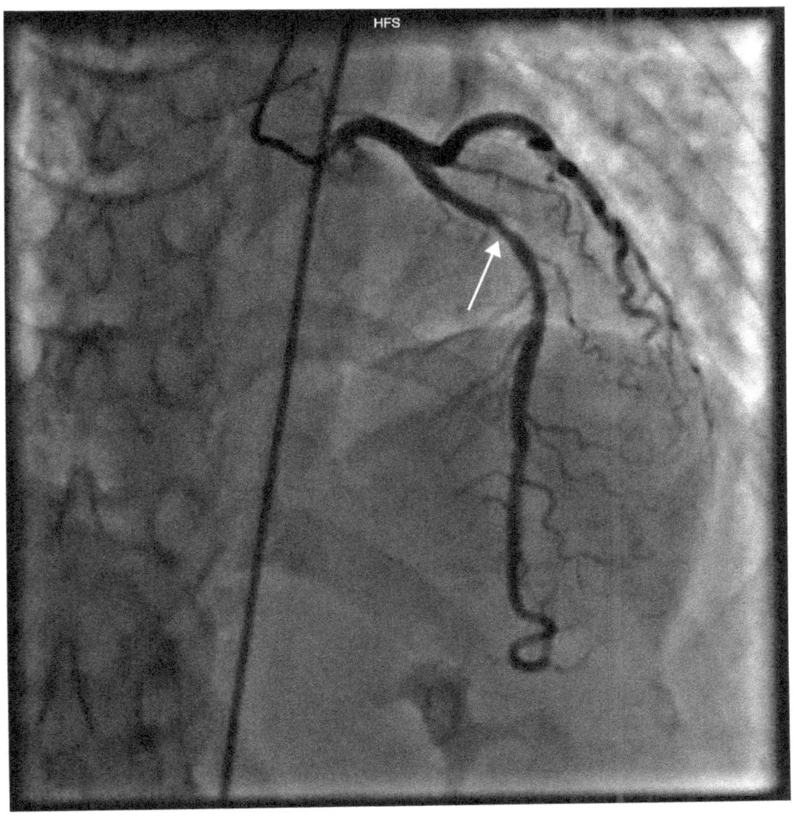

(d)

FIGURE 2: (a) Normal right coronary artery. (b) Normal left main and circumflex artery. (c, d) Left anterior descending artery.

Although vasospastic angina rarely presents as ventricular arrhythmias, patients are at higher risk of sudden cardiac death or, in our patient's case, ASCD if they have the following risk factors: hypertension, hyperlipidemia, multivessel spasm, and spasm involving the left anterior descending artery [17]. Recent retrospective review of patients with vasospastic angina with and without aborted sudden cardiac death demonstrated that patients with aborted sudden cardiac death have a higher incidence of cardiac and all-cause mortality [17–19].

In our case, this young healthy female presented with her first attack after starting a marathon, which may have been the inducing factor for her spasm. She would subsequently have recurrent events in the absence of a clear inciting event, including following correction of her hypokalemia, with ECGs suggesting alternating coronary artery involvement not consistent with her very mild single atherosclerotic LAD artery lesion. Her episodic angina and associated nonsustained ventricular tachycardia at rest were resistant to calcium channel blockers alone. She did respond, however, to combination therapy with the addition of a long-acting nitrate and demonstrated stability for discharge. In light of her initial presentation and these recurring events, she was determined to be at high risk for recurrent sudden cardiac death. Arrangements for a LifeVest as a bridge to ICD placement was coordinated.

VSA is an uncommon diagnosis but should be considered for atypical presentations of angina and ECG changes that are not attributed to obstructive coronary artery disease or unstable plaque rupture. This is true for patients, such as ours, in which the presentation is also associated with documented ventricular dysrhythmias and sudden cardiac death. As a diagnosis of exclusion, evaluation for other causes needs to be completed. Pharmaceutical treatment also needs to be individualized and tailored. Additionally, many reports have highlighted the difficulty in predicting the risk of recurrent events. Given the potentially high mortality associated with these arrhythmias, ICD implantation in these patients should be considered. The decision for ICD implantation in patients who experience a significant ventricular arrhythmia should be individualized, taking into consideration known and potentially reversible risk factors for future adverse events, as well as the patient's preferences.

References

[1] M. J. Hung, C. W. Cheng, N. I. Yang, M. Y. Hung, and W. J. Cherng, "Coronary vasospasm-induced acute coronary syndrome complicated by life-threatening cardiac arrhythmias in patients without hemodynamically significant coronary artery disease," *International Journal of Cardiology*, vol. 117, no. 1, pp. 37–44, 2007.

[2] J. R. Kapoor, E. T. Price, J. R. Nijmeh, and S. B. Williams, "Multivessel coronary artery spasm and cardiac arrest following single vessel stenting," *International Journal of Cardiology*, vol. 129, no. 1, pp. e35–e36, 2008.

[3] J. C. Kaski, A. Maseri, M. Vejar, F. Crea, and D. Hackett, "Spontaneous coronary artery spasm in variant angina is caused by a local hyperreactivity to a generalized constrictor stimulus," *Journal of the American College of Cardiology*, vol. 14, no. 6, pp. 1456–1463, 1989.

[4] J. C. Kaski, F. Crea, D. Meran et al., "Local coronary supersensitivity to diverse vasoconstrictive stimuli in patients with variant angina," *Circulation*, vol. 74, no. 6, pp. 1255–1265, 1986.

[5] M. Nakamura, A. Takeshita, and Y. Nose, "Clinical characteristics associated with myocardial infarction, arrhythmias, and sudden death in patients with vasospastic angina," *Circulation*, vol. 75, no. 6, pp. 1110–1116, 1987.

[6] S. R. Meisel, A. Mazur, I. Chetboun et al., "Usefulness of implantable cardioverter-defibrillators in refractory variant angina pectoris complicated by ventricular fibrillation in patients with angiographically normal coronary arteries," *The American Journal of Cardiology*, vol. 89, no. 9, pp. 1114–1116, 2002.

[7] J. F. Beltrame, F. Crea, J. C. Kaski et al., "International standardization of diagnostic criteria for vasospastic angina," *European Heart Journal*, vol. 38, no. 33, pp. 2565–2568, 2017.

[8] M. Slavich and R. S. Patel, "Coronary artery spasm: current knowledge and residual uncertainties," *IJC Heart & Vasculature*, vol. 10, pp. 47–53, 2016.

[9] A. Da Costa, K. Isaaz, E. Faure, S. Mourot, A. Cerisier, and M. Lamaud, "Clinical characteristics, aetiological factors and long-term prognosis of myocardial infarction with an absolutely normal coronary angiogram; a 3-year follow-up study of 91 patients," *European Heart Journal*, vol. 22, no. 16, pp. 1459–1465, 2001.

[10] Y. Igarashi, Y. Tamura, K. Suzuki et al., "Coronary artery spasm is a major cause of sudden cardiac arrest in survivors without underlying heart disease," *Coronary Artery Disease*, vol. 4, no. 2, pp. 177–185, 1993.

[11] G. A. Lanza, A. Sestito, G. A. Sgueglia et al., "Current clinical features, diagnostic assessment and prognostic determinants of patients with variant angina," *International Journal of Cardiology*, vol. 118, no. 1, pp. 41–47, 2007.

[12] K. Takaoka, M. Yoshimura, H. Ogawa et al., "Comparison of the risk factors for coronary artery spasm with those for organic stenosis in a Japanese population: role of cigarette smoking," *International Journal of Cardiology*, vol. 72, no. 2, pp. 121–126, 2000.

[13] M. C. Kim, Y. Ahn, K. H. Park et al., "Clinical outcomes of low-dose aspirin administration in patients with variant angina pectoris," *International Journal of Cardiology*, vol. 167, no. 5, pp. 2333-2334, 2013.

[14] R. M. Robertson, A. J. Wood, W. K. Vaughn, and D. Robertson, "Exacerbation of vasotonic angina pectoris by propranolol," *Circulation*, vol. 65, no. 2, pp. 281–285, 1982.

[15] Y. Matsue, M. Suzuki, M. Nishizaki, R. Hojo, Y. Hashimoto, and H. Sakurada, "Clinical implications of an implantable cardioverter-defibrillator in patients with vasospastic angina and lethal ventricular arrhythmia," *Journal of the American College of Cardiology*, vol. 60, no. 10, pp. 908–913, 2012.

[16] A. Ishihara, T. Tanaka, Y. Otsu et al., "Prognosis of patients with coronary vasospasm after successful resuscitation from ventricular fibrillation," *Journal of Arrhythmia*, vol. 28, no. 2, pp. 105–110, 2012.

[17] J. M. Ahn, K. H. Lee, S. Y. Yoo et al., "Prognosis of variant angina manifesting as aborted sudden cardiac death," *Journal*

of the American College of Cardiology, vol. 68, no. 2, pp. 137–145, 2016.

[18] A. Kundu, A. Vaze, P. Sardar, A. Nagy, W. S. Aronow, and N. F. Botkin, "Variant angina and aborted sudden cardiac death," *Current Cardiology Reports*, vol. 20, no. 4, p. 26, 2018.

[19] M. Slavich, C. Ballarotto, D. Margonato et al., "Coronary reactivity testing in vasospastic angina leading to cardiac arrest and coronary dissection," *International Journal of Cardiology*, vol. 210, pp. 10–13, 2016.

13

Primary Cardiac Lymphoma Manifesting as Complete Heart Block

Courtney R. Usry, Andrew S. Wilson, and Kelvin N. V. Bush

Division of Cardiology, San Antonio Military Medical Center, 3551 Roger Brooke Dr. San Antonio, TX 78234, USA

Correspondence should be addressed to Courtney R. Usry; courtneyrwvr@gmail.com

Academic Editor: Domingo A. Pascual-Figal

Primary cardiac tumors are exceedingly rare with variable clinical manifestations. This case involves a patient presentation of symptomatic complete heart block and cardiac imaging revealing a right atrial mass invading the myocardium consistent with Burkitt lymphoma on histopathology. The patient received definitive bradytherapy with a pacemaker and chemotherapy for the primary cardiac lymphoma. After three cycles of chemotherapy, the right atrial mass regressed significantly with restoration of atrioventricular conduction and no pacing burden. Primary cardiac lymphomas infrequently manifest as atrioventricular block and this case highlights cardiac masses as a potential etiology when evaluating new conduction disturbances and bradyarrhythmias.

1. Introduction

Primary cardiac tumors are exceedingly rare with a reported prevalence of 0.02% [1]. Primary cardiac lymphomas (PCL) are a subset of extranodal lymphomas where the primary tumor develops from the heart and/or the pericardium [2]. The incidence of PCL is 1-2% of primary cardiac tumors [3]. Secondary involvement of the heart is more common and reported to represent 16-28% of extracardiac lymphomas [4, 5]. Primary and secondary cardiac tumors are an important but often overlooked pathology to include in the differential diagnosis for patients presenting with bradyarrhythmias.

2. Case

An 80-year-old high-functioning female with a history of hypertension presented to the emergency department for evaluation of new onset dyspnea. Vital signs were significant for a heart rate of 40 beats per minute in the absence of being treated with atrioventricular (AV) nodal blocking agents. Physical examination was remarkable for bradycardic heart sounds. The electrocardiogram (ECG) demonstrated sinus rhythm, complete heart block with a junctional escape rhythm (Figure 1). During admission, the junctional rhythm degraded to a ventricular escape rhythm and transvenous pacing was acquired via right internal jugular venous access. Chest X-ray showed looping of the lead in the right atrium while pacing the right ventricular apex (Figure 2). Transthoracic echocardiography revealed a hyperechoic dense structure in the right atrium (Figure 3). To further characterize the findings on echocardiography, additional imaging was pursued. Cardiac magnetic resonance imaging (MRI) from a multidisciplinary discussion was deemed to not be safe due to the presence of the temporary transvenous pacing wire. Therefore, cardiac computed topography angiography (CCTA) was performed and characterized the right atrial mass measuring $6.6 \times 4.8\,cm$ with Hounsfield units similar to myocardium without vascularization (Figure 4). The right atrial mass involved the tricuspid annulus, extending medially to the interatrial septum and inlet ventricular septum. Imaging of the coronaries, mediastinum, great vessels, abdomen, and osseous structures was noncontributory. Fluoroscopic-guided endomyocardial tissue biopsy of the mass was performed and revealed findings consistent with C-MYC positive, EBV-negative, Burkitt lymphoma with very high Ki-67 proliferation index (>95%), and positive for CD10 and CD20. The patient underwent implantation of a single ventricular lead pacemaker. For treatment of the PCL, systemic chemotherapy with rituximab plus cyclophosphamide, doxorubicin, vincristine, and prednisone (R-CHOP) was

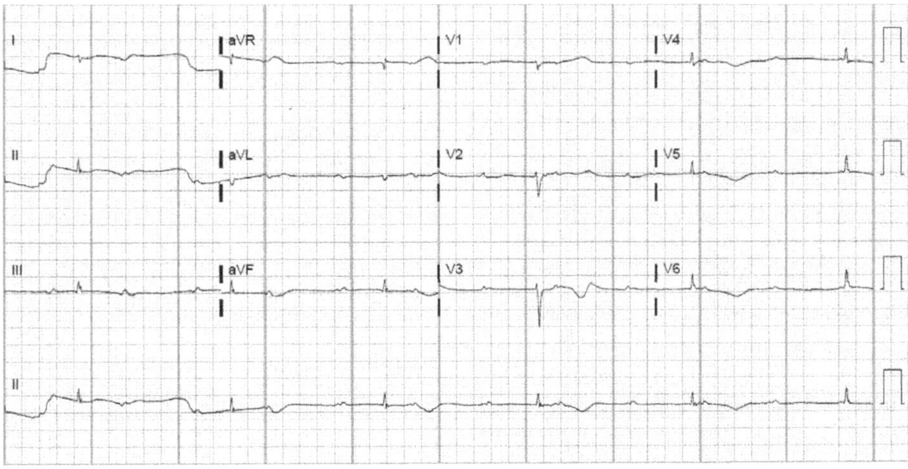

FIGURE 1: Electrocardiogram on presentation shows sinus rhythm, complete heart block with junctional escape rhythm.

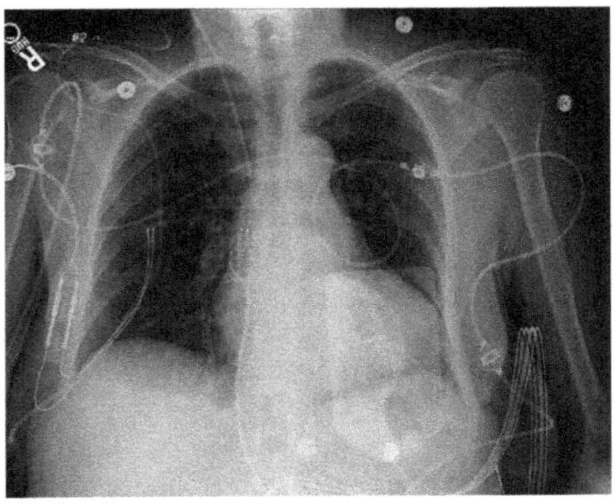

FIGURE 2: Chest X-ray single view with right jugular transvenous pacing wire with lead terminating in the right ventricle. There is a loop of the transvenous pacing wire seen within the right atrium.

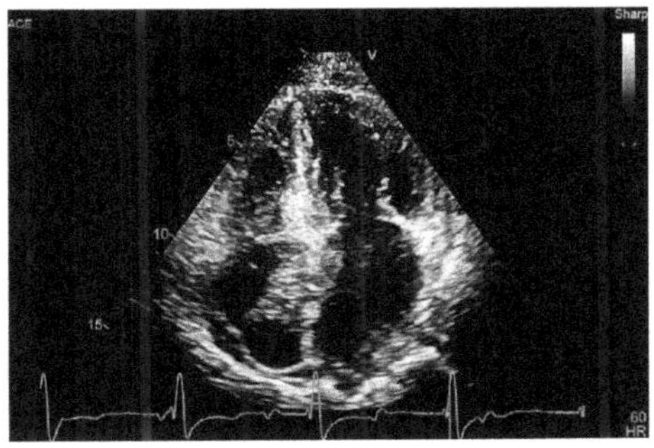

FIGURE 3: Apical four chamber from the transthoracic echocardiogram demonstrating a mass in the right atrium approximately 3-4 cm in size involving the interatrial septum.

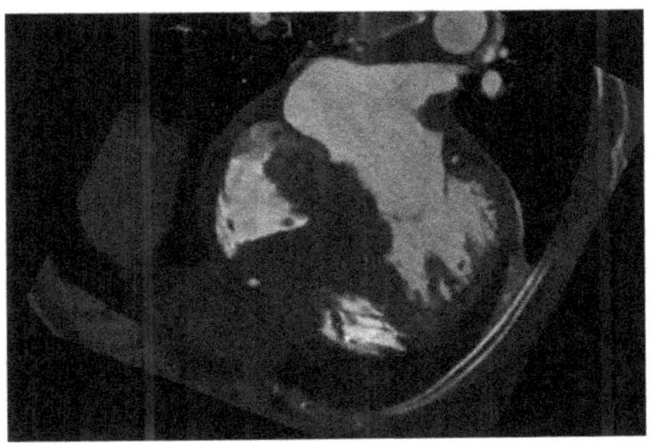

FIGURE 4: Four chamber view from the cardiac computed tomography angiogram demonstrating the mass invading the interatrial septum and inlet ventricular septum, and extending into the tricuspid annulus as well.

initiated. After three cycles of chemotherapy, native AV conduction was recovered with no pacing burden and the right atrial mass was decreased in size to $1 \times 1\, cm$ on repeat echocardiogram.

3. Discussion

PCL usually presents after the fifth decade of life and most often involves the right heart chambers [6]. Heart failure and pericardial effusions are the two most commonly reported clinical presentations of PCL [4]. AV block and ventricular tachycardia account for approximately 27% of the clinical manifestations of PCL and are secondary to direct infiltration of the conduction system or by irritation of the myocardium itself [7–9]. The CCTA in this case was instrumental in showing invasion of the atrial septum and inlet ventricular septum by the PCL.

The incidence of PCL has been on the rise in association with acquired immunodeficiency syndromes and transplant recipients receiving immunosuppressive therapy [9]. PCL has been a rarely reported malignancy in immunocompetent individuals and is often not diagnosed until there are advanced clinical manifestations [10]. A cardiac neoplasm was not suspected as the cause for our immunocompetent patient's complete heart block until imaging was obtained.

Echocardiographic findings concerning PCL or tumor invasions are recommended to be supported with a complementary imaging technique, either cardiac CT or MRI [11]. Cardiac MRI is a superior imaging modality with a higher sensitivity when compared to cardiac CT in identifying PCL, 90% versus 73%, respectively [8]. The presence of the temporary pacing wire excluded safe use of cardiac

MRI in this case due to the risk of significant heating or dislodgement.

Development of various arrhythmias during chemotherapy has been described and highlights the importance of ongoing arrhythmia surveillance as the tumor substrate changes with treatment [6]. Other reported cases of AV block secondary to PCL with subsequent pacemaker implantation have reported resolution of heart blocks after initiation of chemotherapy without continued pacing requirements [4].

In the majority of patients with PCL, chemotherapy with CHOP has reigned as the treatment of choice [12, 13]. Adjunctive use of rituximab with CHOP for patients with B-cell lymphoma as described by Coiffier et al. has proven higher complete response rates in comparison to those who received CHOP alone, 76% versus 63%, respectively [7, 14]. Risk of death secondary to tissue necrosis can occur after the first cycle of chemotherapy, particularly in patients with significant myocardial infiltration [12]. For refractory cases of PCL, autologous stem cell transplantation and radiotherapy has had promising outcomes in few described cases [7, 15, 16].

Research by Dunleavy et al. has suggested that DA-EPOCH-R (dose-adjusted etoposide, prednisone, vincristine, cyclophosphamide, doxorubicin, and rituximab) may be a useful option in low-risk adult patients with Burkitt lymphoma. Additionally, in frail elderly patients with advanced Burkitt lymphoma, this regimen may be considered as an alternative treatment in an effort to reduce toxicity [17]. Additional studies are necessary to examine responses in biologic subtypes and risk subgroups to determine the optimal chemotherapy regimen to be utilized upfront [18–20]. Our patient had return of preserved AV conduction with R-CHOP, regression of the cardiac mass, and tolerated chemotherapy without subsequent cardiotoxicity.

Malignant cardiac tumors should be considered in the differential diagnosis when evaluating new conduction abnormalities or bradyarrhythmias. This case describes an immunocompetent patient presenting with complete heart block as the main clinical manifestation of a PCL. Early imaging and prompt histopathologic diagnosis is essential in diagnosing PCL, directing chemotherapy, and alleviating burden of AV block.

Disclosure

The view(s) expressed herein are those of the author(s) and do not reflect the official policy or position of San Antonio Military Medical Center, the U.S. Army Medical Department, the U.S. Army Office of the Surgeon General, the Department of the Air Force, the Department of the Army or the Department of Defense, or the U.S. Government.

References

[1] K. Reynen, "Frequency of primary tumors of the heart," *The American Journal of Cardiology*, vol. 77, no. 1, p. 107, 1996.

[2] H. Á. McAllister and J. J. Fenoglio, "Tumors of the cardiovascular system," in *Atlas of tumor pathology*, p. 99, Armed Forces Institute of Pathology, Washington DC, 2nd edition, 1978.

[3] C. Chim, A. Chan, Y. Kwong, and R. Liang, "Primary cardiac lymphoma," *American Journal of Hematology*, vol. 54, no. 1, pp. 79–83, 1997.

[4] C.-J. Tai, W.-S. Wang, M.-T. Chung et al., "Complete atrioventricular block as a major clinical presentation of the primary cardiac lymphoma: a case report," *Japanese Journal of Clinical Oncology*, vol. 31, no. 5, pp. 217–220, 2001.

[5] C. R. Curtsinger, M. J. Wilson, and K. Yoneda, "Primary cardiac lymphoma," *Cancer*, vol. 64, no. 2, pp. 521–525, 1989.

[6] K.-W. Chen, J.-H. Chang, S.-P. Yeh, and C.-R. Lu, "Primary cardiac B-cell lymphoma with atrioventricular block and paroxysmal ventricular tachycardia," *Journal of Cardiothoracic Surgery*, vol. 7, no. 1, 2012.

[7] C. E. Miguel and R. B. Bestetti, "Primary cardiac lymphoma," *International Journal of Cardiology*, vol. 149, no. 3, pp. 358–363, 2011.

[8] G. Faganello, M. Belham, R. Thaman, J. Blundell, T. Eller, and P. Wilde, "A case of primary cardiac lymphoma: analysis of the role of echocardiography in early diagnosis," *Echocardiography*, vol. 24, no. 8, pp. 889–892, 2007.

[9] L. M. Shapiro, "GENERAL CARDIOLOGY: Cardiac tumours: diagnosis and management," *Heart*, vol. 85, no. 2, pp. 218–222, 2001.

[10] C. Montanaro, F. Loiacono, G. Fragasso, F. D. Cobelli, M. Foppoli, and A. Margonato, "Primary cardiac lymphoma in an immunocompetent 71-year-old man," *Texas Heart Institute Journal*, vol. 42, no. 6, pp. 561–564, 2015.

[11] T. A. Dorsay, V. B. Ho, M. J. Rovira, M. A. Armstrong, and M. D. Brissette, "Primary cardiac lymphoma: CT and MR findings," *Journal of Computer Assisted Tomography*, vol. 17, no. 6, pp. 978–981, 1993.

[12] G. Rolla, M. T. Bertero, G. Pastena et al., "Primary lymphoma of the heart. A case report and review of the literature," *Leukemia Research*, vol. 26, no. 1, pp. 117–120, 2002.

[13] S.-M. Kang, S.-J. Rim, H.-J. Chang et al., "Primary cardiac lymphoma diagnosed by transvenous biopsy under transesophageal echocardiographic guidance and treated with systemic chemotherapy," *Echocardiography*, vol. 20, no. 1, pp. 101–103, 2003.

[14] B. Coiffier, E. Lepage, J. Brière et al., "CHOP chemotherapy plus rituximab compared with CHOP alone in elderly patients with diffuse large-B-cell lymphoma," *New England Journal of Medicine*, vol. 346, no. 4, pp. 235–242, 2002.

[15] A. Nonami, K. Takenaka, K. Kamezaki et al., "Successful treatment of primary cardiac lymphoma by rituximab-CHOP and high-dose chemotherapy with autologous peripheral blood stem cell transplantation," *International Journal of Hematology*, vol. 85, no. 3, pp. 264–266, 2007.

[16] T. Miyashita, I. Miyazawa, T. Kawaguchi et al., "A case of primary cardiac B cell lymphoma associated with ventricular tachycardia, successfully treated with systemic chemotherapy and radiotherapy: a long-term survival case," *Japanese Circulation Journal*, vol. 64, no. 2, pp. 135–138, 2000.

[17] K. Dunleavy, "Approach to the diagnosis and treatment of adult Burkitt's lymphoma," *Journal of Oncology Practice/ American Society of Clinical Oncology*, vol. 14, no. 11, pp. 665–671, 2018.

[18] K. Dunleavy, A. Noy, J. S. Abramson et al., "Risk-adapted therapy in adults with Burkitt lymphoma: preliminary report of a

multicenter prospective phase II study of DA-EPOCH-R," *Blood*, vol. 126, no. 23, p. 342, 2015.

[19] K. Dunleavy, R. F. Little, and W. H. Wilson, "Update on Burkitt lymphoma," *Hematology/Oncology Clinics of North America*, vol. 30, no. 6, pp. 1333–1343, 2016.

[20] N. L. Bartlett, W. H. Wilson, S. H. Jung et al., "Dose-adjusted EPOCH-R compared with R-CHOP as frontline therapy for diffuse large B-cell lymphoma: clinical outcomes of the phase III intergroup trial alliance/CALGB 50303," *Journal of Clinical Oncology*, vol. 37, no. 21, pp. 1790–1799, 2019.

14

Pseudo Myocardial Infarction in a Patient with Severe Diabetic Ketoacidosis and Mild Hyperkalemia

Edgar Francisco Carrizales-Sepúlveda,[1] Ángel Noé del Cueto-Aguilera,[1] Raúl Alberto Jiménez-Castillo,[1] Olga Norali de la Cruz-Mata,[1] Mariana Fikir-Ordoñez,[1] Raymundo Vera-Pineda,[1] Dalí Alejandro Hernández-Guajardo,[1] Alejandro Ordaz-Farías,[2] and Ramiro Flores-Ramírez[1,2]

[1]*Internal Medicine Department, Hospital Universitario, Universidad Autónoma de Nuevo León, Monterrey, Nuevo León, Mexico*
[2]*Echocardiography Laboratory, Cardiology Service, Hospital Universitario, Universidad Autónoma de Nuevo León, Monterrey, Nuevo León, Mexico*

Correspondence should be addressed to Edgar Francisco Carrizales-Sepúlveda; edgar.carri_89@hotmail.com

Academic Editor: Man-Hong Jim

A 48-year-old male with a prior diagnosis of diabetes mellitus presented to the emergency department with malaise and nausea. On work-up, he was found with hyperglycemia and high anion gap metabolic acidosis, with a blood pH < 6.94. A diagnosis of severe diabetic ketoacidosis was established; serum electrolyte analysis showed mild hyperkalemia. On work-up, a 12-lead electrocardiogram was obtained, and it showed an ST-segment elevation on anterior leads that completely resolved with diabetic ketoacidosis treatment. ST-segment elevation myocardial infarction can be a precipitant factor for diabetic ketoacidosis, and evaluation of diabetic patients with suspected myocardial infarction can be challenging since they can present with atypical or little symptoms. Hyperkalemia, which usually accompanies diabetic ketoacidosis, can cause electrocardiographic alterations that are well described, but ST-segment elevation is uncommon. A pseudomyocardial infarction pattern has been described in patients with diabetic ketoacidosis; of note, most of these patients presented severe hyperkalemia. We believe this is of great importance for clinicians because they must be able to recognize those patients that present with electrocardiographic abnormalities secondary to the metabolic alterations and those that can be experiencing actual ongoing ischemia, in order to establish an appropriate and prompt treatment.

1. Introduction

Heart tissue is particularly prone to the effects of systemic acidosis and hyperkalemia [1, 2]. Acidosis decreases myocardial contractibility by affecting the excitation-contraction coupling [1], and hyperkalemia causes depolarization of the cardiac-cell resting membrane potential, shortening of the action potential duration, and alterations in the conduction velocity [2]. Diabetic ketoacidosis (DKA) is considered one of the most serious acute complications of diabetes mellitus; it is characterized by hyperglycemia, metabolic acidosis, and increased total body ketone concentrations [3]. Despite volume depletion seen in DKA secondary to vomiting and reduced oral intake, serum potassium levels are typically high at presentation; this is because lack of insulin and the presence of acidosis cause a shift of potassium from the intracellular space to extracellular space which usually resolve with DKA treatment [3, 4]. Thus, as a consequence of the acid-base and potassium derangements, patients with DKA can present electrocardiographic alterations than can be transient and resolve with treatment.

2. Case Report

A 48-year-old male presented to the emergency department with complaints of malaise and nausea. The past medical

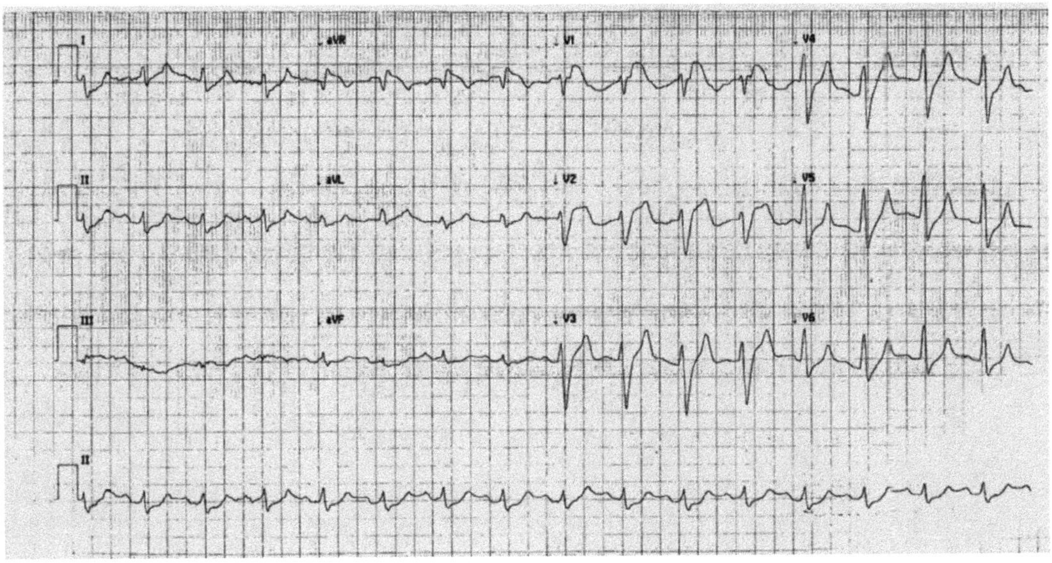

FIGURE 1: A twelve-lead electrocardiogram showing ST-segment elevation of 4 millimeters in leads V1 and V2, 1 millimeter in aVR, and QRS complex widening, which raised the suspicion of a possible acute coronary syndrome.

record was relevant for type 2 diabetes mellitus that was treated at the time with neutral protamine Hagedorn insulin. On initial examination, he had signs of severe dehydration and was polypneic; blood pressure was 80/60 mmHg, and heart rate was 125 bpm, with an oxygen saturation of 95% at room air. The capillary glucose level was 620 mg/dL; venous blood gases showed a metabolic acidosis with pH < 6.94 and HCO_3^- of 4.1 mEq/L. A severe DKA was diagnosed, and treatment was started with aggressive hydration and IV insulin. Initial electrolytes were Na^+ 119.6 mEq/L, Cl^- 95 mEq/L, and K^+ 5.7 mEq/L, and serum creatinine was 2.6 mg/dL; the anion gap was high, with 21 mmol/L. A 12-lead electrocardiogram (ECG) was performed and showed an ST-segment elevation of 4 millimeters in V1 and V2 leads and 1 millimeter elevation in aVR lead; also, there was a QRS complex widening and tall T-waves in V3-V5 (Figure 1). Concerns were raised of possible myocardial infarction as the precipitant factor for the DKA. A cardiology consult was required, and a point-of-care cardiac ultrasound was performed, which showed a normal left ventricular ejection fraction and no regional wall motion abnormalities, cardiac troponins where ordered and reported within the normal range. The patient continued on management. After 1 hour and 30 minutes of treatment for DKA, a subsequent ECG was performed, and it showed a complete resolution of the ST-segment elevation (Figure 2). DKA was resolved, and the patient was admitted for monitoring, with a favorable evolution.

3. Discussion

Myocardial infarction is a known precipitant factor for DKA; it is responsible of about 1% of the cases, and along with congestive heart failure, it accounts for 28% of deaths in DKA [5]. According to clinical guideliness for diagnosis and treatment of myocardial infarction, ST-segment elevation is considered suggestive of acute coronary obstruction if present in at least two contiguous leads (≥2.5 mm in men < 40 years, ≥2 mm inmen ≥ 40 years, or ≥1.5 mm in women in leads V2-V3) and/or ≥1 mm in any other lead [6]. In the proper clinical context, patients with ST-segment elevation are candidates for reperfusion therapy, which must be instituted promptly since delay in treatment is associated with worst prognosis [6]. Evaluation of suspected myocardial infarction can be particularly challenging in diabetic patients, since they are more likely to present with atypical or little symptomatology [7].

Electrocardiographic alterations related to hyperkalemia are well described [8]. Their presence and presentation depend on the potassium level and also on the rate of raise, acid-base status, other electrolyte disturbances, and medications [8, 9]. Tall, tent-shaped T-waves are the earliest manifestations with mild hyperkalemia (5.5–6.5 mEq/L). With moderate hyperkalemia (6.5–8 mEq/L), a prolonged PR interval, decreased P-wave amplitude, and widening of the QRS complex can be seen. With severe hyperkalemia (>8 mEq/L) there is absence of P-wave, intra- and interventricular conduction blocks, progressive widening of the QRS complex and eventually ventricular fibrillation and asystole. A pseudomyocardial infarction pattern has been described in patients with DKA and hyperkalemia [9–13]. Bellazzini and Meyer reviewed 24 cases of pseudomyocardial infarction in DKA with hyperkalemia reported in the literature [9]. They found that an anteroseptal pattern is the most common presentation (79.2%), followed by a combination of anteroseptal and inferior distribution (12.5%). Of note, 23 of the 24 cases presented with a mean potassium concentration of 8.1 mEq/L. In all these cases, there was no echocardiographic or angiographic finding suggestive of real myocardial ischemia, and there was a complete resolution of electrocardiographic abnormalities after metabolic improvement. There is only one case described in the literature that presented with

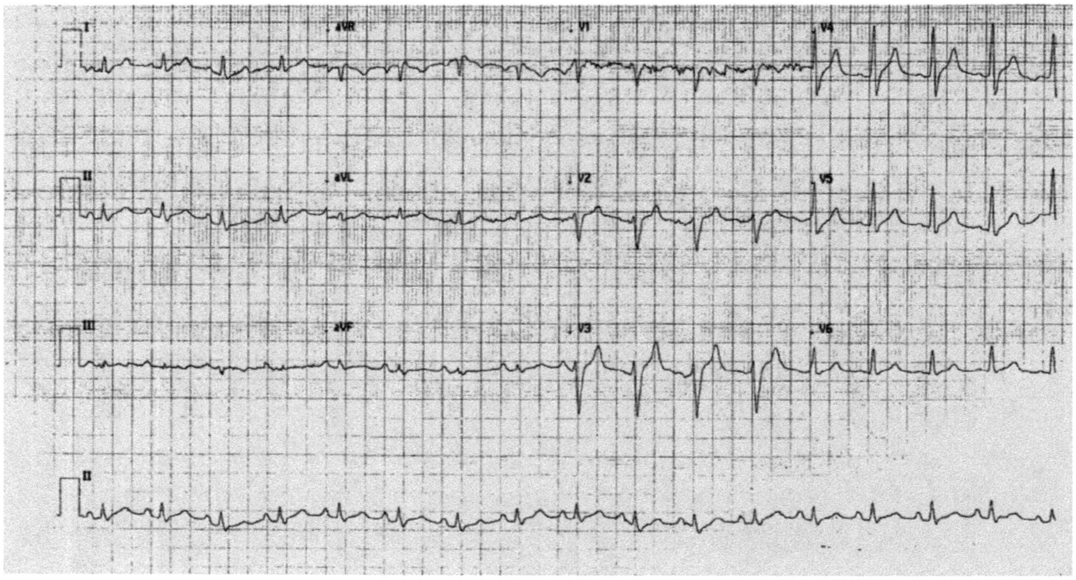

FIGURE 2: A twelve-lead electrocardiogram performed 1 hour and thirty minutes after initiation of DKA treatment showing complete resolution of ST-segment abnormalities.

a pseudomyocardial infarction pattern and normal potassium levels [10]. According to our literature review, no cases of a pseudomyocardial infarction pattern in DKA with mild hyperkalemia have been reported. Possible explanations for the presence of ST-segment elevation in the absence of severe hyperkalemia are the concomitant acid-base disturbances present in our patient, other electrolyte alterations, and possibly a slow coronary blood flow secondary to elevated blood viscosity as a consequence of hyperglycemia [14].

4. Conclusion

We present an uncommon electrocardiographic alteration in a patient with severe DKA. Myocardial infarction should always be considered as a possible precipitant of DKA in diabetic patients, but clinicians must be able to recognize when electrocardiographic abnormalities suggestive of myocardial ischemia are related to metabolic derangements in order to avoid unnecessary diagnostic procedures and treatments and also to promptly recognize those patients with actual ongoing ischemia that may benefit from a coronary percutaneous intervention or IV thrombolysis. Normal levels of myocardial necrosis biomarkers, the absence of echocardiographic and angiographic alterations suggestive of myocardial ischemia, and resolution of electrocardiographic alterations with the metabolic control can be reassuring, but close monitoring of the patient during treatment and after resolution is crucial.

Authors' Contributions

All authors had full access to data and a role in the preparation of this manuscript.

References

[1] C. H. Orchard and J. C. Kentish, "Effects of changes of pH on the contractile function of cardiac muscle," *American Journal of Physiology-Cell Physiology*, vol. 258, no. 6, pp. C967–C981, 1990.

[2] J. N. Weiss, Z. Qu, and K. Shivkumar, "Electrophysiology of hypokalemia and hyperkalemia," *Circulation: Arrhythmia and Electrophysiology*, vol. 10, no. 3, 2017.

[3] A. E. Kitabchi, G. E. Umpierrez, J. M. Miles, and J. N. Fisher, "Hyperglycemic crises in adult patients with diabetes," *Diabetes Care.*, vol. 32, no. 7, pp. 1335–1343, 2009.

[4] M. Fayfman, F. J. Pasquel, and G. E. Umpierrez, "Management of hyperglycemic crises: diabetic ketoacidosis and hyperglycemic hyperosmolar state," *Medical Clinics of North America*, vol. 101, no. 3, pp. 587–606, 2017.

[5] P. K. Moulik, C. Nethaji, and A. A. Khaleeli, "Misleading electrocardiographic results in patient with hyperkalaemia and diabetic ketoacidosis," *BMJ*, vol. 325, no. 7376, pp. 1346-1347, 2002.

[6] B. Ibanez, S. James, S. Agewall et al., "2017 ESC Guidelines for the management of acute myocardial infarction in patients presenting with ST-segment elevation: the Task Force for the management of acute myocardial infarction in patients presenting with ST-segment elevation of the European Society of Cardiology (ESC)," *European Heart Journal*, vol. 39, no. 2, pp. 119–177, 2018.

[7] C. Junghans, N. Sekhri, M. J. Zaman, H. Hemingway, G. S. Feder, and A. Timmis, "Atypical chest pain in diabetic patients with suspected stable angina: impact on diagnosis and coronary outcomes," *European Heart Journal - Quality of Care and Clinical Outcomes*, vol. 1, no. 1, pp. 37–43, 2015.

[8] A. Mattu, W. J. Brady, and D. A. Robinson, "Electrocardiographic manifestations of hyperkalemia," *The American Journal of Emergency Medicine*, vol. 18, no. 6, pp. 721–729, 2000.

[9] M. A. Bellazzini and T. Meyer, "Pseudo-myocardial infarction in diabetic ketoacidosis with hyperkalemia," *The Journal of Emergency Medicine*, vol. 39, no. 4, pp. e139–e141, 2010.

[10] E. Aksakal, T. Ulus, E. Bayram, and H. Duman, "Acute inferior pseudoinfarction pattern in a patient with normokalemia and diabetic ketoacidosis," *The American Journal of Emergency Medicine*, vol. 27, no. 2, pp. 251.e3–251.e5, 2009.

[11] J. Ruiz-Morales, C. Canha, F. Al-Saffar, and S. Ibrahim, "Anterior myocardial pseudoinfarction in a patient with diabetic ketoacidosis," *Journal of geriatric cardiology*, vol. 15, no. 3, pp. 238–240, 2018.

[12] E. Sharma, S. Dahal, P. Sharma, D. K. C. Ghimire, and S. Dahal, "A case of pseudoinfarction pattern in diabetic ketoacidosis: a diagnostic and therapeutic dilemma," *Cardiology Research*, vol. 9, no. 4, pp. 250–252, 2018.

[13] A. Ziakas, C. Basagiannis, and I. Stiliadis, "Pseudoinfarction pattern in a patient with hyperkalemia, diabetic ketoacidosis and normal coronary vessels: a case report," *Journal of Medical Case Reports*, vol. 4, no. 1, p. 115, 2010.

[14] C. Irace, C. Carallo, F. Scavelli, M. S. De Franceschi, T. Esposito, and A. Gnasso, "Blood viscosity in subjects with normoglycemia and prediabetes," *Diabetes Care*, vol. 37, no. 2, pp. 488–492, 2014.

15

Clinical Paradox: Anterior Wall Myocardial Infarction with Predominant Inferior ST Elevation and No Variation in Coronary Anatomy in a PAI-1 Homozygote

Marko Perčić ,[1] Tea Friščić ,[1] Jasna Čerkez Habek ,[1] Dean Strinić ,[1] Ninoslav Rudman ,[2] and Jozica Šikić [1]

[1]*Department of Cardiology, Clinic of Internal Medicine, "Sveti Duh" University Hospital, Zagreb, Croatia*
[2]*Department of Radiology, "Sveti Duh" University Hospital, Zagreb, Croatia*

Correspondence should be addressed to Tea Friščić; friscictea1@gmail.com

Academic Editor: Assad Movahed

Changes of the ST segment are commonly used as predictors of the culprit vessel during an acute myocardial infarction. In case of combined ST elevation in both inferior and anterior leads, these changes can be due to a distal occlusion of a "wrapped" left anterior descending artery (LAD) or a two-vessel disease. Our case of anterior wall myocardial infarction with inferior ST elevation and anterior ST depression shows that electrocardiographic changes during acute myocardial infarction cannot always be explained by logical sequelae of the injury current, vessel anatomy, and their irrigation territory.

1. Introduction

ST segment changes, whether elevation or depression, as well as their distribution are commonly used as predictors of the culprit vessel during an acute myocardial infarction. ST elevation in inferior leads suggests an acute occlusion of the right coronary artery (RCA) or the left circumflex coronary artery (LCx). In case of combined ST elevation in both inferior and anterior leads, these changes can be due to a distal occlusion of a "wrapped" left anterior descending artery (LAD) or a two-vessel disease [1]. There are several studies and case reports presenting the "wrapped" LAD being the cause of ST elevation in inferior and anterior leads, defining the "wrapped" LAD as a LAD from a postreperfusion coronary angiogram that perfuse at least one-fourth of the inferior wall of the left ventricle in the right anterior oblique projection [2–8]. According to a recent study, hereditary thrombophilia was the most frequently encountered atypical etiology for acute myocardial infarction in young people, accounting for 15% of cases [9]. We report a rare case of ST elevation in inferior leads following proximal LAD occlusion without coronary anatomy deviation and subsequent anterior wall myocardial infarction in a patient with PAI-1 mutation.

2. Case Presentation

A 30-year-old male patient with no previous history of cardiovascular disease, cardiovascular risk factors, or family history of cardiovascular disease presented in emergency department with retrosternal chest pain not related to exertion that had started four hours before. There was no pain radiation, nausea, or vomiting. He had no recent history of infectious disease (as a pericarditis/myocarditis trigger). On physical examination, there were no abnormal findings. The initial electrocardiogram (ECG) showed 2 mm ST segment elevation in leads II, III, and aVF; 1 mm in V6; and horizontal ST depression in aVL and V1-3 (Figure 1(a)). His blood pressure was 180/105 mmHg, his heart rate was 65/minute, and he was afebrile. The patient was administered acetylsalicylic acid 300 mg and ticagrelor 180 mg orally and then admitted to coronary intensive care unit (ICU) where the second ECG showed more prominent ST elevation in leads II, III, aVF, and V5-6 and ST denivelation in aVL

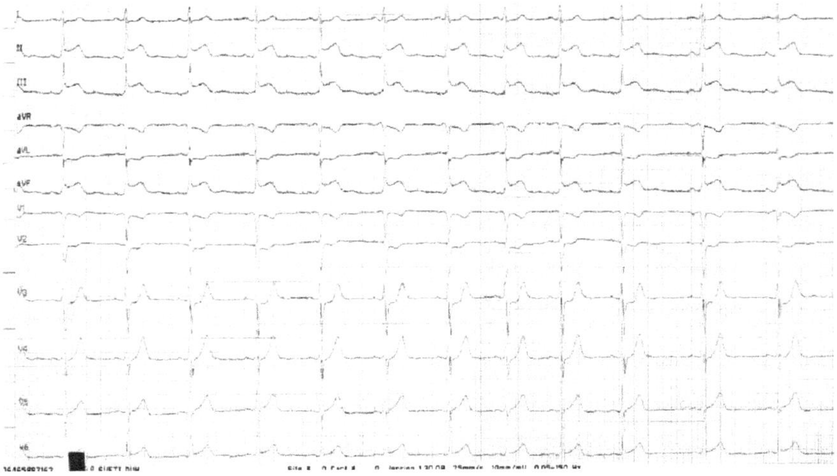

(a)

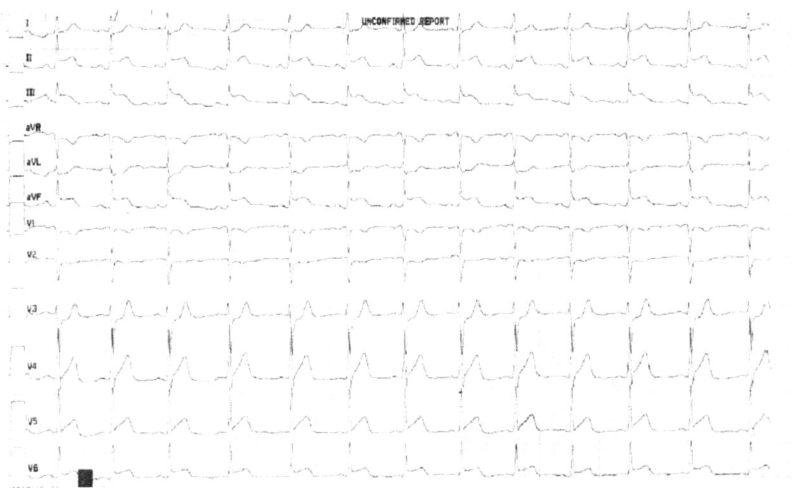

(b)

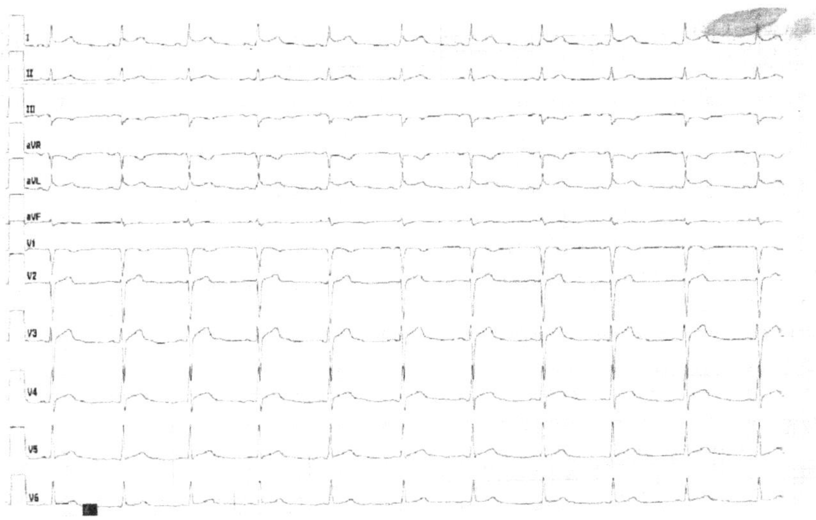

(c)

FIGURE 1: Continued.

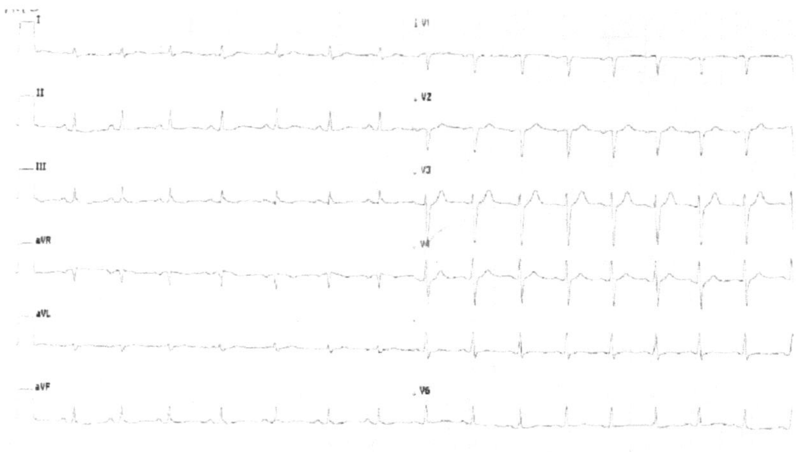

(d)

FIGURE 1: (a) ECG in the emergency department. (b) ECG at the admission to the ICU. (c) ECG taken 12 h after pPCI. (d) ECG taken 4 months after pPCI.

and V1-3 (Figure 1(b)). Initial troponin on presentation was 41 ng/L (referent value < 40 ng/L). He was taken up for coronary angiography immediately after admission to the ICU. Coronary angiogram showed right-dominant system (Figure 2). LAD had a microathero/thrombotic subocclusion of the proximal segment with initial TIMI 2 flow and a small embolus in the distal segment. RCA showed slow flow phenomenon with no signs of stenosis. Primary percutaneous coronary intervention (pPCI) was preformed, and one drug-eluting stent (4.0 × 15mm) in LAD has been implanted. ECG taken 12 hours after pPCI showed 1.5 mm ST elevation in leads I and aVL and formed Q with inversed T wave in lead III (Figure 1(c)). The laboratory test showed LDL levels of 2.85 mmol/L and total cholesterol of 4.79 mmol/L. All the other results were within normal range, including electrolyte levels, and the peak troponin level was 22845 ng/L. There were no postprocedural complication, and the patient had stable hemodynamics and rhythm until discharge. The therapy he received was according to the latest European guidelines for the treatment of acute coronary syndrome. Three days after pPCI, echocardiographic global longitudinal strain was -13.8% with reduced strain in basal anteroseptolateral segments of the left ventricle, while inferior and posterior segments remained intact (Figure 3). Three months after myocardial infarction, multislice computed tomography (MSCT) coronary angiography was performed, showing no variations in coronary anatomy (including "wrapped" LAD), no abnormal heart rotation, and no signs of stenosis (Figure 4). Thrombophilia testing was also performed, and the results came in negative for factor V Leiden (R506Q) and factor II prothrombin (G20210A), with no antithrombin III or protein S deficiency, or increase in lupus anticoagulant, MTHFR (C677T) heterozygote, and PAI-1 (4G/5G) homozygote 4G. Patient has been asymptomatic since the discharge and is on regular follow-up. ECG taken 4 months after the acute myocardial infarction shows Q in V1-2, with no Q in inferior leads.

3. Discussion

During acute anterior wall myocardial infarction, elevation of the ST segment is usually seen in the anterior leads. ST segment depression is sometimes observed simultaneously in the inferior leads which is generally considered to be a reciprocal change of ST elevation in aVL related to anterolateral extension of the ischaemia of D1 branch irrigation territory [7].

Inferior ST elevation during acute anterior myocardial infarction is unusual but explainable when the "wrapped" LAD is occluded distal to its first diagonal branch, appearing with a combination of a transmural ischaemic myocardium in the anterobasal and anterolateral wall of a lesser degree together with transmural ischaemic myocardium in the inferior wall [10].

Sapin et al. explained the ST segment changes in "anterior-inferior" myocardial infarction with the distal occlusion in the LAD which allows the more proximal patent branch vessels to perfuse the anterior wall resulting in a smaller mass of ischemic anterior wall myocardium, thus smaller anterior wall injury current and less reciprocal inferior ST segment depression. Inferior wall injury current, as a result of occluded "wrapped" LAD, must be combined with the weak reciprocal of a smaller anterior injury current to generate the ST elevation in the inferior leads [4]. Sasaki et al. had drawn a similar conclusion [8].

Our case describes a rare form of anterior myocardial infarction with inferior ST elevation with no deviation in coronary anatomy and right-dominant system. Also, there was no inferior wall myocardial infarction and no ST elevation in anterior leads. The patient is a PAI-1 4G homozygote, which some authors consider as an independent risk factor for acute myocardial infarction in young patients [11]. To our knowledge, there is no relationship between PAI-1, patient age, and ECG changes. We stressed the age of the patient and PAI-1 because the reason for

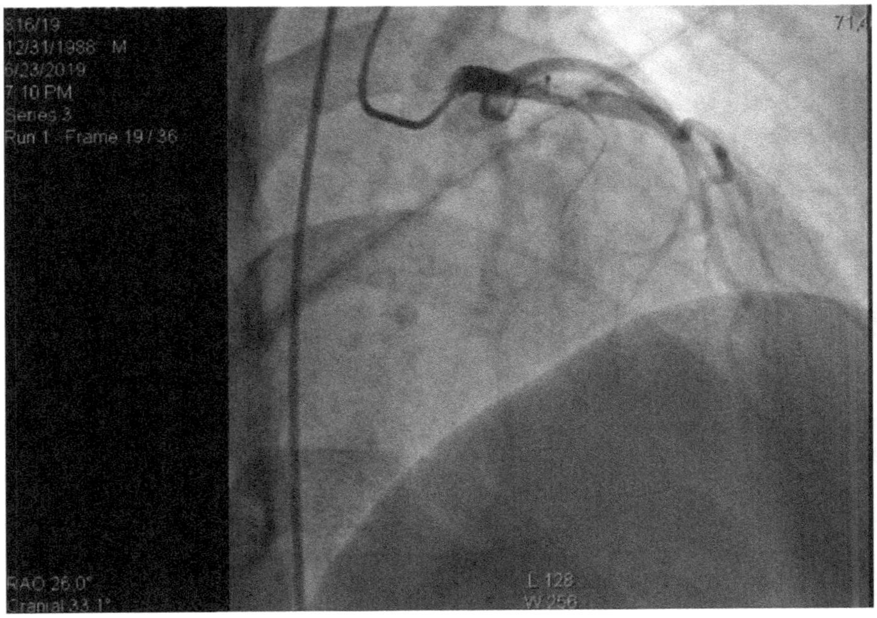

(a)

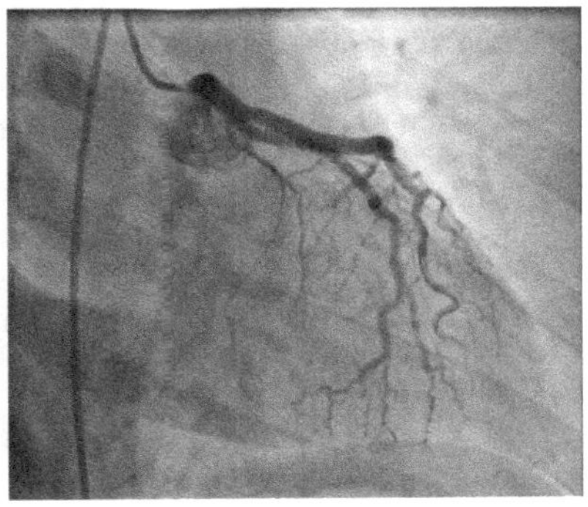

(b)

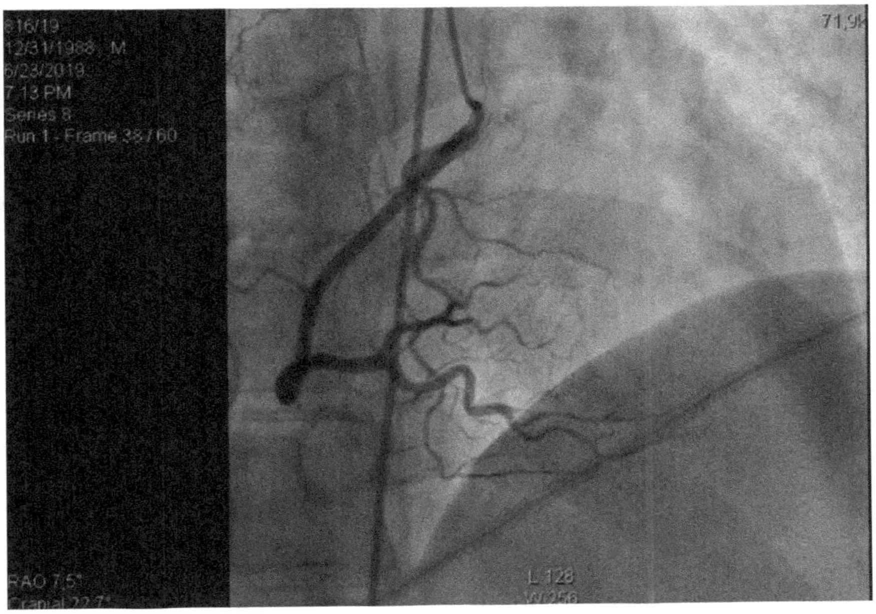

(c)

Figure 2: Continued.

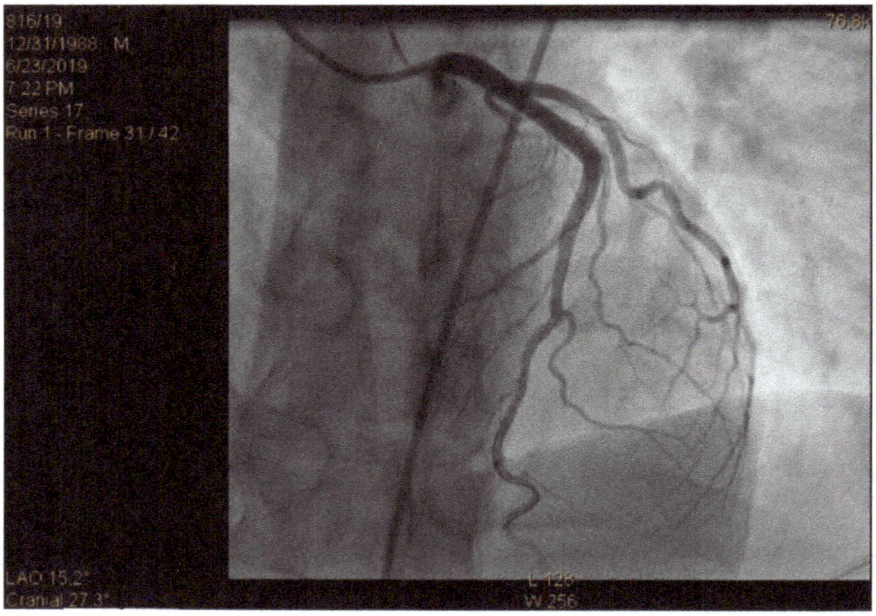

(d)

FIGURE 2: (a) Left anterior descending artery—proximal segment subocclusion. (b) Left anterior descending artery—RAO. (c) Right coronary artery. (d) Left anterior descending artery after pPCI with drug eluting stent (4×15mm).

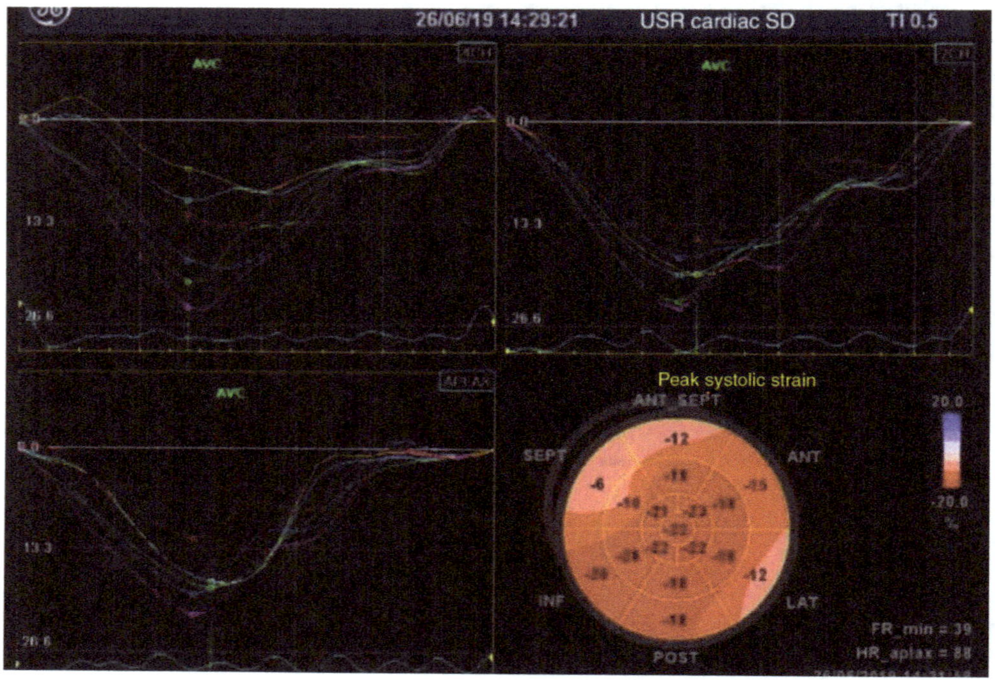

FIGURE 3: Peak longitudinal strain 3 days after myocardial infarction showing reduced strain in basal anteroseptolateral segments while inferior and posterior segment remained intact.

LAD subocclusion was probably embolism and not a rupture of atherosclerotic plaque. These changes of the ST segment are hard to explain, especially with the results of the peak systolic strain which shows no reduction in inferior segments and a significant strain reduction in anterior segments. Also, in the ECG taken 4 months after pPCI, there was Q in septal leads. One of the possible explanations could be a spontaneous recanalization of the RCA.

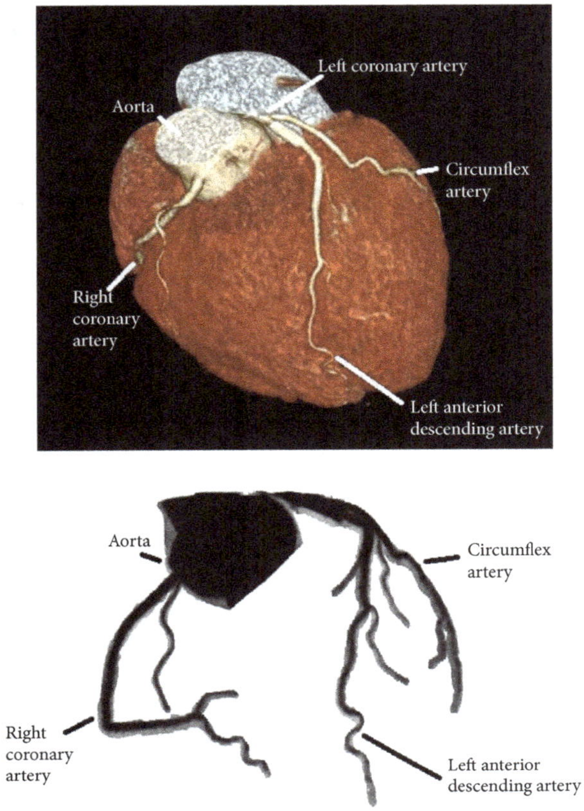

FIGURE 4: MSCT coronary angiography showed no signs of stenosis and no variations in coronary anatomy.

4. Conclusion

Inferior ST elevation in an acute myocardial infarction of anterior wall is usually combined with anterior ST elevation. Both of the electrocardiographic changes are caused by occlusion of a "wrapped" LAD distal to D1 branch. Our case of anterior wall myocardial infarction with inferior ST elevation and anterior ST depression shows that electrocardiographic changes during acute myocardial infarction cannot always be explained by logical sequelae of the injury current, vessel anatomy, and their irrigation territory.

Acknowledgments

Research did not receive specific funding but was performed as part of the employment of the authors with the employer University hospital Sveti Duh.

References

[1] M. H. Jim, A. O. Chan, M. O. Tang, C. W. Siu, S. W. Lee, and C. P. Lau, "Angiographic and clinical implications of combined ST-segment elevation in anterior and inferior leads in acute myocardial infarction," *Clinical Cardiology*, vol. 32, no. 1, pp. 21–27, 2009.

[2] T. Honda, K. Fujimoto, Y. Miyao, H. Koga, and M. Ishii, "Acute myocardial infarction caused by left anterior descending artery occlusion presenting as inferior ST elevation and anterior ST depression," *Journal of Cardiology Cases*, vol. 9, no. 2, pp. 67–70, 2014.

[3] T. N. S. Roy, J. S. Nagham, and R. A. Kumar, "Acute inferior wall myocardial infarction due to occlusion of the wrapped left anterior descending coronary artery," *Case Reports in Cardiology*, vol. 2013, Article ID 983943, 2013.

[4] P. M. Sapin, D. R. Musselman, G. J. Dehmer, and W. E. Cascio, "Implications of inferior ST-segment elevation accompanying anterior wall acute myocardial infarction for the angiographic morphology of the left anterior descending coronary artery morphology and site of occlusion," *The American journal of cardiology*, vol. 69, no. 9, pp. 860–865, 1992.

[5] O. Skakun, S. Fedorov, O. Verbovska, and I. Martyniv, "Acute inferior myocardial infarction caused by left anterior descending artery occlusion," *Critical Care Innovations*, vol. 2, no. 2, pp. 32–37, 2019.

[6] M. Kosuge and K. Kimura, "Clinical implications of electrocardiograms for patients with anterior wall ST-segment elevation acute myocardial infarction in the interventional era," *Circulation Journal*, vol. 76, no. 1, pp. 32–40, 2012.

[7] R. Akdimir, H. Gunduz, H. Ozhan, M. Yazici, E. Erbilen, and C. Uyan, "Simultaneous anterior and inferior myocardial infarction due to occlusion of the left anterior descending coronary artery," *Turkish Journal Of Medical Sciences*, vol. 34, pp. 121–126, 2004.

[8] K. Sasaki, M. Yotsukura, K. Sakata, H. Yoshino, and K. Ishikawa, "Relation of ST-segment changes in inferior leads during anterior wall acute myocardial infarction to length and occlusion site of the left anterior descending coronary artery," *American Journal of Cardiology*, vol. 87, no. 12, pp. 1340–1345, 2001.

[9] S. Puricel, C. Lehner, M. Oberhänsli et al., "Acute coronary syndrome in patients younger than 30 years – aetiologies, baseline characteristics and long-term clinical outcome," *Swiss Medical Weekly*, vol. 143, 2013.

[10] A. Tamura, H. Kataoka, K. Nagase, Y. Mikuriya, and M. Nasu, "Clinical significance of inferior ST elevation during acute anterior myocardial infarction," *British Heart Journal*, vol. 74, no. 6, pp. 611–614, 1995.

[11] I. Isordia-Salas, A. Leaños-Miranda, I. M. Sainz, E. Reyes-Maldonado, and G. Borrayo-Sánchez, "Asociación entre el polimorfismo 4G/5G en el gen del inhibidor del activador del plasminógeno-1 (PAI-1) y el infarto agudo de miocardio con elevación del ST en pacientes jóvenes," *Revista Espanola de Cardiologia*, vol. 62, no. 4, pp. 365–372, 2009.

16

Polymorphic Ventricular Tachycardia Associated with High-Dose Methadone Use

Weng-Chio Tam, U-Po Lam, Toi-Meng Mok, Tou Chang, Wa Ho, and Mario Alberto De Brito Lima Evora

Department of Cardiology, Centro Hospitalar Conde São Januário, Macau, SAR, China

Correspondence should be addressed to Weng-Chio Tam; chio_2001_2@hotmail.com

Academic Editor: Kathleen Ngu

Methadone is a well-tolerated drug that has been used for pain control and the treatment of opioid addiction. However, some fatal cardiac side effects have been reported previously, including ventricular arrhythmia, stress cardiomyopathy, and coronary artery disease. We reported a middle-aged woman receiving high-dose methadone whom was presented with QT prolongation and torsade de pointes. We replaced the methadone with benzodiazepine and gave lidocaine use simultaneously. Thus, QT interval was shortened within the normal limit. Methadone-induced torsade de pointes is a rare but serious event, and QT interval should be monitored periodically to prevent this fatal adverse event, especially some patients with high-dose methadone use.

1. Introduction

Long QT syndromes can be categorized as either congenital or acquired etiologies. QT prolongation is manifested by the delayed cardiac repolarization phase resulting from transmembrane potassium, sodium, and calcium ion current alteration [1]. These may cause fatal ventricular arrhythmia and sudden cardiac death. Acquired long QT syndrome is known to be associated with some antibiotics, antihistamines, electrolyte imbalance, and metabolic disorders. Methadone is a synthetic opiate most commonly used for the pain control and treatment of heroin addiction. It may also block the cardiac potassium ion current and induce QT prolongation and dispersion, especially high-dose methadone [2]. The prevalence of methadone-induced QT prolongation and torsade de pointes may also be underestimated clinically. Therefore, we investigate the association of high-dose methadone and fatal ventricular arrhythmia in this report.

2. Case Presentation

A 44-year-old female patient presented herself with sudden onset of impaired consciousness at our emergency room. She had an underlying disease of microcytic anemia. She was also a methadone user for opioid addiction, receiving 130 mg/day. She initiated methadone use about 6 months ago. Otherwise, she denied any other medication use. On arrival, physical examination showed body weight: 55 kg, body temperature: 36.5°C, blood pressure: 114/70 mmHg, and pulse: 124/min. 12-lead electrocardiography (ECG) revealed sinus rhythm with frequent premature ventricular contractions (PVCs) (Figure 1(a)). The result of chest X-ray showed cardiomegaly with pulmonary edema. Echocardiography revealed preserved left ventricle systolic function with mild tricuspid regurgitation and grade III diastolic dysfunction. The level of potassium, calcium, and magnesium were within normal limit (potassium: 3.7 mmol/L (3.4-4.5), calcium: 2.16 mmol/L (2.15-2.5), and magnesium: 0.8 mmol/L (0.66-0.99)).Recurrent conscious disturbance was found about several minutes after the first episode. ECG monitor showed polymorphic PVCs, R on T, and QT prolongation, suggestive of torsade de pointes (TdP) with unstable hemodynamic status (Figures 1(b) and 1(c)). After three times of 200 J biphasic cardioversion defibrillation, ECG rhythm was converted to sinus rhythm spontaneously by herself (Figure 1(d)). Intravenous magnesium sulfate was used.

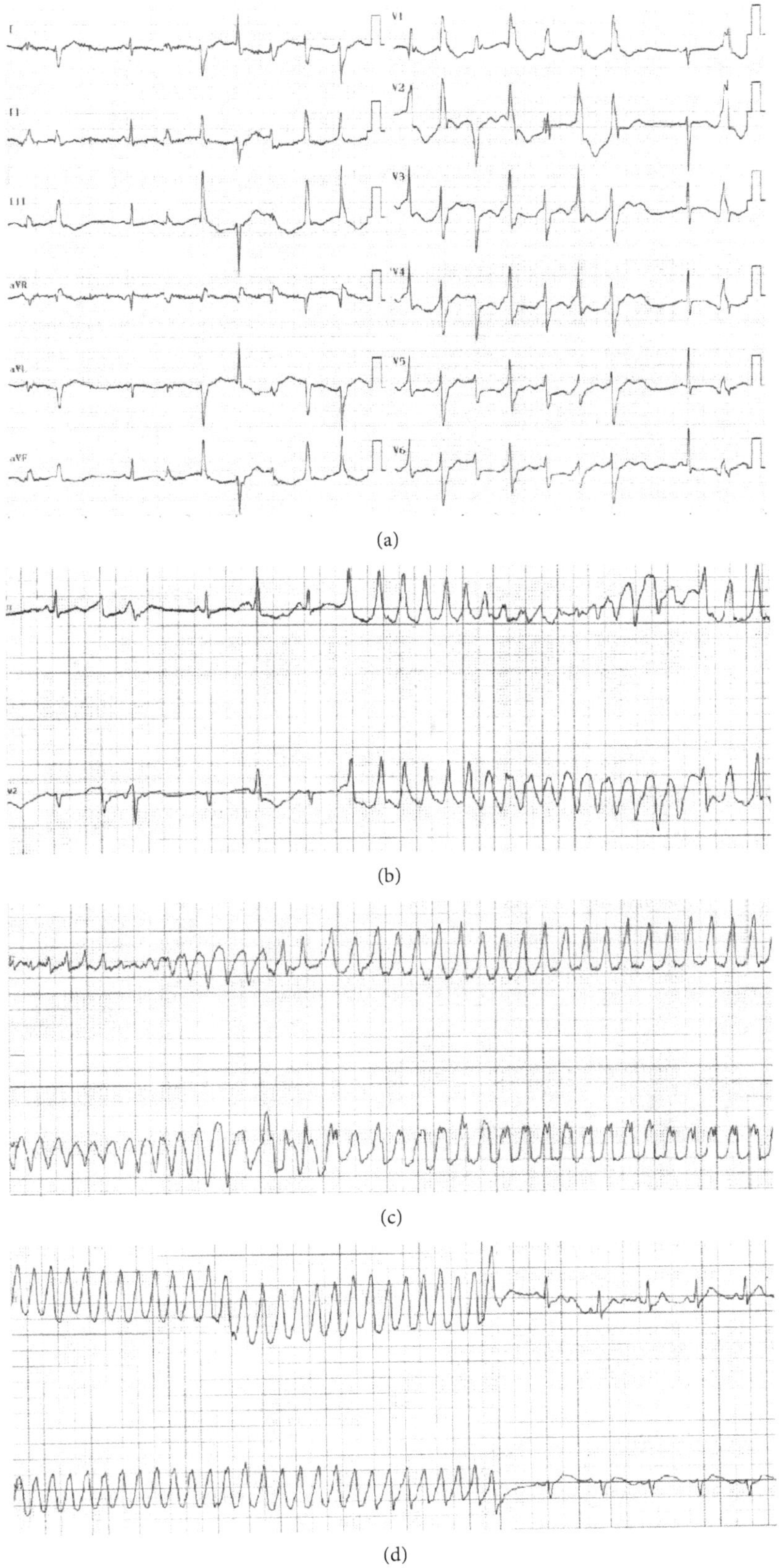

FIGURE 1: (a) 12-lead ECG revealed sinus rhythm with frequent PVCs. (b) Telemetry showed polymorphic premature ventricular contractions and R on T, and TdP was initiated. (c) QRS amplitude varied, and QRS complexes appeared to twist around the baseline, suggestive of TdP. (d) Self-termination of TdP.

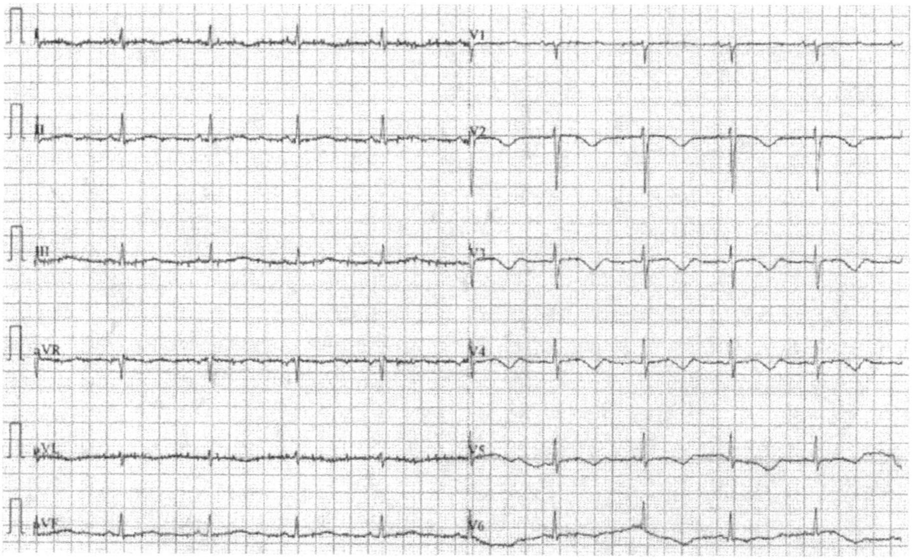

(a)

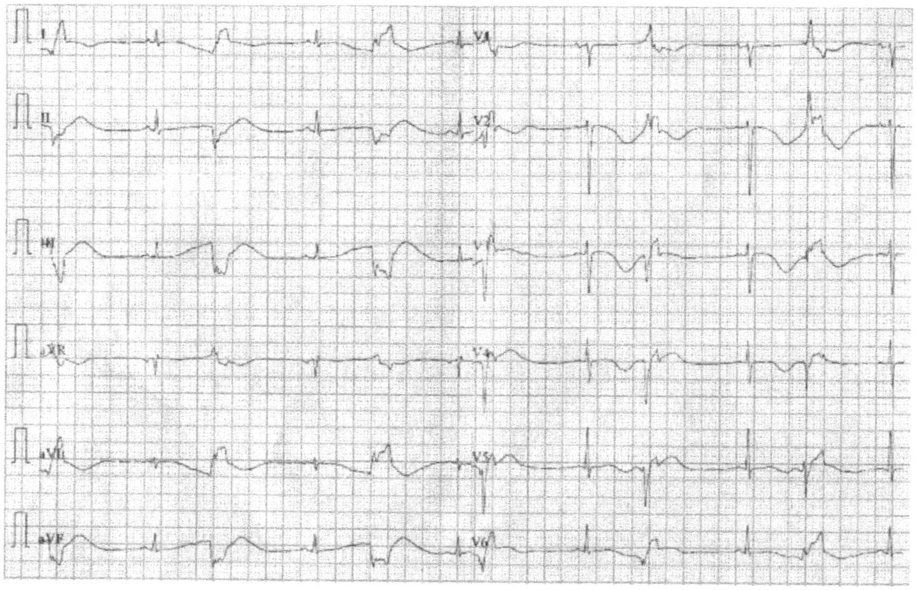

(b)

FIGURE 2: (a) After termination of TdP, repeated ECG revealed sinus rhythm with significant QT prolongation and QT interval was about 600 milliseconds. (b) ECG showed sinus rhythm with bigeminy PVC and R on T.

Repeated ECG showed sinus rhythm with obvious QT prolongation (QT interval > 600 milliseconds) (Figure 2(a)) and intermittent bigeminy PVC with R on T (Figure 2(b)). We gave her lidocaine to treat the potentially fatal ventricular arrhythmia because of its class IB antiarrhythmic effect. We gave magnesium and potassium supplements to prevent hypokalemia and hypomagnesemia, simultaneously to suppress early afterdepolarizations. We reviewed her medical and family history. She denied any history of syncope or premature family history of sudden death. Moreover, the previous ECG without methadone use was documented about 2 years ago (Figure 3(a)). It showed sinus rhythm with normal QT interval. According to the QT interval of documented ECG and medical background of high-dose methadone use, acquired long QT syndrome was suspected eventually. We discontinued the methadone and replaced it with benzodiazepine. Acute coronary syndrome was excluded because coronary computed tomography showed insignificant coronary artery disease with eccentric plaque over the left anterior descending artery. No recurrence of ventricular arrhythmia was noted after discontinuation of methadone use. QT interval was shortened to near 460 milliseconds within 2 weeks (Figure 3(b)).

3. Discussion

Methadone is a synthetic opiate which has been commonly used for the pain management. It is a mu-receptor and may

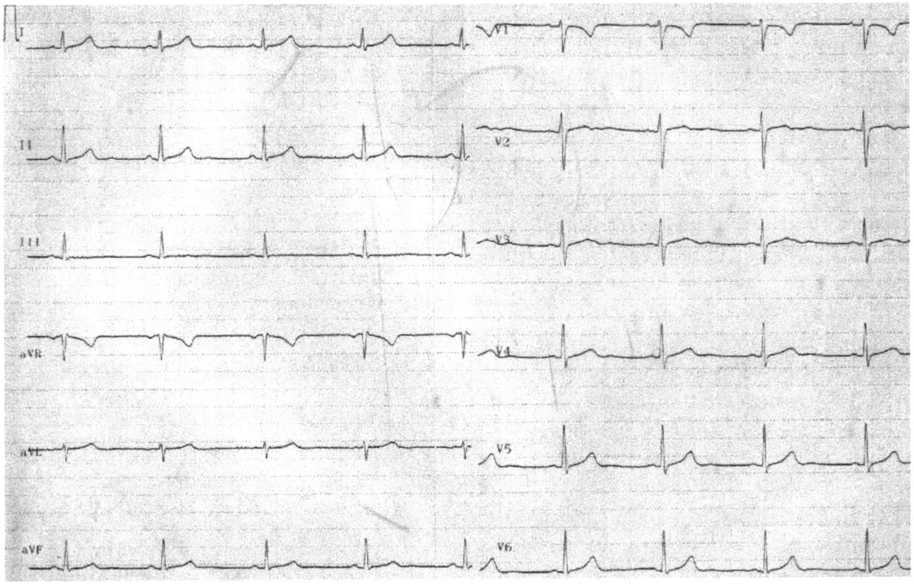

(a)

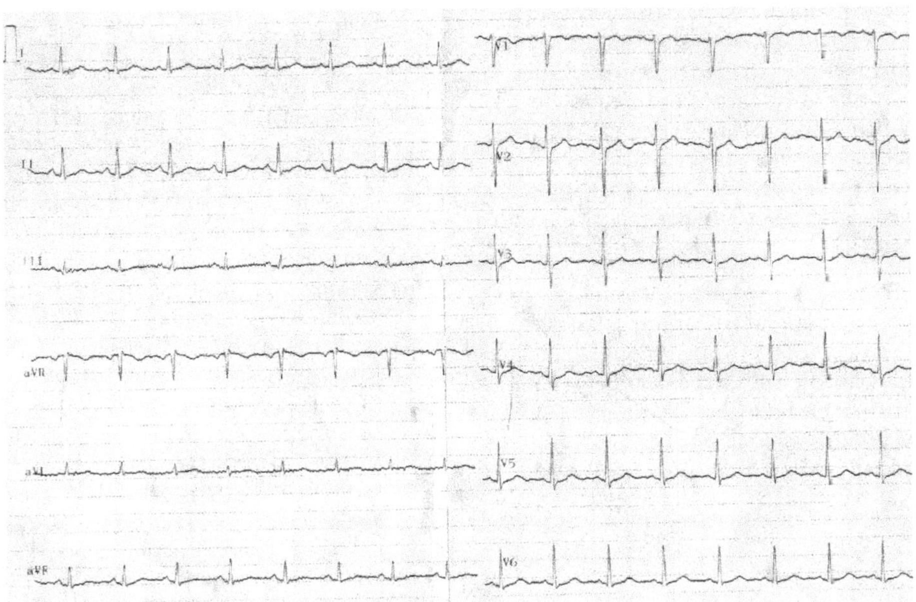

(b)

FIGURE 3: (a) The ECG without methadone use showed normal QT interval. (b) After discontinuation of methadone use, QT interval was shortened to near 460 milliseconds.

act as antagonist at the NMDA receptor. Physicians also use this medication either for opiate detoxification or maintenance to help people with opioid dependence. However, there are similar side effects to those of opioids, commonly including dizziness, sleepiness, vomiting, and sweating. More serious risks include respiratory depression and fatal cardiac arrhythmia. The incidence of adverse effect increases with higher doses [3], and high dose was defined as >100 mg daily methadone use [4]. Unexpected death could be associated with methadone which had lead to clinical safety concern by the U.S. Food and Drug Administration in 2006 [5]. Furthermore, recent studies indicated that methadone may be associated with polymorphic ventricular tachycardia and QT prolongation-induced TdP [3, 6]. The incidence of methadone-associated TdP was about 0.06/100 patient-years [7]. Patients with QT prolongation while using methadone should be cautioned and focused by clinicians as this could be one necessary precondition for the result of sudden cardiac death.

Methadone inhibits the human ether-a-go-go-related gene (hERG1) encoding for a potassium channel protein that regulates Ikr. This Ikr blockage may cause prolonged duration of the phase III of the ventricular action potential. It finally delays repolarization and represents as QT interval prolongation [8]. Moreover, it can trigger early afterdepolarizations due to the activation of L-type calcium channels and sodium-calcium exchange channel. According to the triggered activity from the early afterdepolarization, ectopic beats and premature ventricular extrasystoles can be generated to initiate TdP [9]. In addition to its effect of channelopathy, methadone use may be associated with the development of bradycardia because of its anticholinesterase properties. Increased QT dispersion and negative chronotropy has also been proven to be possible mechanism of methadone-induced TdP [10]. Moreover, other risk factors include hypokalemia, hypomagnesemia, hypocalcemia, and female. It is worth noting that concomitant use of psychiatric medication or anti-HIV medication can affect the drug-drug interaction and predispose the effect of QT prolongation from methadone [9].

The treatment of methadone cardiotoxicity depends on the patient's symptoms and signs. For asymptomatic patients, correction of electrolytes imbalance should be considered. Dose reduction or substitution of methadone is also reasonable. Some alternatives of methadone may also be considered including buprenorphine, naltrexone, or slow releasing morphine [11]. For patients with ventricular tachyarrhythmia, in addition to cessation of offending agents and electrolyte correction, magnesium sulfate is the first-line therapy. Temporary pacing or intravenous isoproterenol may be considered to prevent bradycardia. Intravenous lidocaine or oral mexiletine is also an alternative medication for some patients with recurrence of tachyarrhythmia [12].

In conclusion, although methadone is commonly used for the treatment of pain and opioid addiction, its cardiotoxicity, especially fatal ventricular arrhythmia, should be treated with caution. For some patients with hypokalemia or combination of medication that prolong the QT interval, physicians should monitor the QT interval before and during the methadone use, especially when high-dose methadone is prescribed.

Consent

Informed consent was obtained from all individual participants included in the study.

Acknowledgments

The authors would like to acknowledge Macau Cardiology Association.

References

[1] P. J. Schwartz, L. Crotti, and R. Insolia, "Long-QT syndrome: from genetics to management," *Circulation: Arrhythmia and Electrophysiology*, vol. 5, no. 4, pp. 868–877, 2012.

[2] B. A. Martell, J. H. Arnsten, M. J. Krantz, and M. N. Gourevitch, "Impact of methadone treatment on cardiac repolarization and conduction in opioid users," *The American Journal of Cardiology*, vol. 95, no. 7, pp. 915–918, 2005.

[3] M. J. Krantz, L. Lewkowiez, H. Hays, M. A. Woodroffe, A. D. Robertson, and P. S. Mehler, "Torsade de pointes associated with very-high-dose methadone," *Annals of Internal Medicine*, vol. 137, no. 6, pp. 501–504, 2002.

[4] A. Fareed, J. Casarella, M. Roberts et al., "High dose versus moderate dose methadone maintenance: is there a better outcome?," *Journal of Addictive Diseases*, vol. 28, no. 4, pp. 399–405, 2009.

[5] M. Faul, M. Bohm, and C. Alexander, "Methadone prescribing and overdose and the association with medicaid preferred drug list policies-United States, 2007-2014," *Morbidity and Mortality Weekly Report*, vol. 66, no. 12, pp. 320–323, 2017.

[6] D. Justo, "Methadone-induced long QT syndrome vs methadone-induced torsades de pointes," *Archives of Internal Medicine*, vol. 166, no. 20, pp. 2288–2290, 2006.

[7] A. R. Magnano, N. B. Talathoti, R. Hallur et al., "Effect of acute cocaine administration on the QTc interval of habitual users," *The American Journal of Cardiology*, vol. 97, no. 8, pp. 1244–1246, 2006.

[8] A. Gupta, A. T. Lawrence, K. Krishnan, C. J. Kavinsky, and R. G. Trohman, "Current concepts in the mechanisms and management of drug-induced QT prolongation and torsade de pointes," *American Heart Journal*, vol. 153, no. 6, pp. 891–899, 2007.

[9] P. J. Kannankeril and D. M. Roden, "Drug-induced long QT and torsade de pointes: recent advances," *Current Opinion in Cardiology*, vol. 22, no. 1, pp. 39–43, 2007.

[10] S. Mujtaba, J. Romero, and C. C. Taub, "Methadone, QTc prolongation and torsades de pointes: current concepts, management and a hidden twist in the tale?," *Journal of Cardiovascular Disease Research*, vol. 4, no. 4, pp. 229–235, 2013.

[11] G. Walton, S. Nolan, C. Sutherland, and K. Ahamad, "Sustained release oral morphine as an alternative to methadone for the treatment of opioid-use disorder post torsades de pointes cardiac arrest," *BML Case Reports*, vol. 2015, 2015.

[12] M. Badri, A. Patel, C. Patel et al., "Mexiletine prevents recurrent torsades de pointes in acquired long QT syndrome refractory to conventional measures," *JACC: Clinical Electrophysiology*, vol. 1, no. 4, pp. 315–322, 2015.

17

A Patient Infected with SARS-CoV-2 Presenting with Complete Heart Block

Bindu Gyawali,[1] Bikash Baral,[1] Sangam Shah ,[1] Sutap Yadav,[2] and Chandra Mani Poudel[2,3]

[1]*Maharajgunj Medical Campus, Institute of Medicine, Tribhuvan University, Maharajgunj, 44600, Nepal*
[2]*Department of Cardiology, Manmohan Cardiothoracic Vascular and Transplant Center, Nepal*
[3]*Maharajgunj Medical Campus, Institute of Medicine, Tribhuvan University, Maharajgunj 44600, Nepal*

Correspondence should be addressed to Sangam Shah; sangam.shah.1997@gmail.com

Academic Editor: Assad Movahed

Complete heart block is a rare presentation in a patient with COVID-19 infection that may result when the virus enters the myocardial cell by the angiotensin-converting enzyme-2 receptor. Here, we report a case of forty-nine-year male with COVID-19 with complete heart block (CHB).

1. Introduction

COVID-19 is a serious illness caused by severe acute respiratory syndrome coronavirus-2 (SARS-CoV-2) which has symptoms that range from asymptomatic to moderate respiratory symptoms and can develop to potentially fatal cardiovascular and pulmonary problems. Cardiac complications include acute myocardial infarction (MI), arrhythmias, heart block, and cardiomyopathy [1]. Although respiratory problems have been widely documented in coronavirus infection, evidences suggest that cardiac involvement may result in poor outcomes [2]. The exact mechanism of this poor outcome is not understood; however, it is believed that the virus enters cardiac and vascular cells through the angiotensin-converting enzyme-2 (ACE-2) receptor. This increases the risk of direct injury to the conduction system, which might result in heart block [3]. We report a case of a forty-nine-year male with COVID-19 with complete heart block (CHB) and COVID-19.

2. Case Presentation

A forty-nine-year male with a history of hypertension was admitted to our hospital with chief complaints of fatigue, palpitation, uneasiness, and chest heaviness on exertion for nine days. He had no history of syncope, edema, and shortness of breath, fever, and cold intolerance. He was an occasional smoker and used to consume alcohol. He was suspected with the provisional diagnosis of suspected COVID-19 infection. He had no history of taking herbal or over-the-counter medications.

He was conscious, cooperative, and well oriented to time, place, and person at the time of presentation. On examination, his blood pressure was 100/60 mm of Hg, pulse rate was 48 beats/min which was regular with low volume, respiratory rate was 14 breaths/min, oxygen saturation was 96% in room air, and axillary temperature was 36.5°C. Systemic examination was unremarkable.

His laboratory investigations revealed hemoglobin 11.9 gram % and packed cell volume 35.9%. He had an elevated level of alanine aminotransferase (ALT) (86 units per liter). His renal function test and thyroid function test were normal. Cardiac markers were within the normal range (creatinine kinase-MB (17 units per liter) and Troponin I (<0.012 nanograms per milliliter)). C-reactive protein (CRP) was positive (++) and Erythrocyte Sedimentation Rate (ESR) was 20/1st hour. On serological examination, Hepatitis B Surface Antigen (HBsAg) immunochromatography was nonreactive. COVID-19 was confirmed positive by Reverse Transcriptase Polymerase Chain Reaction (RT-PCR). His ECG showed a wide QRS complex with no relation between the successive P wave and the QRS complex (Figure 1). The rate of the P

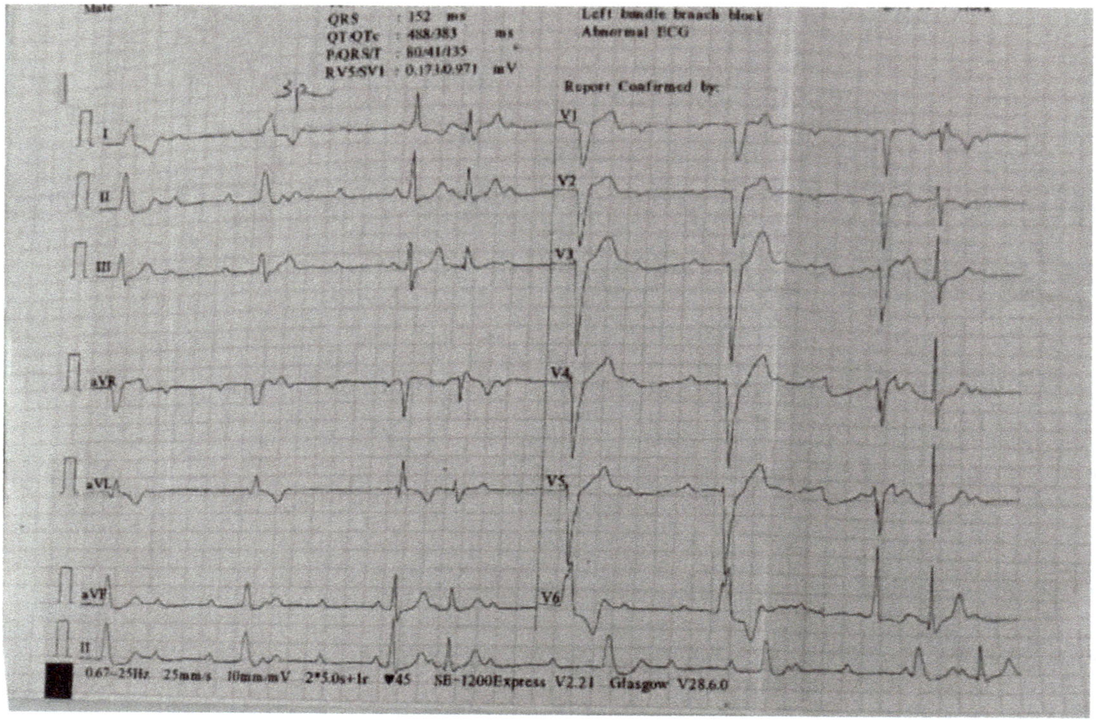

FIGURE 1: ECG of the patient done at the time of admission. ECG showed a wide QRS complex with no relation between the P wave and QRS complex.

wave was 100 beats/min, and the rate of the QRS complex was 38 beats/min which was suggestive of complete heart block.

Diagnosis of third-degree complete heart block with COVID-19 was made. His echocardiogram findings were normal with a left ventricle ejection fraction of 60%. The patient was admitted to the isolation ward for the symptomatic medical management. A repeat COVID-19 RT-PCR test after 10 and 12 days of admission was confirmed negative. Dual chamber permanent pacemaker implantation was done after 14 days without procedural complications (Figure 2). After insertion of a permanent pacemaker, there was a significant improvement in his symptoms (Figures 3 and 4), and following this, he was discharged from the hospital on oral medications.

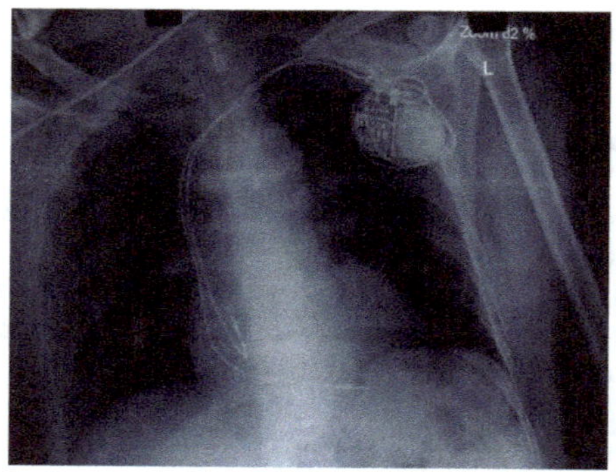

FIGURE 2: Chest X-ray showing dual-chamber permanent pacemaker (pulse generator with leads in right atrium and right ventricle).

3. Discussion

COVID-19 infection's ability to induce cardiac damage has been the subject of considerable discussion. Hypoxemia, electrolyte abnormalities, microthrombi, an inflammatory surge from the cytokine storm, and direct invasion of the cardiomyocytes are some of the probable causes causing cardiac injury [4]. Inflammatory cells and the SARS-CoV-2 virus, if found in autopsy results, imply direct cardiac invasion. A fifty-year male patient with COVID-19 showed interstitial mononuclear inflammatory cells suggesting an inflammatory process typical of myocarditis in one of the case reports [5].

Ischemic heart disease, thyroid dysfunction, drugs, and infections are thought to be the cause of the new-onset AV node disease [6]. In our case, there was no derangement of the cardiac marker or thyroid markers; no medications before hospitalization were given that ruled out these etiologies. Thus, either focal involvement or secondary cause of AV block causing critical illness could be the probable cause in our patient. Besides, injury to the conduction system can be related to direct virus invasion. High-degree heart block caused by an infectious organism is rare. Complete heart block caused by a virus is noted in few studies. SARS and MERS have no reported cases of atrioventricular block among infected patients [7]. In this case, COVID-19 may have induced subclinical myocarditis, which resulted in high-degree AV block; this is the most likely mechanism. ACE-2 receptors are present in macrophages, endothelial cells, smooth muscle cells, and cardiomyocytes [8]. In animal models, ACE-2 receptors were found in sinoatrial nodal cells

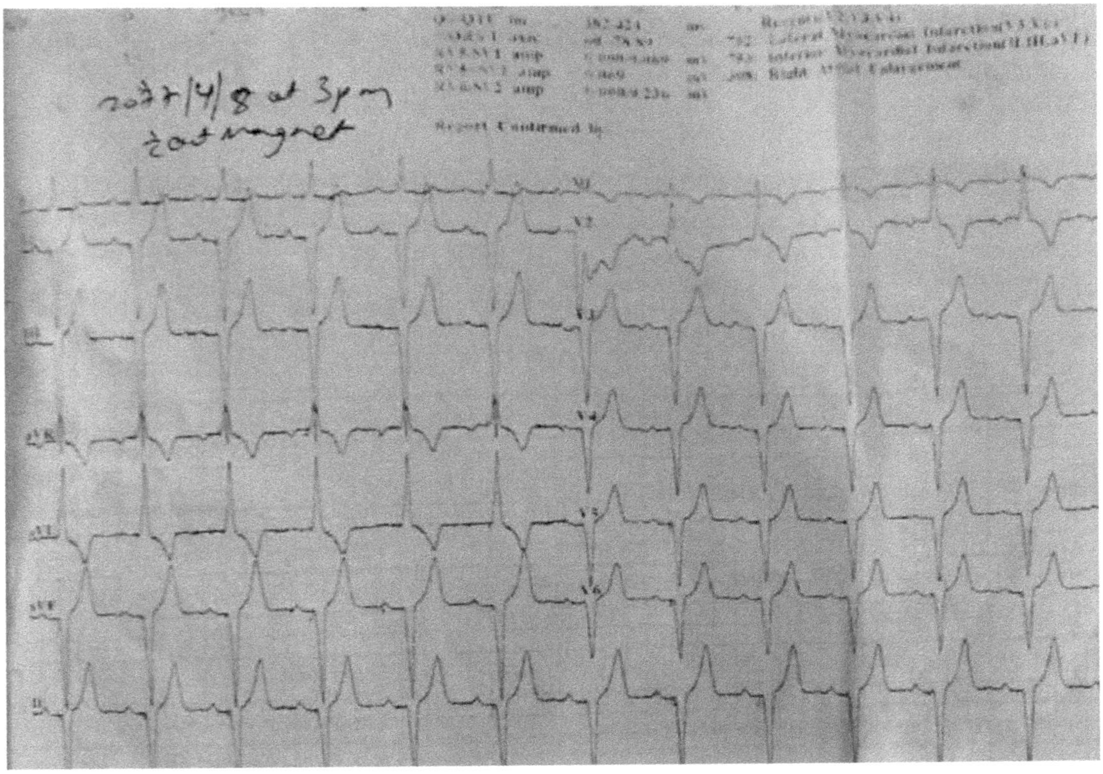

FIGURE 3: ECG of patient without magnet done after pacemaker insertion showing AsVP (atrial-sensed and ventricular-paced beats).

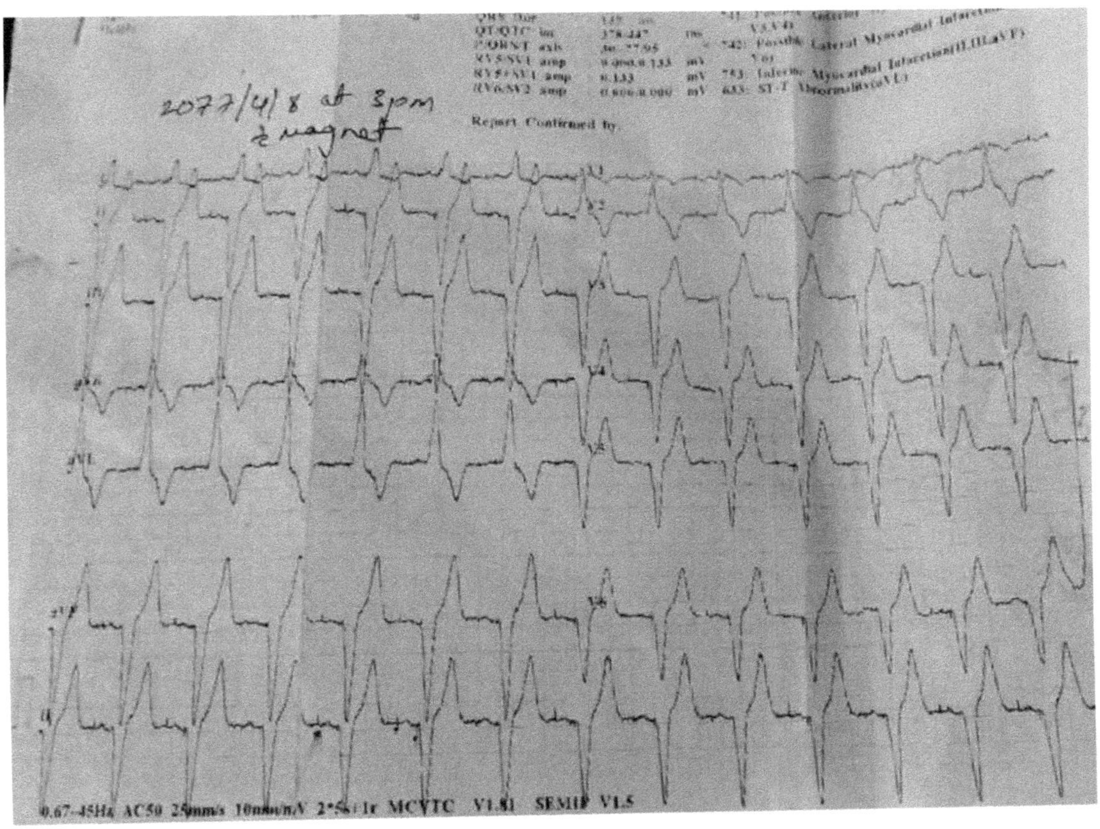

FIGURE 4: ECG of the patient with magnet after pacemaker implantation showing ApVp (both atrial- and ventricular-paced beats).

in rats, and their overexpression caused conduction problems and ventricular fibrillation [9, 10]. Another potential is SARS-CoV-2 infection of the AV node and infra-Hisian conduction pathway, resulting in AV block. Some studies suggest the role of hydroxychloroquine used in the treatment of COVID-19 as the probable cause of AV block. Hydroxychloroquine can lead to prolongation of QT intervals, and a notable side effect is the fascicular block which consequently results in an atrioventricular block.

We believe the patient was originally infected with the coronavirus, and the systemic inflammatory response to multiple organ systems may have damaged the heart's conduction system, resulting in total heart block. Complete heart block in this patient may just be an incidental finding without symptom in a patient with COVID-19 infection.

4. Conclusion

COVID-19's spectrum is broadening. SARS-CoV-2 viral RNA has been discovered in the heart, raising the possible risk of direct harm to the cardiac conduction system and cardiac myocytes. This may form a basis for the manifestation of complete heart block in the COVID-19 patient with cardiac involvement. However, it should be emphasized that CHB may be a rare consequence of the coronavirus infection. Furthermore, the link between CHB and coronavirus should be explored.

Consent

This article is published with the written consent of the patient.

Authors' Contributions

SS conceptualized the study and reviewed and edited the manuscript; BG and BB wrote the original and reviewed and edited the manuscript; BG, BB, SS, SY, and CMP were in charge of the case and reviewed the manuscript.

References

[1] B. Long, W. J. Brady, A. Koyfman, and M. Gottlieb, "Cardiovascular complications in COVID-19," *American Journal of Emergency Medicine*, vol. 38, no. 7, pp. 1504–1507, 2020.

[2] G. Aghagoli, B. Gallo Marin, L. B. Soliman, and F. W. Sellke, "Cardiac involvement in COVID-19 patients: risk factors, predictors, and complications: a review," *Journal of Cardiac Surgery*, vol. 35, no. 6, pp. 1302–1305, 2020.

[3] G. Y. Oudit, Z. Kassiri, C. Jiang et al., "SARS-coronavirus modulation of myocardial ACE2 expression and inflammation in patients with SARS," *European Journal of Clinical Investigation*, vol. 39, no. 7, pp. 618–625, 2009.

[4] M. Bansal, "Cardiovascular disease and COVID-19," *Diabetes Metab Syndr Clin Res Rev*, vol. 14, no. 3, pp. 247–250, 2020.

[5] G. Tse, J. M. Yeo, Y. W. Chan, E. T. H. Lai, and B. P. Yan, "What is the arrhythmic substrate in viral myocarditis? Insights from clinical and animal studies," *Frontiers in Physiology*, vol. 7, 2016.

[6] M. ZOOB and K. SMITH, "The Aetiology of complete heart-block," *BMJ*, vol. 2, no. 5366, pp. 1149–1153, 1963.

[7] M. Madjid, P. Safavi-Naeini, S. D. Solomon, and O. Vardeny, "Potential effects of coronaviruses on the cardiovascular system: a review," *JAMA Cardiology*, vol. 5, no. 7, pp. 831–840, 2020.

[8] L. S. Zisman, "ACE and ACE2: a tale of two enzymes," *European Heart Journal*, vol. 26, no. 4, pp. 322–324, 2005.

[9] A. J. Ferreira, P. L. Moraes, G. Foureaux, A. B. Andrade, R. A. S. Santos, and A. P. Almeida, "The angiotensin-(1-7)/mas receptor axis is expressed in sinoatrial node cells of rats," *Journal of Histochemistry & Cytochemistry*, vol. 59, no. 8, pp. 761–768, 2011.

[10] U. Danilczyk and J. M. Penninger, "Angiotensin-converting enzyme II in the heart and the kidney," *Circulation Research*, vol. 98, pp. 463–471, 2006.

18

First Reported Case of *Candida dubliniensis* Endocarditis Related to Implantable Cardioverter-Defibrillator

Nooraldin Merza,[1] **John Lung**,[2] **Taryn B. Bainum**,[3] **Assad Mohammedzein**,[1] **Shanna James**,[3] **Mazin Saadaldin**,[1] **and Tarek Naguib**[1]

[1]*Department of Internal Medicine, Texas Tech University Health Sciences Center, Amarillo, TX, USA*
[2]*School of Medicine, Texas Tech University Health Sciences Center, Amarillo, TX, USA*
[3]*Department of Pharmacy Practice, Texas Tech University Health Sciences Center Jerry H. Hodge School of Pharmacy, Amarillo, TX, USA*

Correspondence should be addressed to Mohammad Ali Zakeri; mazakeri@rums.ac.ir

Academic Editor: Hajime Kataoka

A 36-year-old male presented to the ED with acute chronic hyponatremia found on routine weekly lab work with one-week history of generalized weakness, confusion, nausea/vomiting, and diarrhea. The patient has nonischemic cardiomyopathy of unknown etiology diagnosed in his teens with an AICD device placed 8 years ago and receiving milrinone infusion 3 years ago via peripherally inserted central catheter (PICC) line. Two sets of blood cultures grew *Candida dubliniensis*. The patient was started on micafungin and the PICC line was removed and replaced with a central line. A transthoracic echocardiogram (TEE) showed findings consistent with AICD lead involvement. The patient was continued on treatment for fungal infective endocarditis and transferred to another hospital where he had successful AICD lead extraction. Blood cultures upon transfer back to our facility were positive for methicillin-sensitive *Staphylococcus aureus* (MSSA). This bacteremia was thought to be secondary to right-sided internal jugular (IJ) central line and resolved with line removal and initiation of intravenous (IV) cefazolin. The patient was discharged on IV cefazolin and IV micafungin. He had a LifeVest® until completion of his antibiotic course and a new AICD was placed.

1. Introduction

Automatic implantable cardioverter-defibrillator (AICD) devices are used for a wide variety of cardiac conditions including secondary prevention of sudden cardiac death for patients with a previous cardiac arrest who have sustained ventricular tachycardia, coronary artery disease, nonischemic dilated cardiomyopathy, hypertrophic cardiomyopathy, and genetic arrhythmia syndromes. AICDs can also be used for the primary prevention of sudden cardiac death. [1].

Complications of AICD implantation include infections that may include vegetations on the leads or valves [2, 3]. Estimates of the rate of infection postimplantation range from 0.13% [4] to 19.9% [5]. Pocket infections related to AICD devices usually involve staphylococci and occur within weeks of implantation.

Systemic AICD device infections were less common, presented later, and typically involve a wider range of microbes compared to pocket infections. Current guidelines call for AICD removal with TEE demonstrating valve or lead vegetation, presence of pocket infection, or positive blood cultures with *S. aureus*, coagulase-negative staphylococci, *Cutibacterium*, *Candida* species, or other high-grade bacteremia without alternative source [6]. Antimicrobial treatment without device removal has a high reinfection and failure rate [7]. In most cases, the long-term harm to the patient of repeated infections and mortality outweigh the risks of immediate extraction with other approaches like device retention and antibiotic therapy having a higher risk of mortality [8, 9].

Candida-related ICD infection is extremely rare and there are only 23 *Candida* device-associated endocarditis cases published in the literature (Table 1) [10–13]. The

Table 1: MIC concentrations for *Candida dubliniensis*. Susceptibility results were not published in the report due to the lack of outcomes data for less common species including *C. dubliniensis*.

Antifungal	MIC (μg/mL)
Amphotericin B	0.25
Caspofungin	0.06
Fluconazole	0.25
Flucytosine	0.06
Itraconazole	0.06
Ketoconazole	0.015
Voriconazole	0.008

majority of patients are over age 60 and had an infection with a time postimplantation ranging from less than a month to 16 years [14].

We report on a unique case of AICD-related fungemia complicated by simultaneous use of a chronic milrinone infusion. We describe the rare infection, the path to diagnosis, treatment, and postoperative complications observed prior to discharge.

We report the first case of *Candida dubliniensis* as a source of ICD fungemia in the English language literature. *Candida dubliniensis* is an opportunistic pathogen that was originally isolated from AIDS patients, but since then, it has been isolated from both immunocompetent and immunocompromised individuals [15, 16]. Furthermore, invasive infections by *C. dubliniensis* have increased considerably in recent years in immunocompromised/immunosuppressed individuals [16].

2. Case Presentation

A 36-year old male presented to the ED with generalized weakness, confusion, and fatigue starting one week prior. The symptoms were associated with some episodes of nausea, vomiting, and loose semisolid stools. The patient reported shortness of breath that had progressed to rest over the past weeks. He denied any fever but reported some chills. He denied any chest pain, palpitations, lower extremity swelling, abdominal pain, or other complaints. The patient has routine weekly labs which showed hyponatremia (sodium = 122 mmol/dL, baseline 130 mmol/dL) so he was sent for evaluation to the emergency room by his cardiologist. The patient has a past medical history of nonischemic cardiomyopathy diagnosed at age 16. A transthoracic echocardiogram done about 9 months prior showed a left ventricular ejection fraction of less than 20% and severe concentric left ventricular hypertrophy. The patient had an automatic implantable cardioverter-defibrillator (AICD) placement 8 years prior for primary prevention of sudden cardiac death. The patient had been on a chronic milrinone infusion delivered through a peripherally inserted central catheter (PICC) line for the past 3 years. This was initiated as a bridge to transplant. However, during transplant evaluation, he was noted to have secondary pulmonary hypertension and would need a combined heart and lung transplant, and no transplant center in the state would accept his insurance for a combined transplant. Besides cardiomyopathy, he also has a history of chronic atrial fibrillation, congenital hydrocephalus with ventriculoperitoneal shunt (since the age of 2), and spinal stenosis. Of note, the patient was taking apixaban, bumetanide, magnesium oxide, allopurinol, digoxin, metolazone, eplerenone, and carvedilol.

On exam, the patient had a red, swollen left upper extremity at the site of his PICC and white nail beds on the left hand and cool extremities, but no lower extremity edema. The patient was afebrile, had an elevated heart rate of 109 beats per minute (bpm), an elevated respiratory rate of 26 breaths per minute, and SpO2 was 96% on 2 L nasal cannula. All other vitals were within normal limits.

Labs on admission are as follows: WBC: 10.9×10^3/mcL; sodium: 123 mmol/L; potassium: 4.7 mmol/L; chloride: 90 mmol/L; bicarbonate: 22; BUN: 27 mg/dL; creatinine: 0.9 mg/dL; glucose: 102 mg/dL; INR: 1.56; total bilirubin: 4.12 mg/dL; alkaline phosphatase: 166 units/L; AST: 44 units/L; and ALT: 27 units/L. The patient was initially diagnosed with viral gastroenteritis and his symptoms of nausea, vomiting, and diarrhea resolved within 2 days. As the team was preparing to discharge the patient, 2 sets of blood cultures taken at admission came back positive for *Candida dubliniensis*. The patient's WBC count increased from 11.0 to 15.2 with continued stability in his vital signs other than an increase in his heart rate to 120 s bpm. A chest X-ray on admission showed no acute abnormalities, stable cardiomegaly, and an AICD in place. An electrocardiogram (EKG) showed atrial flutter. CT scan of the head showed a left VP shunt with mild ventriculomegaly of the lateral and third ventricles unchanged since 2017. No evidence of intracranial hemorrhage was found. A lumbar puncture obtained clear CSF that was sent to microbiology. The CSF cultures had no growth. The patient was started on empiric micafungin 100 mg IV daily and vancomycin.

A blood culture of the PICC line and a culture of the catheter tip was positive for *Candida dubliniensis* as determined by matrix-assisted laser desorption/ionization time-of-flight (MALDI-TOF) mass spectrometry. Minimum inhibitory concentrations (MICs) for antifungals are listed in Table 1.

The PICC line was removed and a right-sided internal jugular vein (IJV) central line was placed. Vancomycin was discontinued after one day once the culture grew yeast. A negative blood culture of *C. dubliniensis* was drawn 4 weeks after the first positive culture. Micafungin was continued for a total of 6 weeks after the initial positive culture.

Transesophageal echocardiogram (TEE) (Figure 1) showed a new finding of echogenicity of one of the three leads consistent with lead vegetation. Consistent with a TEE done 8 months ago, there was minimal thickening of the aortic valve, mild thickening of the mitral valve with moderate to severe mitral regurgitation, and moderate to severe tricuspid regurgitation. One of the leads had a mobile echodensity measuring 0.4 × 1.3 cm, consistent with lead vegetation. No valvular vegetations were identified on TEE. The findings of the TEE were consistent with AICD fungal septicemia. An AICD lead extraction was done one week after admission at

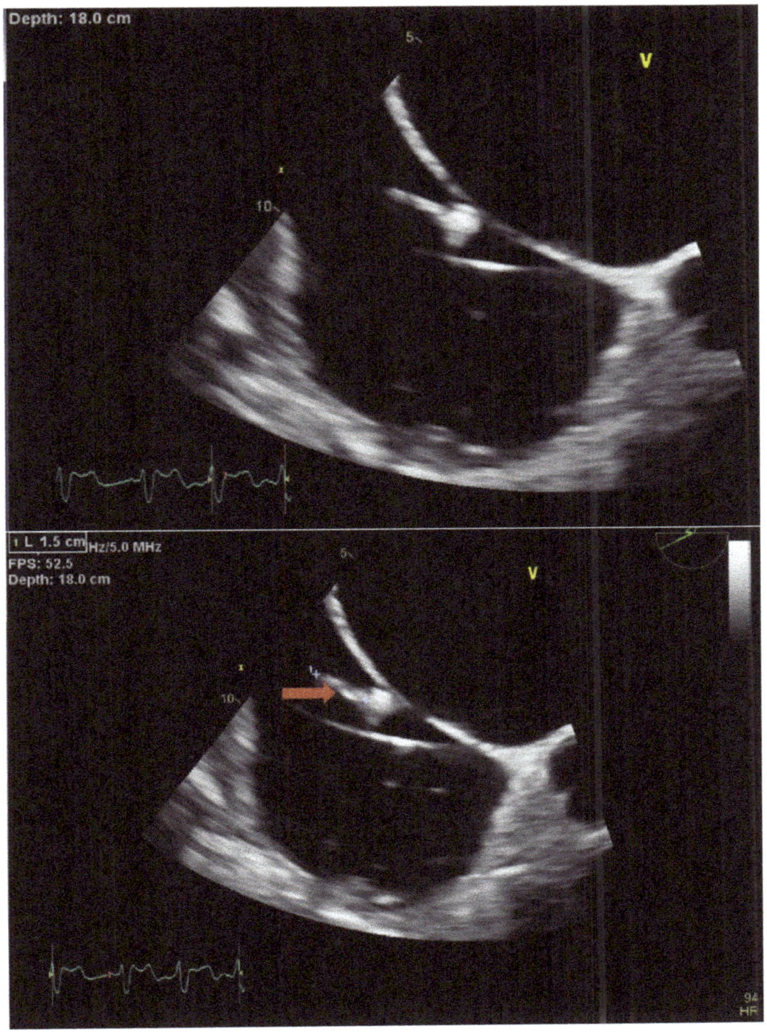

FIGURE 1: Echogenicity of one of the three leads consistent with lead vegetation measuring 0.4 × 1.3 cm. The transesophageal echocardiogram did not identify any significant valvular vegetations.

an outside facility with a temporary transcutaneous pacer placed, after which the patient returned to our inpatient facility for placement of a replacement AICD two weeks later. Blood cultures done at the outside facility were negative. Blood cultures from the right and left arms done at our facility after AICD implantation returned *Staphylococcus aureus* on 2/2 sets sensitive to cefazolin, oxacillin, tetracycline, and trimethoprim/sulfamethoxazole. The right-side IJV central line was removed and a left-side IJV central line was placed with negative blood cultures after placement. The micafungin was recommended to be continued for four weeks after new AICD placement and cefazolin was started for two weeks due to the right-sided IJV central line MSSA infection. A vascular surgeon was consulted for optimal line access with the least infectious risk. The vascular surgeon recommended a PICC line. A replacement PICC line was placed three weeks later and the patient was discharged the next day with a PICC line for milrinone, cefazolin, and micafungin infusion.

3. Discussion

With the increasing use of AICD devices for the secondary and primary prevention of cardiac death, clinicians should be vigilant of the possibility of infection caused by AICD placement. Risk factors that can increase infection rates include heart failure, diabetes, renal disease, immunosuppressed state, oral anticoagulation, chronic lung disease, and recent device modifications [10, 17]. Our patient had several comorbidities that increased his risk of an infection including use of oral anticoagulation, a history of heart failure, and pulmonary hypertension. His primary risk factor, however, was chronic PICC line for milrinone infusion, despite PICC being exchanged about every 6 months and the patient practicing adequate PICC care at home.

Our patient's scenario was unique because, to our knowledge, it is the first reported case of *C. dubliniensis*-ICD fungemia with sepsis, in the English-language literature. He denied fever which was not uncommon in candidemia. Additionally,

TABLE 2: Summary of the reported cases of *Candida*-associated ICD septic fungemia.

Case	Age (yrs)	Gender	Illnesses	Device type	Length of device use before infection	Symptoms	Echo result	Culture results	Management/outcome
Davis et al. 1969	71	Male	Diabetes, obstructive uropathy, UTI, CHF	Permanent pacemaker	9 months	Fever, confusion, leukocytosis	Not reported	Blood: no growth; urine: yeast	Broad-spectrum antibacterials. Patient expired.
Cole et al. 1986	65	Male	CVA, IV catheter-related *Candida albicans* fungemia 6 months prior	Permanent pacemaker	8 years	Fever, confusion, urine/fecal incontinence	5 × 2 × 2 cm shaggy mass attached to pacer wire extending from RA to RV	Initial blood and urine cultures: no growth. Subsequent blood culture: *Candida albicans*	Broad-spectrum antibacterials followed by amphotericin B. Thoracotomy. Expired at surgery.
Wilson et al. 1993	56	Male	Heart block	Permanent pacemaker	5 years	Fever, cough, dyspnoea, leukocytosis	Multiple large RA masses prolapse into RV. Possible adherence to pacer wire. (TTE)	Blood: *Candida albicans*	Amphotericin B (2 g total). Right atriotomy and pulmonary arteriotomy. Removed leads and fungus ball from left main PA. Recovered, well after 2 years
Shmuely et al. 1997	75	Male	Diabetes, sick sinus syndrome	Permanent pacemaker	2 years	Blurred vision, endophthalmitis	3 cm vegetation on pacer wire below TV, within RV (TEE)	Blood: *Candida tropicalis*	Amphotericin B+5-flucytosine. Refused surgery to remove PPM. Expired with multiorgan failure
Joly et al. 1997	56	Male	Chronic bronchitis, sinus dysfunction	Permanent pacemaker	4 years: old PPM wires, 3 months: new PPM	Fever, dyspnoea	RA mass (TEE)	Initial blood culture: no growth. Blood then positive for *Candida albicans*. Wires and vegetation: *Candida albicans*	Right atriotomy: removed vegetation, wires, and PPM. Amphotericin B+5-flucytosine, then oral fluconazole × 7 months. Recovered
Cacoub et al. 1998	56	Male	Sick sinus syndrome	Permanent pacemaker	Not reported	Fever, dyspnoea	Vegetation on pacer lead	Blood and pacer lead: *S. epidermidis*, *Candida albicans*	Antibiotic. Surgical removal of PPM. Survived.
Victor et al. 1999	72	Male	Bradycardia, tachycardia syndrome	Permanent pacemaker	<1 month	Not reported	Vegetation on TV	Lead culture: *Candida glabrata*	Endovascular extraction of PPM. Expired after 2 months with active Candida endocarditis
Kurup et al. 2000	77	Male	Diabetes, coronary artery disease, sick sinus syndrome	Permanent pacemaker	5 months	Fever, dyspnoea, lethargy	TV vegetation (TTE)	Blood, vegetation: *Candida tropicalis*	Amphotericin B. Thoracotomy: vegetation on TV and PPM lead. Removed PPM and vegetations. Expired with multiorgan failure after surgery.
Roger et al. 2000	87	Male	CML, renal neoplasm, prosthetic AV	Permanent pacemaker	16 years	Fever, renal insufficiency	7 cm vegetation on pacer wire (TTE+TEE)	Blood, vegetation: *Candida albicans* and *Candida glabrata*	Fluconazole. Not a surgical candidate. Expired with fatal stroke

Table 2: Continued.

Case	Age (yrs)	Gender	Illnesses	Device type	Length of device use before infection	Symptoms	Echo result	Culture results	Management/outcome
Brown et al. 2001	49	Male	Diabetes, coronary artery disease, CHF, ventricular tachycardia	Implanted cardioverter defibrillator	12 months	Fever, dyspnoea, cough, leukocytosis	3.5 cm vegetation on defibrillator lead (TTE)	Blood and vegetation: *Candida albicans*	Amphotericin B × 8 weeks, then fluconazole 400 mg P.O. daily. Explanted device by thoracotomy. Clinically stable 6 months later
Hindupur and Muslin 2005	63	Male	Coronary artery disease, CHF, ventricular tachycardia	Implanted cardioverter-defibrillator	10 months	Fatigue	Vegetations on atrial ICD lead (largest: 1.6 cm) (TTE+TEE)	Blood, ICD lead and pocket: *Candida albicans*	Removed generator, percutaneous extraction of ICD lead. Lead fractured, embolised with vegetation into left PA. Received fluconazole, then amphotericin B. improved, then expired with P. aeruginosabacteraemia
Ho et al. 2006	56	Male	Rheumatic heart disease, cardiomyopathy, ventricular tachycardia	Implanted cardioverter-defibrillator	12 years; generator change 1 week before	Fever, sweat, hypotension, ICD pocket dehisced	1.8 cm mobile vegetation on intracardiac lead (TEE)	Blood: *Candida parapsilosis*	Fluconazole IV × 6 weeks, then oral fluconazole 400 mg da: 1 lifelong. Explanted device. Survived
Talarmin et al. 2009	76	Male	Colorectal cancer	Permanent pacemaker	Not reported	Not reported	Not reported	Blood: *Candida parapsilosis*	Removed PPM: found vegetations on leads. Received fluconazole for 42 days. Expired secondary to abdominal surgery complications
Falcone et al. 2009	38	Male	Previous aortic valve replacement	Permanent pacemaker	3 months	Fever	Vegetations on pacer lead	Lead culture: *Candida parapsilosis*	Removed PPM. Received caspofungin for 6 weeks, then 12 weeks oral fluconazole and posaconazole. Cured at 14 months follow-up
Durante-Mangoni and Nappi 2010	19	Male	Complete heart block	Permanent pacemaker	1 year	Fever, cough, hemoptysis	Massive, mobile structure on pacer lead	Blood: *Candida albicans*	Caspofungin and fluconazole × 8 weeks, removal and replacement of ICD. Recovered.
Halawa et al. 2011	80	Male	Coronary artery disease, COPD, atrial fibrillation, complete heart block	Permanent pacemaker	12 years	Chills, confusion	0.5 × 0.5 cm mobile mass on pacer wire, fibrinous strands on TV	Blood and pacer vegetation: *Candida parapsilosis*	Amphotericin B, maintained for 3 weeks after PPM removed. PPM explantation and percutaneous lead extraction, no infection at 1 year follow-up.
Grunberg et al. 2013	62	Male	CHF, diabetes, coronary artery disease, hepatitis C infection	Implanted cardioverter-defibrillator	11 months	Fever, dyspnea on exertion, chest pressure	4 cm mass on ICD lead	Blood: *Candida albicans*	Fluconazole IV, ICD removal. Plan 6 weeks of fluconazole before ICD reimplantation.
Tascini et al. 2013	75	Female	Symptomatic bradycardia	Permanent pacemaker	6 years	Fever × 2 weeks	2 cm vegetation adherent to the	Blood: *Candida albicans*	IV fluconazole × 10 days, then IV micafungin × 75 days. Survived.

Table 2: Continued.

Case	Age (yrs)	Gender	Illnesses	Device type	Length of device use before infection	Symptoms	Echo result	Culture results	Management/outcome
							atrial lead of the bicameral PM		
Rivera et al. 2014	60	Female	HF with reduced EF, sarcoidosis, and diabetes	Implanted cardioverter defibrillator	2 years, 2 months	Fevers, chills, sweats, cough	Mobile 2.09 cm × 4.49 cm mass associated with ICD wire	Blood: *Candida albicans*	Removed ICD. Micafungin × 2 weeks, then fluconazole × 6 weeks. Survived.
Bandyopadhyay et al. 2015	86	Male	Diabetes	Permanent pacemaker	3 years	Weakness, fever	Vegetation on the pacemaker electrode in right atrium and ventricle	Blood: *Candida tropicalis*	IV caspofungin × 10 days, then IV fluconazole ×15 days, then oral fluconazole × 2 months. Survived.
Glavis-Bloom et al. 2015	70	Female	CHF, diabetes, chronic kidney disease	Implanted cardioverter-defibrillator	13 months	Fever, nausea, vomiting, fatigue	Multiple ICD lead masses and 0.7 cm mobile aortic valve mass	Blood and urine: *Candida glabrata*	Caspofungin IV × 3 days, then micafungin IV and flucytosine IV. Expired with multiorgan failure 1 month later.
Jain et al. 2018	60	Female	Diabetes, ischemic cardiomyopathy, pancytopenia	Implanted cardioverter-defibrillator	Not reported	Fever, altered mental status	Mass attached to the tricuspid valve	Blood: *Candida parapsilosis*	Amphotericin B, removed ICD and leads, removed tricuspid valve vegetations. Survived.
Jones et al. 2018	25	Female	Obesity, hypertension, diabetes, nonischemic cardiomyopathy	Implanted cardioverter-defibrillator	2 years, 9 months	Not reported	Large vegetation above the tricuspid valve, 2.1 cm × 1.6 cm echodensity within the right atrium	Blood: *Candida albicans*	AngioVac aspiration and laser sheath extraction of ICD lead, suppressive fluconazole. Survived.

UTI: urinary tract infection; CHF: congestive heart failure; CVA: cerebral vascular accident; PPM: permanent pacemaker; TEE: transesophageal echocardiogram; HF: heart failure; EF: ejection fraction.

Table 3: Case reports of infection with *Candida dubliniensis*.

Case report	Patient age and sex	Patient comorbidities	Site of infection
[19]	74, M	Chronic lymphocytic leukemia, COPD, CAD, hypertension	Blood
	30, F	End-stage liver disease, alcohol and drug abuse	Blood
	39, M	End-stage liver disease, lymphadenopathy, diabetes mellitus	Blood
	37, F	Intravenous drug use, chronic DVTs, valvular heart disease	Blood
[20]	46, F	End-stage liver disease, liver transplant	Blood, abdominal wound, tracheal aspirate
[21]	30, M	Intravenous drug user, hepatitis C	Blood
[22]	71, M	End-stage liver cirrhosis	Sputum
[23]	38, M	No past medical history	Endophthalmitis
[24]	53, M	Alcohol abuse	Fungal bezoar encapsulating a calculus in right upper kidney
[25]	62, F	Rheumatic heart disease, mitral valve replacement, thyroid papillary carcinoma, congestive heart failure	Central venous catheter and blood
	71, M	Bladder cancer	Central venous catheter and blood
[26]	31, M	Intravenous drug use	Blood, sputum, endophthalmitis
[27]	75, F	Laryngeal cancer, tuberculosis	Pneumonia
[28]	49, M	Hepatitis C, cirrhosis, substance use disorder, recent exposure to IV antibiotics	Meningitis
[29]	56, M	Diabetes mellitus type 2	Right hand abscess
[30]	59, M	COPD, diabetes mellitus type 2, ulcerative colitis	Pneumonia
[31]	45, F	None reported	Keratitis

his age was younger than the average of the other case reports which were related to AICD-*Candida* infection (see Table 2); he has nonischemic cardiomyopathy diagnosed at age 16 and has multiple comorbidities that complicate diagnosis and treatment.

Candida dubliniensis was first recovered postmortem from a lung specimen of a patient who expired in the United Kingdom in 1957. This organism was originally misidentified as *C. stellatoidea*. This species was discovered to be unique from other *Candida* species in the city of Dublin, resulting in the name *Candida dubliniensis*. This organism was found in mainly oral cavities, primarily those of HIV-infected individuals. Though this species has been found in oral cavities of healthy individuals and has been implicated infections in healthy individuals, it is rare for this organism to produce infection in immunocompetent adults. It appears that diminished T-cell activity, such as that seen in HIV, could allow overgrowth of *C. dubliniensis* [15, 18].

This species only accounts for a small percentage of Candida infections [15]. However, infections associated with this species have been reported (Table 3). While the table represents many of the cases in which this organism was implicated, it is by no means an exhaustive list. In reviewing these cases, it seems *C. dubliniensis* is most commonly found in those with some degree of immunocompromise. In particular, many reported cases have occurred in patients with liver disease and/or substance abuse. Understanding the population at risk for this infection can help clinicians identify this organism in a timely manner.

C. dubliniensis has demonstrated resistance to antifungal agents, specifically fluconazole. While these resistant strains do not account for the majority of strains, caution should be exercised when prescribing empiric therapy. In addition, fluconazole resistance is easily developed in vitro. This further highlights the need for caution and utilization of other antifungal agents if *C. dubliniensis* is found [15, 17].

Although our patient had some signs of sepsis including an elevated heart rate and respiratory rate, he was afebrile and appeared to have viral gastroenteritis. After a WBC count spike and *Candida* growth 2 days later, our team suspected sepsis, but did not know the source. The possibilities included the PICC line for milrinone infusion, an AICD infection, and an infection from the left VP shunt. The TEE identified a clear AICD lead infection and a CT head without contrast combined with negative CSF cultures ruled out a VP shunt infection. Additionally, the TEE detected no valvular vegetations which lowered the possibility of a PICC line-related infective endocarditis. The TEE and microbiology results made a strong case for *Candida dublinesis* infective endocarditis related to the AICD leads. The AICD device was removed at an outside facility due to patient preference with implantation of a new AICD device 5 days later. Finally, an MSSA infection related to the right-side IJV line placed in the hospital for antibiotic infusion delayed the patient's discharge further.

The patient was on IV micafungin for treatment of *Candida dubliniensis*. Recommendations from the Infectious Disease Society of America recommend the use of echinocandin (such as micafungin), amphotericin B, or amphotericin B with 5-flucytosine for treatment of *Candida* endocarditis with or without an ICD device [32, 33]. Regardless of the medication chosen, resolution of the fungemia usually occurs with ICD device removal, although one case report describes resolution of *Candida* endocarditis with medical management and no surgical intervention [34]. In our patient, treatment was continued for 4-6 weeks after ICD device removal.

3.1. Learning Points/Take Home Messages

(i) *Candida dubliniensis* is an opportunistic pathogen originally isolated from AIDS patients but can be isolated from immunocompetent individuals

(ii) We report the first case in literature of *Candida dubliniensis*-ICD sepsis with fungemia and multiple possible sources of infection including a VP shunt and an indwelling PICC for milrinone infusion

(iii) Clinicians should do a full sepsis workup for all patients admitted to the hospital with an ICD device, tachycardia, and tachypnea even in absence of fever and leukocytosis

References

[1] C. M. Tracy, A. E. Epstein, D. Darbar et al., "2012 ACCF/AHA/HRS focused update incorporated into the ACCF/AHA/HRS 2008 guidelines for device-based therapy of cardiac rhythm abnormalities: a report of the American College of Cardiology Foundation/American Heart Association task force on practice guidelines and the Heart Rhythm Society," *Journal of the American College of Cardiology*, vol. 61, no. 3, pp. e6–e75, 2013.

[2] F. Victor, C. de Place, C. Camus et al., "Pacemaker lead infection: echocardiographic features, management, and outcome," *Heart*, vol. 81, no. 1, pp. 82–87, 1999.

[3] J. G. Voet, Y. R. Vandekerckhove, L. L. Muyldermans, L. H. Missault, and L. J. Matthys, "Pacemaker lead infection: report of three cases and review of the literature," *Heart*, vol. 81, no. 1, pp. 88–91, 1999.

[4] E. F. Conklin, S. Giannelli Jr., and T. F. Nealon Jr., "Four hundred consecutive patients with permanent transvenous pacemakers," *The Journal of Thoracic and Cardiovascular Surgery*, vol. 69, no. 1, pp. 1–7, 1975.

[5] G. Bluhm, "Pacemaker infections," *Acta Medica Scandinavica*, vol. 218, no. S699, pp. 1–62, 1985.

[6] F. M. Kusumoto, M. H. Schoenfeld, B. L. Wilkoff et al., "2017 HRS expert consensus statement on cardiovascular implantable electronic device lead management and extraction," *Heart Rhythm*, vol. 14, no. 12, pp. e503–e551, 2017.

[7] M. Koutentakis, S. Siminelakis, P. Korantzopoulos et al., "Surgical management of cardiac implantable electronic device infections," *Journal of Thoracic Disease*, vol. 6, 2014.

[8] E. Athan, V. H. Chu, P. Tattevin et al., "Clinical characteristics and outcome of infective endocarditis involving implantable cardiac devices," *JAMA*, vol. 307, no. 16, pp. 1727–1735, 2012.

[9] U. A. R. Chaudhry, L. Harling, H. Ashrafian et al., "Surgical management of infected cardiac implantable electronic devices," *International Journal of Cardiology*, vol. 203, pp. 714–721, 2016.

[10] N. T. Rivera, N. Bray, H. Wang, K. Zelnick, A. Osman, and R. Vicuña, "Rare infection of implantable cardioverter-defibrillator lead with Candida albicans: case report and literature review," *Therapeutic Advances in Cardiovascular Disease*, vol. 8, no. 5, pp. 193–201, 2014.

[11] A. G. Jain, J. Guan, and J. D'Souza, "Candida parapsilosis: an unusual cause of infective endocarditis," *Cureus*, vol. 10, no. 11, article e3553, 2018.

[12] C. Garzoni, V. A. Nobre, and J. Garbino, "Candida parapsilosis endocarditis: a comparative review of the literature," *European Journal of Clinical Microbiology & Infectious Diseases*, vol. 26, no. 12, pp. 915–926, 2007.

[13] S. Hindupur and A. J. Muslin, "Septic shock induced from an implantable cardioverter-defibrillator lead-associated Candida albicans vegetation," *Journal of Interventional Cardiac Electrophysiology*, vol. 14, no. 1, pp. 55–59, 2005.

[14] A. Halawa, P. D. Henry, and F. A. Sarubbi, "Candida endocarditis associated with cardiac rhythm management devices: review with current treatment guidelines," *Mycoses*, vol. 54, no. 4, pp. e168–e174, 2011.

[15] D. Sullivan and D. Coleman, "Candida dubliniensis: characteristics and identification," *Journal of Clinical Microbiology*, vol. 36, no. 2, pp. 329–334, 1998.

[16] Z. Khan, S. Ahmad, L. Joseph, and R. Chandy, "Candida dubliniensis: an appraisal of its clinical significance as a bloodstream pathogen," *PLoS One*, vol. 7, no. 3, article e32952, 2012.

[17] J. M. Prutkin, M. R. Reynolds, H. Bao et al., "Rates of and factors associated with infection in 200 909 Medicare implantable cardioverter-defibrillator implants," *Circulation*, vol. 130, no. 13, pp. 1037–1043, 2014.

[18] J. Gutiérrez, P. Morales, M. A. González, and G. Quindós, "Candida dubliniensis, a new fungal pathogen," *Journal of Basic Microbiology*, vol. 42, no. 3, pp. 207–227, 2002.

[19] M. E. Brandt, L. H. Harrison, M. Pass et al., "Candida dubliniensis fungemia: the first four cases in North America," *Emerging Infectious Diseases*, vol. 6, no. 1, pp. 46–49, 2000.

[20] G. S. Gottlieb, A. P. Limaye, Y.-C. Chen, and W. C. Van Voorhis, "*Candida dubliniensis* fungemia in a solid organ transplant patient: case report and review of the literature," *Medical Mycology*, vol. 39, no. 6, pp. 483–485, 2001.

[21] M. J. Carr, S. Clarke, F. O'Connell, D. J. Sullivan, D. C. Coleman, and B. O'Connell, "First reported case of endocarditis caused by Candida dubliniensis," *Journal of Clinical Microbiology*, vol. 43, no. 6, pp. 3023–3026, 2005.

[22] R. Tsuruta, Y. Oda, H. Mizuno et al., "Candida dubliniensis isolated from the sputum of a patient with end-stage liver cirrhosis," *Internal Medicine*, vol. 46, no. 9, pp. 597–600, 2007.

[23] R. W. Sedeek, M. Shah, R. Gentile, and C. M. Samson, "First case report of Candida dubliniensis endogenous endophthalmitis," *Investigative Ophthalmology & Visual Science*, vol. 49, no. 13, p. 952, 2008.

[24] D. O'Kane, A. Kiosoglous, and K. Jones, "Candida dubliniensis encrustation of an obstructing upper renal tract calculus," *Case Reports*, vol. 2013, no. 1, article bcr2013009087, 2013.

[25] C. C. Lai, H. Y. Tsai, T. C. Chang, and P. R. Hsueh, "Catheter-related fungemia caused by Candida dubliniensis," *Journal of Microbiology, Immunology and Infection*, vol. 46, no. 4, pp. 306–308, 2013.

[26] E. Rosenberger, D. A. Youssef, S. Safdar, C. R. Larzo, and J. Myers, "Third case of Candida dubliniensis endogenous endophthalmitis in North America: case report and review of the literature," *International Ophthalmology*, vol. 34, no. 4, pp. 945–950, 2014.

[27] L. A. Petty, A. J. Gallan, J. A. Detrick, J. P. Ridgway, J. Mueller, and J. Pisano, "Candida dubliniensis pneumonia: a case report and review of literature," *Mycopathologia*, vol. 181, no. 9-10, pp. 765–768, 2016.

[28] A. Yamahiro, K. H. V. Lau, D. R. Peaper, and M. Villanueva, "Meningitis caused by Candida dubliniensis in a patient with cirrhosis: a case report and review of the literature," *Mycopathologia*, vol. 181, no. 7-8, pp. 589–593, 2016.

[29] E. Y. Chang, S. Fatima, S. Balan et al., "Candida dubliniensis abscess: a clinical case and a review of the literature," *Medical Mycology Case Reports*, vol. 21, pp. 41–43, 2018.

[30] J. K. T. Dermawan, S. Ghosh, M. K. Keating, K. V. Gopalakrishna, and S. Mukhopadhyay, "Candida pneumonia with severe clinical course, recovery with antifungal therapy and unusual pathologic findings: a case report," *Medicine*, vol. 97, no. 2, article e9650, 2018.

[31] T. D. Oostra, L. R. Schoenfield, and T. F. Mauger, "Candida dubliniensis: a novel cause of fungal keratitis," *IDCases*, vol. 14, article e00440, 2018.

[32] C. Tascini, M. G. Bongiorni, E. Tagliaferri et al., "Micafungin for Candida albicans pacemaker-associated endocarditis: a case report and review of the literature," *Mycopathologia*, vol. 175, no. 1-2, article 9591, pp. 129–134, 2013.

[33] P. G. Pappas, C. A. Kauffman, D. R. Andes et al., "Clinical practice guideline for the management of candidiasis: 2016 update by the Infectious Diseases Society of America," *Clinical Infectious Diseases*, vol. 62, no. 4, pp. e1–50, 2016.

[34] S. Bandyopadhyay, P. K. Tiwary, S. Mondal, and S. Puthran, "Pacemaker lead Candida endocarditis: is medical treatment possible?," *Indian Heart Journal*, vol. 67, pp. S100–S102, 2015.

Early Disseminated Lyme Carditis Inducing High-Degree Atrioventricular Block

Connor C. Kerndt,[1] John A. Bills,[2] Zaid J. Shareef,[2] Alexander M. Balinski,[3] Daniel F. Summers,[1] and Jose M. Tan[1,4]

[1]*Department of Internal Medicine, Spectrum Health Butterworth Hospital, Grand Rapids, Michigan, USA*
[2]*Michigan State University College of Osteopathic Medicine, East Lansing, Michigan, USA*
[3]*Oakland University William Beaumont School of Medicine, Rochester, Michigan, USA*
[4]*Department of Cardiovascular Disease, Spectrum Health Butterworth Hospital, Grand Rapids, Michigan, USA*

Correspondence should be addressed to Connor C. Kerndt; kerndtconnor@gmail.com

Academic Editor: Assad Movahed

Lyme disease is the most common tick-borne illness in the United States due to *Borrelia burgdorferi* infection. This case demonstrates a 20-year-old male patient presenting with complaints of annular skin rash, malaise, fever, and lightheadedness after significant outdoor exposure. Physical exam revealed multiple large targetoid lesions on the back and extremities. The rash had raised borders and centralized clearing consistent with erythema migrans chronicum. Electrocardiogram (ECG) revealed a high-degree atrioventricular (AV) block. The patient was started on intravenous ceftriaxone due to clinical suspicion for Lyme carditis. ELISA and Western blot tests were reactive for Lyme IgM and IgG, confirming the diagnosis. The AV block resolved by hospital day four and the patient was discharged with outpatient follow-up. Early identification of disease allowed for effective treatment with no adverse outcomes or sequelae.

1. Introduction

Lyme disease is the most common tick-borne illness in the United States [1]. Infection is caused by the spirochete *Borrelia burgdorferi* which is transmitted to humans via an Ixodes tick bite [2]. Lyme disease most commonly manifests during the late spring and summer months in the Northeastern United States and Wisconsin with exposure to wooded outdoor areas [3, 4]. Early intervention is critical to avoid the devastating sequelae of disseminated Lyme disease such as neurological impairment, chronic arthritis, and infection-induced heart block [2, 5, 6].

2. Case Presentation

A 20-year-old male patient with no prior medical history presented to the hospital with complaints of skin rash, malaise, and fever. The patient worked as a summer camp counselor and had recently been camping in Wisconsin. Several weeks after returning from a camping excursion, he noticed a nontender, nonpruritic annular rash on his arm with centralized clearing, absent of pain or pruritus. Three days later, he experienced excessive fatigue and accompanying fever (T-max 101°F). The patient presented to the camp clinic with a characteristic rash raising suspicion for Lyme disease. Given his age, symptomatology, recent outdoor exposure, and distinctive rash, a Suspicious Index in Lyme Carditis (SILC) score of 9 gave high suspicion for early Lyme carditis. The patient was sent to a tertiary care center for further evaluation and management.

Upon admission, the patient developed intermittent symptomatic bradycardia with an average heart rate of 40 bpm one episode of severe bradycardia with a nadir of 15 bpm over a period of five seconds. The patient complained of accompanying generalized fatigue and intermittent lightheadedness. He denied complaints of arthralgia, myalgia,

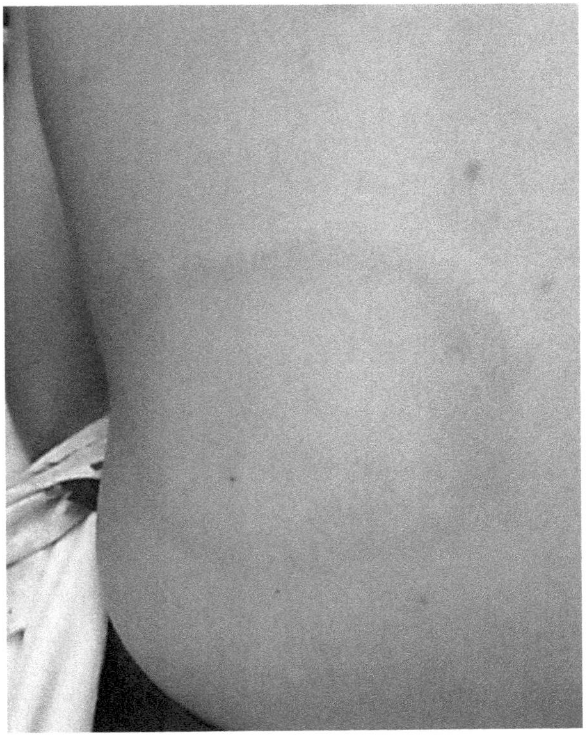

FIGURE 1: Dorsal targetoid lesion with centralized clearing (erythema migrans chronicum).

motor/sensory deficit, headache, altered mental status, or neck pain. Physical exam revealed multiple large targetoid lesions on the lower extremities, upper extremities, and back (Figure 1). The lesions had raised borders with centralized clearing consistent with erythema migrans chronicum.

Presenting electrocardiogram (ECG) revealed a second-degree atrioventricular (AV) block, Mobitz Type I (Figure 2). Inpatient telemetry demonstrated episodes of high-grade AV block (Figure 3). Transthoracic echocardiogram demonstrated a normal ejection fraction of 73% with no regional wall motion abnormalities. The valve anatomy and function were also normal. Antibiotic therapy was initiated with 2 g of intravenous (IV) ceftriaxone due to the characteristic presentation of Lyme carditis. Atropine and transcutaneous pacing were deferred due to relative clinical stability. Follow-up Lyme ELISA was reactive for Lyme IgM and IgG, confirmed by Western blot that showed reactivity of IgM to p23, p39, and p41. IgG was reactive to p18, p23, p39, p41, and p93 (Table 1). Given the ECG findings and serology, the patient was diagnosed with early disseminated Lyme carditis.

Intravenous ceftriaxone was initiated for 28 days, four days inpatient and 24 days outpatient via a peripherally inserted central catheter. After two days of therapy, the annular skin lesions resolved with coinciding resolution of fever and malaise. Heart block also progressively improved from high-grade AV block to second-degree AV block (Mobitz Type I). On the fourth day of treatment, the predominant rhythm was a first-degree AV block maintaining adequate PR interval control measured at 216 ms upon discharge (Figure 4). The patient was discharged on hospital day four. Follow-up appointments with electrophysiology and infectious disease services were arranged for complete resolution of his PR interval and further testing.

On follow-up, the patient reported complete resolution of symptoms and a return to baseline. He did not have any headache, joint pain, fatigue, presyncope, or syncope. Follow-up laboratory panel was also unremarkable with no significant derangement. Patient follow-up ECG showed a normal rate and sinus rhythm with complete resolution of the previous AV block (Figure 5).

3. Discussion

Lyme carditis is the most common vector-borne infection in Northeastern America, yet cardiac manifestations are uncommon [2, 7]. Early localized Lyme disease is caused by systemic infection of *Borrelia burgdorferi*, classically presenting as erythema migrans with or without constitutional symptoms [4]. If left untreated, late systemic disease can create cardiac complications such as reversible AV block, cardiomyopathy, and myocarditis due to spirochete infiltration of cardiac and pericardial structures [8]. Given the cardiac tissue irritation in Lyme carditis, a patient's ECG can exhibit marked derangement including ST-segment changes, t-wave inversion, repolarization abnormalities, and atrioventricular block [3, 9]. First-degree AV block is the most common cardiac arrhythmia of Lyme carditis, but some cases have demonstrated second-degree AV block, third-degree AV block, atrial fibrillation, tachyarrhythmia, and QT prolongation [3, 8–12]. Fluctuations between first-degree and second-degree conduction block have also been reported [2, 9], but first-degree block seldomly fluctuates to the level of complete heart block [13].

Clinical suspicion of early disseminated Lyme carditis is essential in patients presenting with new-onset high-degree AV block. The absence of appropriate treatment can result in progression of disease and worsening symptomatology [14]. Failure to recognize early Lyme carditis is associated with an increased need for permanent pacemaker implantation [14]. To help distinguish etiology of high-degree AV block, an evidence-based scoring system termed the "Suspicious Index in Lyme Carditis" was developed in 2018 [15]. The parameters contributing to this score incorporate common presentations of Lyme disease, including male sex, age less than 50 years, recent outdoor activity or endemic exposure, constitutional symptomology, known tick bite, and classical erythema migrans rash [15]. The cumulative score categorizes patients based on level of suspicion for Lyme disease as the etiologic cause of AV block [15].

Current guidelines for diagnosis and management of Lyme carditis suggest stratifying suspicion of Lyme-induced AV block into low, intermediate, and high-risk categories using an SILC score [10]. SILC scoring reports a sensitivity of nearly 92.9% for intermediate and high suspicion categories, making it a valuable screening tool for decreasing unnecessary laboratory testing and antibiotic use [15]. However, the failure of SILC to confer suspicion based on laboratory and histologic findings may warrant additional diagnostic workup outside of its recommendation [16]. After SILC scoring, individuals with low suspicion receive standard

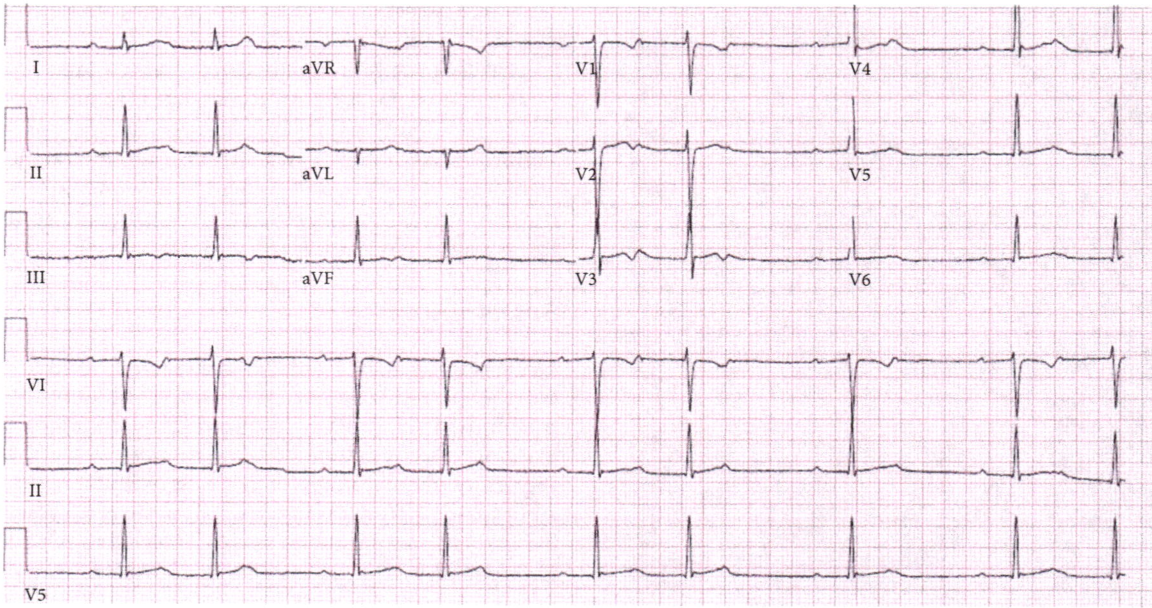

FIGURE 2: ECG demonstrating sinus rhythm with second-degree AV block (Mobitz Type I).

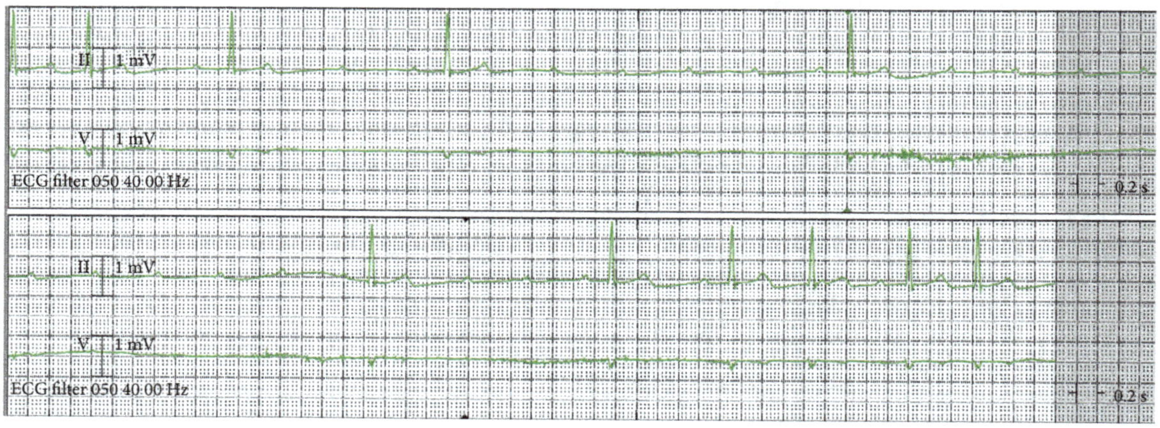

FIGURE 3: Telemetry demonstrating high-grade AV block.

TABLE 1: Lyme serology results.

	Lyme IgG							Lyme IgM			
	WB	p18	p23	p39	p41	p45	p93	WB	p23	p39	p41
Serum	+	+	+	+	+	+	+	+	+	+	+

treatment for AV block and those with intermediate or high suspicion begin empiric IV antibiotic therapy and serologic testing [15]. Patients exhibiting asymptomatic bradycardia are managed with strict cardiac monitoring [10, 17], while symptomatic patients require continuous cardiac telemetry to evaluate the need for transcutaneous pacing or inotropic support due to the risk of ischemia or death with persistent high-grade AV block [13, 17–19].

In this case, the patient obtained a SILC score of 9 due to his status as a young male with classic symptomatology, outdoor activity, and pathognomonic erythema migrans rash. This score placed him within the category of high suspicion of early disseminated Lyme carditis. New-onset heart block in a young patient is exceptionally rare (1/15,000 cases) with widely variable etiologies [20–24]. Electrolyte abnormalities such as hyperkalemia, as well as thyroid dysfunction, may induce heart block and should be considered in these cases [4, 25, 26]. Without the pathognomonic rash, the differential diagnosis may have been significantly confounded in this patient. This emphasizes the importance of a thorough integumentary examination and exposure history in patients with heart block of unidentified etiology [20–24].

In the workup of this case, pending Lyme serology resulted in a comprehensive patient evaluation to assess other possible AV block etiologies. Transthoracic echocardiogram, complete blood count (CBC), complete metabolic panel (CMP), thyroid panel, and autoantibody testing were all

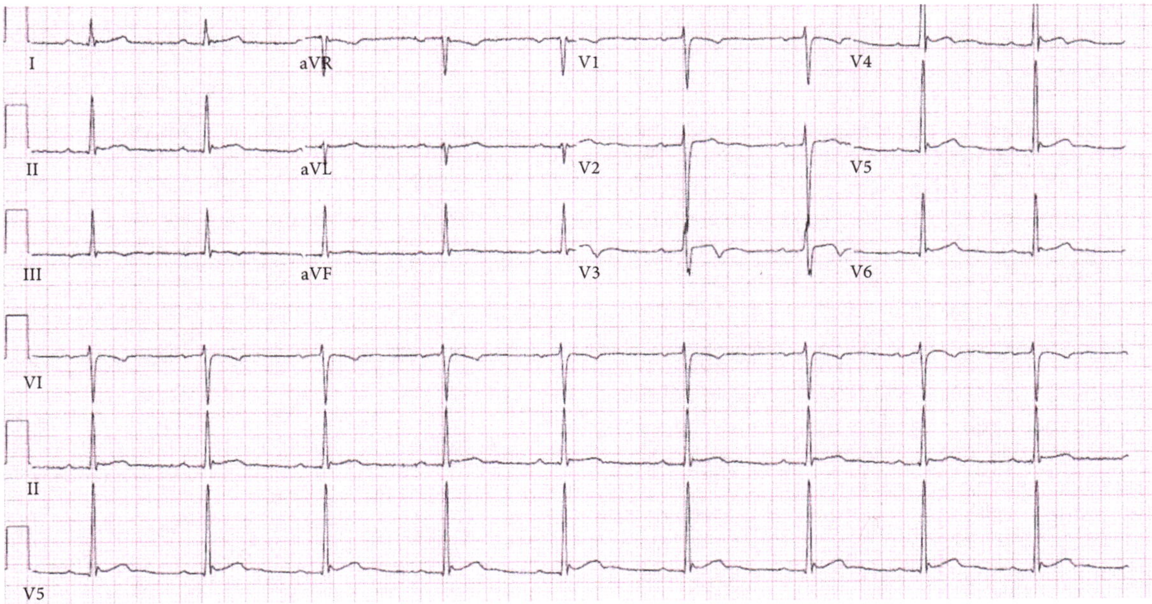

FIGURE 4: ECG demonstrating sinus bradycardia with first-degree AV block.

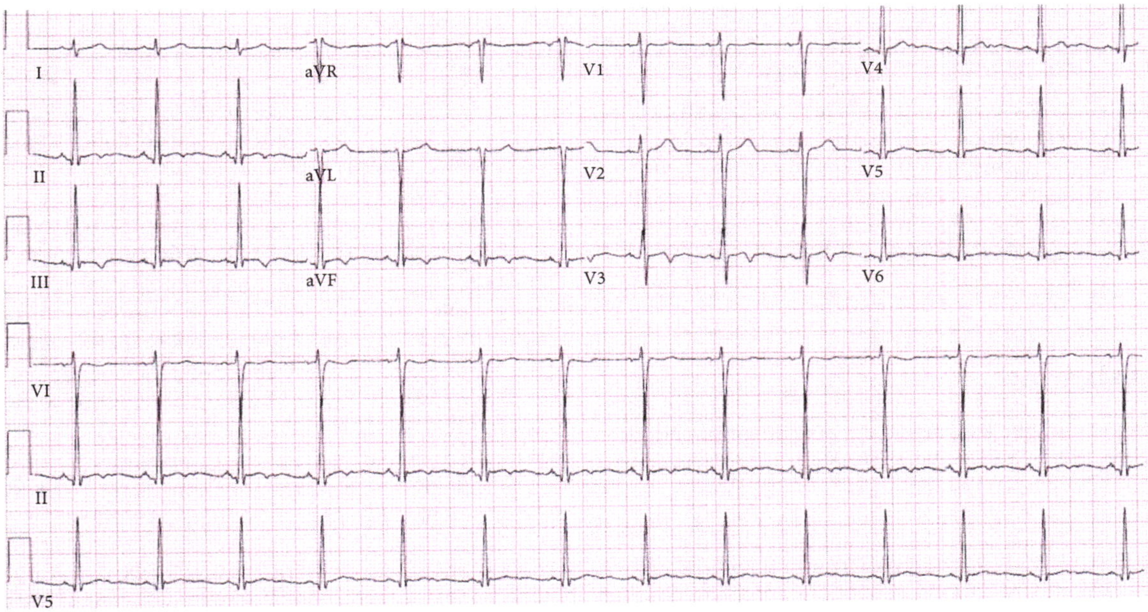

FIGURE 5: Follow-up ECG demonstrating normal sinus rhythm and resolution of AV block.

conducted to rule out the etiology of noninfectious heart block in this patient. Systemic lupus erythematosus (SLE) was also considered [4], but the presence of erythema migrans and absence of renal and hematologic dysfunction were more consistent with Lyme carditis. Inpatient genetic testing was deemed unnecessary for this patient as genetic causes of AV block were ruled out due to the absence of previous personal and/or family cardiac history. Cardiac biopsy for evaluation of infiltrative disease was also deferred given the procedural risk and relative probability of Lyme etiology [4, 27, 28].

With greater than 95 percent specificity, ELISA antibody and Western blot serologic studies were utilized to establish a diagnosis of early disseminated Lyme carditis in this case. Based on the current guidelines, the patient was tested for Lyme serology and started on intravenous ceftriaxone [15, 29]. It is recommended that patients with negative serology proceed to standard high-degree AV block management, while patients with positive serology receive IV ceftriaxone for 10-14 days followed by oral antibiotics (preferably doxycycline) to complete a total course of 14-21 days of antibiotic therapy [10, 30]. For this patient, positive IgM and IgG serologic markers solidified a primary diagnosis of early disseminated Lyme carditis (Table 1) [31] and IV ceftriaxone was continued.

While the CDC recommends an antibiotic course of 14-21 days for Lyme carditis, other manifestations of Lyme disease follow protocols lasting up to 28 days and no clinical trials have been conducted to evaluate appropriate durations of antibiotic treatment [10, 18, 30, 32]. In this case, a 28-day course of ceftriaxone was considered appropriate to ensure clearance of Lyme infection. Furthermore, the patient was not transitioned to oral doxycycline due to a past history of adverse drug reaction [18]. Per current guidelines, the patient obtained a follow-up ECG demonstrating 1 : 1 conduction, but did not receive a stress ECG. This demonstrates a limitation in patient management, as follow-up stress testing is recommended to evaluate AV conduction in a noninvasive manner 4-6 weeks after initial resolution of AV block [10]. Stress ECG testing is critical for appropriate analysis of the point of Wenckebach which can demonstrate cardiac recovery and determine if permanent cardiac pacing, repeat stress testing, or routine ECG follow-up is indicated [17].

4. Conclusion

Lyme carditis is a known etiologic cause of cardiac conduction abnormalities, particularly AV block. SILC scoring can be a useful tool in the evaluation and treatment of suspected Lyme-induced heart block. Stratifying suspicion allows for indicated serologic testing and time-sensitive antibiotic treatment. While patients with early disseminated Lyme carditis carry a good prognosis, delayed management can result in long-term complications and poor cardiac outcomes.

Acknowledgments

The authors would like to thank the Department of Cardiology at Spectrum Health for their assistance with this report.

References

[1] R. Rosenberg, N. P. Lindsey, M. Fischer et al., “Vital signs: trends in reported vectorborne disease Cases — United States and territories, 2004-2016,” *MMWR. Morbidity and Mortality Weekly Report*, vol. 67, no. 17, pp. 496–501, 2018.

[2] D. Semmler, R. Blank, and H. J. Rupprecht, “Complete AV block in Lyme carditis: an important differential diagnosis,” *Clinical Research in Cardiology*, vol. 99, no. 8, pp. 519–526, 2010.

[3] A. E. Fish, Y. B. Pride, and D. S. Pinto, “Lyme carditis,” *Infectious Disease Clinics of North America*, vol. 22, no. 2, pp. 275–288, 2008.

[4] T. Kostić, S. Momčilović, Z. D. Perišić et al., “Manifestations of Lyme carditis,” *International Journal of Cardiology*, vol. 232, pp. 24–32, 2017.

[5] J. L. Sanchez, “Clinical manifestations and treatment of Lyme disease,” *Clinics in Laboratory Medicine*, vol. 35, no. 4, pp. 765–778, 2015.

[6] G. Panic, V. Stanulovic, and T. Popov, “Atrio-ventricular block as the first presentation of disseminated Lyme disease,” *International Journal of Cardiology*, vol. 150, no. 3, pp. e104–e106, 2011.

[7] R. Koene, D. R. Boulware, M. Kemperman et al., “Acute heart failure from Lyme carditis,” *Circulation: Heart Failure*, vol. 5, no. 2, pp. e24–e26, 2012.

[8] L. S. Fuster, E. E. Gul, and A. Baranchuk, “Electrocardiographic progression of acute Lyme disease,” *The American Journal of Emergency Medicine*, vol. 35, no. 7, pp. 1040.e5–1040.e6, 2017.

[9] H. F. McAlister, P. T. Klementowicz, C. Andrews, J. D. Fisher, M. Feld, and S. Furman, “Lyme carditis: an important cause of reversible heart block,” *Annals of Internal Medicine*, vol. 110, no. 5, pp. 339–345, 1989.

[10] C. Yeung and A. Baranchuk, “Diagnosis and treatment of Lyme carditis,” *Journal of the American College of Cardiology*, vol. 73, no. 6, pp. 717–726, 2019.

[11] N. Wenger, C. Pellaton, P. Bruchez, and J. Schläpfer, “Atrial fibrillation, complete atrioventricular block and escape rhythm with bundle-branch block morphologies: an exceptional presentation of Lyme carditis,” *International Journal of Cardiology*, vol. 160, no. 1, pp. e12–e14, 2012.

[12] J. D. Forrester and P. Mead, “Third-degree heart block associated with Lyme carditis: review of published cases,” *Clinical Infectious Diseases*, vol. 59, no. 7, pp. 996–1000, 2014.

[13] A. C. Steere, “Lyme carditis: cardiac abnormalities of Lyme disease,” *Annals of Internal Medicine*, vol. 93, no. 1_Part_1, p. 8, 1980.

[14] D. Wan and A. Baranchuk, “Lyme carditis and atrioventricular block,” *CMAJ*, vol. 190, no. 20, article E622, 2018.

[15] G. Besant, D. Wan, C. Yeung et al., “Suspicious index in Lyme carditis: systematic review and proposed new risk score,” *Clinical Cardiology*, vol. 41, no. 12, pp. 1611–1616, 2018.

[16] N. Scheffold, B. Herkommer, R. Kandolf, and A. E. May, “Lyme carditis,” *Deutsches Ärzteblatt International*, vol. 112, pp. 202–208, 2015.

[17] C. Yeung and A. Baranchuk, “Systematic approach to the diagnosis and treatment of Lyme carditis and high-degree atrioventricular block,” *Healthcare.*, vol. 6, no. 4, p. 119, 2018.

[18] G. P. Wormser, R. J. Dattwyler, E. D. Shapiro et al., “The clinical assessment, treatment, and prevention of Lyme disease, human granulocytic anaplasmosis, and babesiosis: clinical practice guidelines by the Infectious Diseases Society of America,” *Clinical Infectious Diseases*, vol. 43, no. 9, pp. 1089–1134, 2006.

[19] D. Wan, C. Blakely, P. Branscombe, L. Suarez-Fuster, B. Glover, and A. Baranchuk, “Lyme carditis and high-degree atrioventricular block,” *The American Journal of Cardiology*, vol. 121, no. 9, pp. 1102–1104, 2018.

[20] A. E. Baruteau, R. H. Pass, J. B. Thambo et al., “Congenital and childhood atrioventricular blocks: pathophysiology and contemporary management,” *European Journal of Pediatrics*, vol. 175, no. 9, pp. 1235–1248, 2016.

[21] D. Friedman, L. Duncanson, J. Glickstein, and J. Buyon, “A review of congenital heart block,” *Images Paediatric Cardiology*, vol. 5, no. 3, pp. 36–48, 2003.

[22] C. S. Edwards, R. Mootoo, and A. Bhanji, "High grade heart block in association with SLE," *Annals of the Rheumatic Diseases*, vol. 63, no. 5, p. 606, 2004.

[23] B. S. Cevik, A. Cevik, and E. Tavli, "Second degree heart block associated with QT prolongation," *Indian Pacing Electrophysiol J.*, vol. 10, no. 2, pp. 96–98, 2010.

[24] D. Zeltser, D. Justo, A. Halkin et al., "Drug-induced atrioventricular block: prognosis after discontinuation of the culprit drug," *Journal of the American College of Cardiology*, vol. 44, no. 1, pp. 105–108, 2004.

[25] L. Littmann and M. A. Gibbs, "Electrocardiographic manifestations of severe hyperkalemia," *Journal of Electrocardiology*, vol. 51, no. 5, pp. 814–817, 2018.

[26] L. Sataline and G. Donaghue, "Hypercalcemia, heart-block, and hyperthyroidism," *JAMA*, vol. 213, no. 8, p. 1342, 1970.

[27] S. Y. Jang, Y. Cho, J. H. Song et al., "Complication rate of transfemoral endomyocardial biopsy with fluoroscopic and two-dimensional echocardiographic guidance: a 10-year experience of 228 consecutive procedures," *Journal of Korean Medical Science*, vol. 28, no. 9, pp. 1323–1328, 2013.

[28] A. M. From, J. J. Maleszewski, and C. S. Rihal, "Current status of endomyocardial biopsy," *Mayo Clinic Proceedings*, vol. 86, no. 11, pp. 1095–1102, 2011.

[29] J. Shenthar, S. B. Shetty, and D. Krishnamurthy, "Diagnosis not to be missed: Lyme carditis, rare but reversible cause of complete atrioventricular block," *Indian Heart Journal*, vol. 66, no. 6, pp. 723–726, 2014.

[30] S. Muhammad and R. J. Simonelli, "Lyme carditis: a case report and review of management," *Hospital Pharmacy*, vol. 53, no. 4, pp. 263–265, 2017.

[31] M. M. G. Leeflang, C. W. Ang, J. Berkhout et al., "The diagnostic accuracy of serological tests for Lyme borreliosis in Europe: a systematic review and meta-analysis," *BMC Infectious Diseases*, vol. 16, no. 1, 2016.

[32] Centers for Disease Control and Prevention, "Lyme disease treatment," https://www.cdc.gov/lyme/treatment/index.html. March 2020.

20

A Cardiogenic Shock due to an Acute MI with LCA Arising from the Right Coronary Sinus Successfully Treated with PCI

Rayyan Jadeed, Klaus Pethig, and Dirk Böcker

Department of Cardiology, St. Marien Hospital, Hamm, Germany

Correspondence should be addressed to Rayyan Jadeed; jadeedrayyan@yahoo.com

Academic Editor: Expedito E. Ribeiro

Coronary artery anomalies (CAAs) are a diverse group of congenital anomalies with an incidence ranging from 0.17% in autopsy cases to 1.2% in patients undergoing coronary angiography. The left coronary artery (LCA) originating from the right coronary sinus is a very rare CAA with a frequency of 0.03%. We present a very rare case of a cardiogenic shock as a consequence of an acute anterolateral myocardial infarction by a totally occlusive lesion in the long left main stem with a complete LCA arising from the right coronary sinus in an 85-year-old female. This lesion was successfully treated with 2 drug-eluting stents. This is perhaps the first published case about cardiogenic shock due to an acute myocardial infarction associated with this type of coronary anomalies, and it presents a special challenge in the catheter laboratory.

1. Introduction

Coronary artery anomalies (CAAs) are a diverse group of congenital anomalies with an incidence ranging from 0.17% in autopsy cases to 1.2% in patients undergoing coronary angiography [1, 2]. They are so interesting, as they form the second most frequent cause of sudden death in young athletes [3, 4]. It is reported that sudden death due to coronary arteries arising from the opposite sinus (ACAOS) is more frequent in young athletes <35 years than in older patients. It has been suggested that sudden death is less common in the latter group because of the stiffening of the aortic wall [5, 6].

We present a very rare case of a cardiogenic shock resulting from an acute myocardial infarction (MI) with a complete LCA arising from the right coronary sinus. With a frequency of 0.02%-0.05% on angiographic studies, this anomaly is one of the most uncommon coronary anomalies [2, 7].

2. Case Report

An 85-year-old female presented to the emergency department with a three-hour history of a typical anginal chest discomfort associated with shortness of breath, diaphoresis, nausea, and vomiting. The patient denied a history of coronary heart disease and was well anticoagulated for an atrial fibrillation. The patient was afebrile and her heart rate was 123 beats per minute with a blood pressure of 65/40 mmHg. Her oxygen saturation was 92% on 4 l/min via nasal cannula. On physical exam, she was in respiratory distress with a respiratory rate of 30 per minute and had no peripheral edema. On auscultation of the chest, she had diffuse bilateral crackles. The cardiac examination revealed an irregular rhythm without murmurs. Electrocardiogram (ECG) on presentation demonstrated ST elevations in leads I and aVL and ST depressions in leads II, III, aVF, V5, and V6 (Figures 1(a) and 1(b)).

Blood gas analysis (BGA) revealed increased lactate of 4.2 mmol/l.

She underwent an emergency coronary angiography. The left main coronary artery (LMCA) could not be engaged with conventional diagnostic catheters for which an aortic root angiography using a pigtail catheter was performed and raised suspicion that the left coronary artery (LCA) was originating from the right coronary sinus. The injection of contrast in the right coronary sinus demonstrated an anomalous LCA separately arising from the right coronary

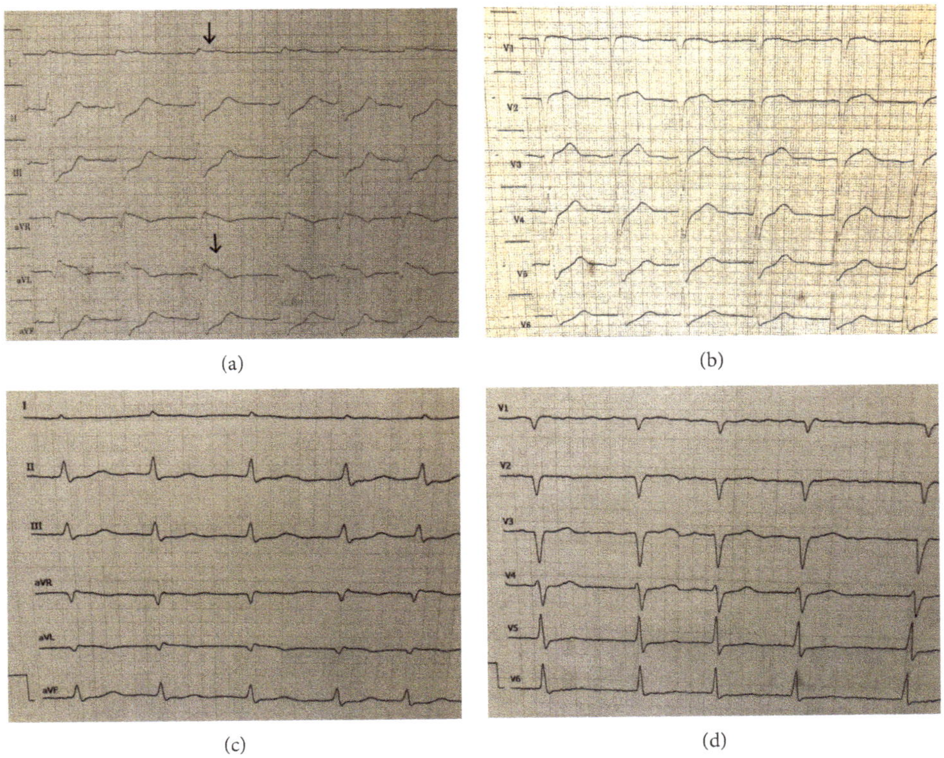

FIGURE 1: ECG findings: (a and b) ST elevations in leads I and aVL on admission. (c and d) After the procedure without elevations or significant depressions.

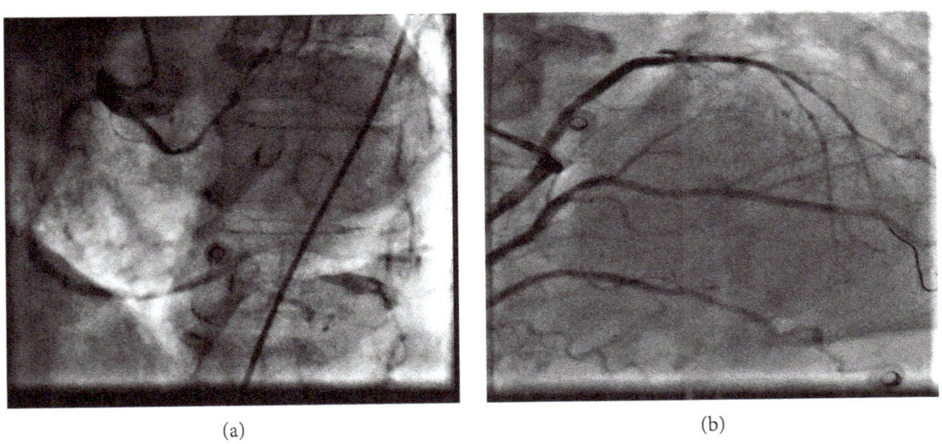

FIGURE 2: Angiographic findings: (a) RAO 40° view illustrates the left coronary artery with a 100% occlusive lesion in the distal LMCA and proximal LAD. (b) Cranial 30° view shows culprit vessel postintervention.

sinus. The culprit lesion was a 100% occlusion in the distal LMCA and proximal left ascending artery (LAD) with grade 0 TIMI flow (Figure 2(a)). For the intervention, a 6F Amplatz right guide catheter (AR-1) was chosen, which engaged the LCA-ostium and provided an acceptable backup. Percutaneous intervention was performed with two drug-eluting stents achieving grade 3 TIMI postintervention without residual stenosis or complications (Figure 2(b)). The left coronary circumflex (LCX) was hypoplastic; therefore, it was ignored in the intervention strategy. The right coronary artery (RCA) was dominant and was divided at the crux of the heart into two large branches and continued posterolaterally as a large posterior lateral branch.

Postintervention ECG showed no significant ST elevations or ST depressions (Figures 1(c) and 1(d)).

During the procedure, a vasopressor was infused in small doses and multiple doses of intravenous diuretics were given.

After that, the patient was transferred to an intensive care unit; she did not require invasive ventilation. In two days, she was weaned off catecholamines and stepped down to the ward in good clinical status.

3. Discussion

The CAAs are classified into anomalies (1) of origin, (2) of courses, and (3) of termination.

The LCA originating from the right coronary sinus is a very unusual CAA.

It is difficult to engage the ostium in this anomaly, which makes an intervention in emergency settings particularly complex. The Amplatz right guide catheter seems to be suitable for this type of coronary anomalies.

To our knowledge, this is the first report of this anomaly with a cardiogenic shock related to a 100% occlusive lesion in the anomalous LCA successfully treated with percutaneous intervention (PCI). One previous case from Korea has described the same anomaly with an acute coronary syndrome by an up-to-90% occlusive lesion in the proximal LAD [8]. Shah et al. reported a similar case which was successfully treated with percutaneous intervention [9].

The clinical implications of CAAs vary depending on the type of anomalous artery and range, from ischemia presenting at an early stage of life to an incidental finding on angiography [10].

Coronary arteries arising from the opposite sinus (ACAOS), like the anomaly in our case, are the second leading cause of sudden cardiac death (SCD) in young athletes in the United States [11].

Although their incidence is low, CAAs should always be taken into consideration by clinicians due to their potentially fatal consequences.

Cardiologists in the catheter laboratory should have the required experience to intervene on such anomalous coronary arteries, especially in the situation of cardiogenic shock.

References

[1] S. Harikrishnan, S. P. Jacob, J. Tharakan et al., "Congenital coronary anomalies of origin and distribution in adults: a coronary arteriographic study," *Indian Heart Journal*, vol. 54, no. 3, pp. 271–275, 2002.

[2] O. Yamanaka and R. E. Hobbs, "Coronary artery anomalies in 126,595 patients undergoing coronary arteriography," *Catheterization and Cardiovascular Diagnosis*, vol. 21, no. 1, pp. 28–40, 1990.

[3] A. D. M. Villa, E. Sammut, A. Nair, R. Rajani, R. Bonamini, and A. Chiribiri, "Coronary artery anomalies overview: the normal and the abnormal," *World Journal of Radiology*, vol. 8, no. 6, pp. 537–555, 2016.

[4] C. Basso, B. J. Maron, D. Corrado, and G. Thiene, "Clinical profile of congenital coronary artery anomalies with origin from the wrong aortic sinus leading to sudden death in young competitive athletes," *Journal of the American College of Cardiology*, vol. 35, no. 6, pp. 1493–1501, 2000.

[5] P. Angelini, "Coronary artery anomalies: an entity in search of an identity," *Circulation*, vol. 115, no. 10, pp. 1296–1305, 2007.

[6] M. D. Cheitlin, "Coronary anomalies as a cause of sudden death in the athlete," in *Sudden Cardiac Death in the Athlete*, N. A. M. Estes, D. N. Salem, and J. J. P. Wang, Eds., pp. 379–391, Futura Publishing Co., Armonk NY, USA, 1998.

[7] D. Flessas, I. Mamarelis, V. Maniatis et al., "An unusual pattern of three major components of the cardiovascular system: multimodality imaging and review of the literature," *Journal of Cardiothoracic Surgery*, vol. 8, no. 1, p. 61, 2013.

[8] J. H. Lee and J. S. Park, "Successful percutaneous coronary intervention in the setting of an aberrant left coronary artery arising from the right coronary cusp in a patient with acute coronary syndrome: a case report," *BMC Cardiovascular Disorders*, vol. 17, no. 1, p. 186, 2017.

[9] N. Shah, V. E. Cheng, N. Cox, and K. Soon, "Percutaneous coronary intervention of an anomalous left main coronary artery arising from the right sinus of Valsalva," *Heart, Lung & Circulation*, vol. 24, no. 8, pp. e123–e126, 2015.

[10] G. Rigatelli, F. Dell Avvocata, N. Van Tan, R. Daggubati, and A. Nanijundappa, "Congenital coronary artery anomalies silent until geriatric age: non-invasive assessment, angiography tips, and treatment," *Journal of Geriatric Cardiology*, vol. 12, pp. 66–75, 2015.

[11] P. P. Agarwal, C. Dennie, E. Pena et al., "Anomalous coronary arteries that need intervention: review of pre- and postoperative imaging appearances," *Radiographics*, vol. 37, no. 3, pp. 740–757, 2017.

21

S. gallolyticus Aortic Valve Endocarditis with Mitral Valve Leaflet Aneurysm

S. Poddi,[1] I. Tropea,[1] G. Faggian,[1] S. De Feo,[2] M. Zordan,[3] and A. Rungatscher[1]

[1]*Division of Cardiac Surgery, University of Verona Medical Center, Verona, Italy*
[2]*Division of Cardiovascular diseases, Pederzoli Hospital, Peschiera del Garda, Italy*
[3]*Division of Pathology, University of Verona Medical Center, Verona, Italy*

Correspondence should be addressed to S. Poddi; poddi.salvatore@gmail.com

Academic Editor: Ertugurul Ercan

S. gallolyticus is one of the pathogenic agents of endocarditis, and mitral valve aneurysm is a rare but potentially devastating complication. We present a case of *S. gallolyticus* aortic valve endocarditis with concomitant anterior mitral valve leaflet aneurysm. Patient underwent surgery before aneurysm perforation, and postoperative course was uneventful. Time of surgery is crucial to avoid severe complications due to aneurysm rupture.

1. Introduction

Streptococcus gallolyticus is one of the etiologic factors of infective endocarditis (IE); it is also associated with colonic neoplasia. Rarely, aortic valve (AV) infection may lead to a specific scenario involving mitral valve (MV) and causing MV anterior leaflet aneurysm. Infection can spread to MV through direct contact between aortic vegetation and MV leaflet, contiguous infection through mitral-aortic fibrosa, and/or regurgitant infectious flow from aortic valve [1, 2]. MV aneurysm is rare but mostly associated with IE; its acute rupture may cause massive mitral regurgitation and subsequent pulmonary edema and/or systemic embolization [3]. According to the current guidelines, indications for surgery in case of IE are uncontrolled infection, abscess or fistula formation, pseudoaneurysm, and large vegetation with embolic potential [4]. In case of MV aneurysm, despite no specific indication in the guidelines, prompt surgery may be indicated to avoid the aforementioned catastrophic complications. To the best of our knowledge, only few cases of endocarditis-related MV aneurysm are described; most of them have been treated by urgent surgery due to aneurysm rupture complications [1, 3, 5–14]. Herein, we present a case of a 78-year-old male with native aortic valve endocarditis with positive blood cultures for *S. gallolyticus* and intraoperative evidence of anterior MV leaflet aneurysm.

2. Case Presentation

IRB approval, consent statement, and clinical trial registration are not applicable for the present study. In January 2022, a 78-year-old male was referred to our center. His past medical history included diabetes mellitus, paroxysmal atrial fibrillation (AF), moderate aortic regurgitation, and moderate ascending aorta dilation. In November 2021, patient experienced dyspnea, high-rate AF, and low-grade fever; he had been admitted in a regional hospital and diagnosis was acute congestive heart failure (HF). Transesophageal echocardiogram (TEE) revealed a tricuspid aortic valve with mild regurgitation (2+/4 +; vena contracta 4 mm) and thin fibrotic striae on the arterial side of the cusps. It also revealed an isoechogenic vegetation-like formation (10 mm) on the atrial side of A2 scallop of the MV, associated with trivial-mild MV regurgitation (1+–2+/4 +). Left ventricular ejection fraction (EF) was preserved. Blood cultures were positive for *S. gallolyticus*. Treatment with ceftriaxone was started, and imaging found no sign of embolization. Patient had been reevaluated 4 weeks later, finding worsened aortic regurgitation (3+/4 +) with regurgitant flow directed to the anterior MV leaflet and confirming the vegetation-like formation on A2 (suspecting now a pseudoaneurysm) with worsened MV regurgitation (3+/4 +) (Figures 1 and 2).

After 8-week intravenous antibiotic therapy, patient was hemodynamically stable and his symptoms improved, but vegetations did not. Patient was then transferred to our center, where he underwent surgery on January. Intraoperatively, a prominent aneurysm was noted on the atrial aspect of A2, with no signs of rupture (Figure 3); apart from that, anterior and posterior MV leaflets were normal. Aortic and mitral valves have been replaced with biological prosthesis (Carpentier-Edwards PERIMOUNT Magna Ease 25 mm and Medtronic Hancock II 27 mm, respectively); left appendage closure was also performed (because of his history of AF). Intraoperative TEE showed excellent prosthesis function with no paravalvular leakage and normal EF. Microscopic evaluation of MV leaflet demonstrated acute IE, important fibrinous exudation and leukocytosis, inflammatory granulation tissue, myxoid degeneration foci, and fibrosis and adipose metaplasia (Figure 4). Postoperative time was uneventful; blood and valve cultures were negative so we stopped the antibiotic regimen. Predischarge echocardiogram showed no signs of IE. Colonoscopy was performed, demonstrating the presence of two polyps, which were later removed endoscopically.

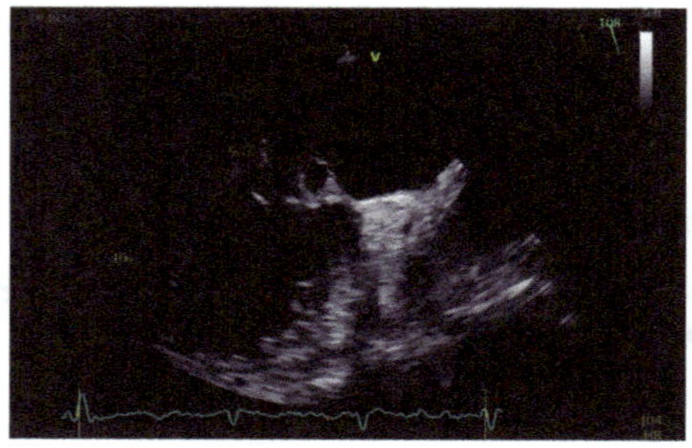

FIGURE 1: Echocardiogram shows anterior mitral valve leaflet aneurysm.

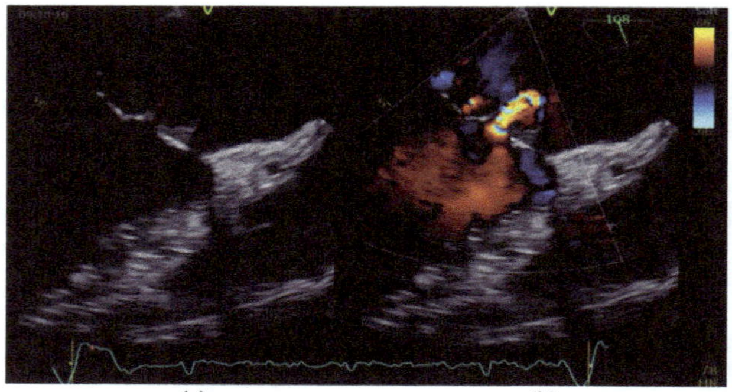

(a) (b)

FIGURE 2: (a) MV aneurysm. (b) Aneurysm-related MV regurgitation.

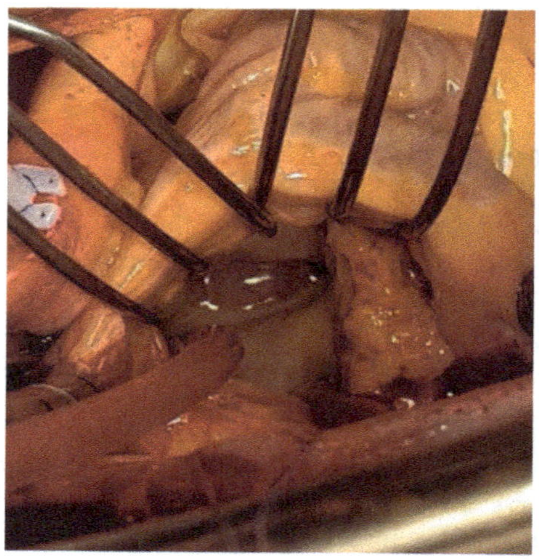

FIGURE 3: Aneurysm on the atrial aspect of the anterior MV leaflet (A2 scallop).

3. Discussion

This is a case of *S. gallolyticus*-related native aortic valve infective endocarditis with concomitant anterior mitral valve leaflet aneurysm. Fortunately, patient underwent surgery before aneurysm rupture. We hypothesize that regurgitant infectious flow from aortic valve played a major role in the present case. Incidence of MV aneurysms is low, and echocardiographic diagnosis is made in just 0.2-0.3% of overall cases. Mostly, aneurysm is related to IE [5, 8, 11]. Mechanisms leading to aneurysm formation are well known; as described by Vilacosta et al., IE progresses to MV; an abscess develops; tissues become more and more weak, having tissue bulging; and eventually aneurysm formation [5]. Few dozens of IE-related MV aneurysms are described. Tomsic et al. did an excellent review documenting perforation in 72% of cases and embolization in 18.2% [13]. Despite that there is no specific guideline regarding surgery and MV aneurysm, we agree with Ruparelia et al.: when aneurysm is demonstrated or highly suspected, surgery should be performed as soon as possible to avoid the severe complications previously described [8]. In our case, TEE showed a vegetation-like formation on the atrial aspect of the MV, with no clear evidence nor specific sign of aneurysm. Preoperative diagnosis could underestimate the real incidence of MV aneurysms, which may mimic vegetation, tumor, prolapse, or billowing. Being IE the most common cause of MV aneurysm, we should always think about this complication. Color flow Doppler usually helps distinguish MV aneurysm from other abnormalities by demonstrating direct communication between aneurysm and left ventricle [15]. The important message we learned is to pay extreme attention on the anatomy of MV leaflets every time we face an endocarditis, always looking for something suspicious for aneurysm. Specifically, in case of AV endocarditis, we should raise suspicion for MV aneurysm. For the same reason, if we see or suspect an MV aneurysm in another clinical scenario (MV prolapse, flail, etc.), always rule out concomitant or previous IE (IE can be clinically subtle). Another debated topic is the comparison between early and late surgery. Late surgery is related with lower morbidity and mortality (preoperative antibiotic leads to reduced inflammation; then, tissues are

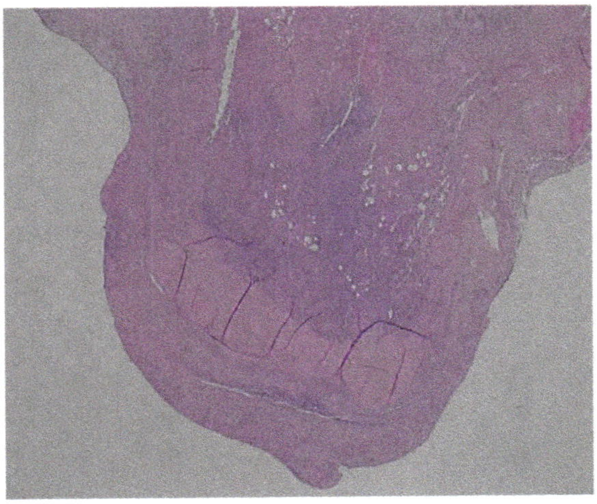

Figure 4: Anterior MV leaflet: slide.

less weak and surgery is easier). Despite that we are in accord with that point, we think it should be imperative to perform serial TEEs to rule out classical complications and unusual ones and plan surgery as soon as possible if aneurysm is present or highly suspected. Tomsic et al. concluded that urgent surgery becomes advisable if signs of HF are present [13]; our patient was stable with no pulmonary edema nor reduced EF. Arguably, delaying surgery may have increased the risk of aneurysm rupture, leading to a more complicated operation and postoperative course. For those reasons, we would suggest urgent surgery should be indicated when evidence or suspect of MV aneurysm is present. Nonetheless, indication must be discussed case by case. Intraoperative evaluation of the MV remains crucial for both diagnosis and treatment. When feasible, MV repair remains the gold standard. In case of IE, however, replacement is often more suitable [16]. Due to not favorable anatomy, we also preferred an MV replacement (bioprosthesis), achieving an excellent outcome. Finally, being *S. gallolyticus* related to colon cancer and colon polyps [17, 18], any blood culture positive for that bacterium must suggest performing a non-urgent colonoscopy. In our patient, colonoscopy was positive for intestinal polyps. There should not be any doubt on planning a colonoscopy every time we deal with *S. gallolyticus*-related IE.

4. Conclusion

Mitral valve aneurysm is rare but mostly associated with infective endocarditis. Transesophageal echocardiogram is crucial to determine vegetation size and mobility but also signs of concomitant abscess, perforation, and valve aneurysm. If aneurysm is present or suspected, surgery is strictly suggested due to high risk of rupture with subsequent deterioration of hemodynamics (massive acute mitral regurgitation) and systemic embolization. If blood culture is positive for *S. gallolyticus*, colonoscopy should be done to rule out colon cancer.

References

[1] M. M. Stechert, J. R. Pletcher, E. E. Tseng, and M. J. London, "Aneurysm of the anterior mitral valve," *Anesthesia and Analgesia*, vol. 114, no. 1, pp. 86–88, 2012.

[2] M. A. Al-Refai, F. M. Oueida, R. C. Lui, S. M. Al-Saif, and H. M. Al-Omran, "Impressive echocardiographic images of a rare pathology: aneurysm of the mitral valve - report of two cases and review of the literature," *Journal of the Saudi Heart Association*, vol. 25, no. 1, pp. 47–51, 2013.

[3] G. Jackson, C. Camargo, L. F. Ling, V. Kalahasti, and C. M. Rimmerman, "The clinical picture: fever, dyspnea, and a new heart murmur," *Cleveland Clinic Journal of Medicine*, vol. 80, no. 9, pp. 559–561, 2013.

[4] G. Habib, B. Hoen, P. Tornos et al., "Guidelines on the prevention, diagnosis, and treatment of infective endocarditis (new version 2009): the task force on the prevention, diagnosis, and treatment of infective endocarditis of the European Society of Cardiology (ESC)," *European Heart Journal*, vol. 30, no. 19, pp. 2369–2413, 2009.

[5] I. Vilacosta, J. A. San Román, C. Sarriá et al., "Clinical, anatomic, and echocardiographic characteristics of aneurysms of the mitral valve," *The American Journal of Cardiology*, vol. 84, no. 1, pp. 110–113, 1999.

[6] P. Marcos-Alberca, M. Rey, J. M. Serrano et al., "Aneurysm of the anterior leaflet of the mitral valve secondary to aortic valve endocarditis," *Journal of the American Society of Echocardiography*, vol. 13, no. 11, pp. 1050–1052, 2000.

[7] C. Gao, C. Xiao, and B. Li, "Mitral valve aneurysm with infective endocarditis," *The Annals of Thoracic Surgery*, vol. 78, no. 6, pp. 2171–2173, 2004.

[8] N. Ruparelia, D. Lawrence, and A. Elkington, "Bicuspid aortic valve endocarditis complicated by mitral valve aneurysm," *Journal of Cardiac Surgery*, vol. 26, no. 3, pp. 284–286, 2011.

[9] V. Subban, V. Krishnamurthy, A. Mohanraj, and M. S. Ajit, "Posterior mitral leaflet aneurysm - a rare cause of mitral regurgitation," *Indian Heart Journal*, vol. 64, no. 4, pp. 402-403, 2012.

[10] R. B. Kharwar, A. Mohanty, A. Sharma, V. S. Narain, and R. Sethi, "Ruptured anterior mitral leaflet aneurysm in aortic valve infective endocarditis-evaluation by three-dimensional echocardiography," *Echocardiography*, vol. 31, no. 3, pp. E72–E76, 2014.

[11] A. Guler, C. Y. Karabay, O. M. Gursoy et al., "Clinical and echocardiographic evaluation of mitral valve aneurysms: a retrospective, single center study," *The International Journal of Cardiovascular Imaging*, vol. 30, no. 3, pp. 535–541, 2014.

[12] M. S. Eiseman, A. R. Schroeder, P. S. Rutkowski, Z. A. Rashid, and P. S. Pagel, "An unusual cause of severe mitral regurgitation in a patient with aortic valve endocarditis," *Journal of Cardiothoracic and Vascular Anesthesia*, vol. 28, no. 5, pp. 1432–1434, 2014.

[13] A. Tomsic, W. W. Li, M. van Paridon, N. R. Bindraban, and B. A. de Mol, "Infective endocarditis of the aortic valve with anterior mitral valve leaflet aneurysm," *Texas Heart Institute Journal*, vol. 43, no. 4, pp. 345–349, 2016.

[14] M. J. Sousa, V. Alves, S. Cabral et al., "Aneurisma da valvula mitral: uma complicaçao grave da endocardite valvular aortica," *Revista Portuguesa de Cardiologia*, vol. 35, no. 11, pp. 621.e1–621.e5, 2016.

[15] F. Muscente, M. Scarano, D. Clemente, F. Pezzuoli, and V. M. Parato, "A ruptured mitral valve aneurysm as complication of

a bicuspid aortic valve endocarditis," *Journal of Cardiovascular Echography*, vol. 27, no. 1, pp. 23–25, 2017.

[16] M. Tariq, I. Zahid, and S. Sami, "Rare aneurysm of anterior mitral valve leaflet-a case report," *Journal of Cardiovascular Echography*, vol. 14, no. 1, p. 204, 2019.

[17] C. Chukwunonso, P. Harish, K. Kishore, E. Ahmed, B. Manoj, and I. Ariyo, "Colon cancer with *Streptococcus gallolyticus* aortic valve endocarditis: a missing link," *Case Reports in Gastrointestinal Medicine*, vol. 2019, Article ID 4205603, 4 pages, 2019.

[18] M. E. Hensler, "Streptococcus gallolyticus, infective endocarditis, and colon carcinoma: new light on an intriguing coincidence," *The Journal of Infectious Diseases*, vol. 203, no. 8, pp. 1040–1042, 2011.

22

Woven Coronary Artery Anomaly: An Incidental Finding and Literature Review

Bdoor Bamousa,[1] **Taher Sbitli**,[1] **Tahir Mohamed**,[2] **Khalid Al Johani**,[3] **and Ali Almasood**[2]

[1]*Department of Medicine, Alfaisal University, Riyadh, Saudi Arabia*
[2]*Heart Center, King Faisal Specialist Hospital & Research Center, Riyadh, Saudi Arabia*
[3]*Cardiac Science Department, King Saud University, Riyadh, Saudi Arabia*

Correspondence should be addressed to Ali Almasood; aalmasood@kfshrc.edu.sa

Academic Editor: Ertugurul Ercan

Woven coronary artery anomaly is a rare description of an epicardial vessel segment that divides into multiple intertwining segments with eventual convergence of the distal vessel. We present our case, a 57-year-old male with an incidental woven coronary artery anomaly found during work-up investigations for a possible lung transplant, and we conduct a literature review on woven anomaly cases reported from 1988 to 2021 and provide a thorough analysis of its diversified clinical presentation. Imaging identification and various treatment modalities are also discussed.

1. Introduction

Woven coronary artery anomaly is a rare and sporadic disorder that has been previously described as a benign pathology. Recently, there has been an increase of reported "malignant" or ischemic forms of this disorder in the literature. This anomaly entails the division of the epicardial coronary artery into multiple channel segments that converge distally. It has been associated with the formation of a thrombus, consequently giving rise to more serious clinical sequelae. Herein, we report a case of a 57-year-old male patient with a woven anomaly of the coronary artery that was treated with percutaneous coronary angioplasty.

2. Case Report

A 57-year-old male, with a known case of idiopathic pulmonary fibrosis, diagnosed 7 years ago, presented to our emergency room due to shortness of breath and productive cough for the last 2 months. He is a previous smoker for 25 years and has quit 2 years ago. He has no history of hypertension, diabetes, or any other coronary artery disease risk factors. During his admission, he underwent work-up for possible lung transplantation. His blood pressure was 114/71 mmHg. An electrocardiogram showed normal sinus rhythm. Echocardiography demonstrated findings of moderately severe pulmonary hypertension, mild dilatation of the right atrium, and normal left ventricular systolic function without any regional wall motion abnormalities, with an ejection fraction of >55%. He underwent a coronary angiogram as a routine procedure prelung transplantation which demonstrated branching of the proximal segment of the right coronary artery (RCA) into thin channels that converge distally into a normal conduit (Figure 1). Optical coherence tomography (OCT) was performed and documented the finding of a braid-like woven coronary with multiple channels within the vessel (Figure 2). Left anterior descending artery (LAD) and left circumflex coronary artery (LCX) vessels had mild ectasia, with otherwise normal Thrombolysis In Myocardial infarction (TIMI) III flow. According to the hospital protocol and for the patient to remain on the lung transplantation listing, coronary intervention had to be done; therefore,

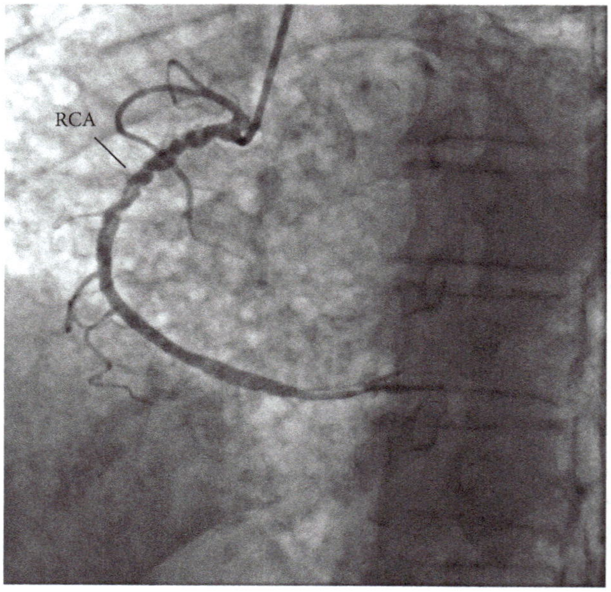

Figure 1: Left anterior oblique (LAO) view of right coronary artery (RCA), demonstrating braid-like lesion.

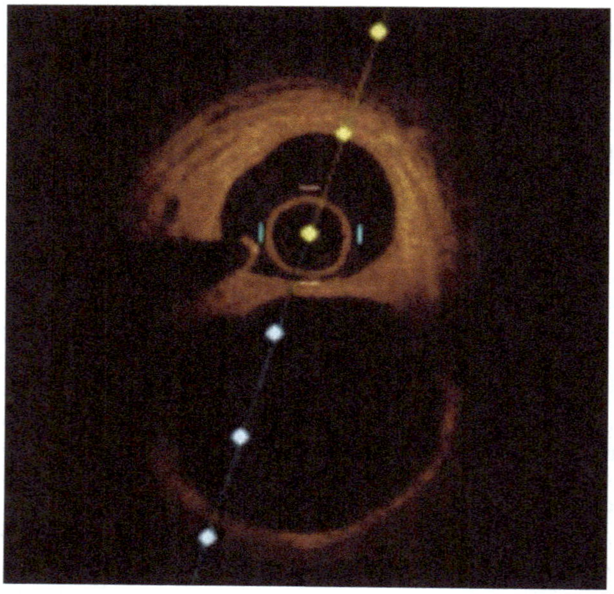

Figure 2: Optical coherence tomography (OCT) of right coronary artery (RCA) showing multiple channels.

percutaneous coronary intervention (PCI) was performed; an Asahi Sion blue wire was used to cross the woven lesion successfully, the lesion was predilated, and a DES stent was placed and deployed successfully (Figure 3). Post PCI, the patient was put on dual antiplatelet therapy. He was reevaluated in 3 months, during which he was admitted for his lung transplant.

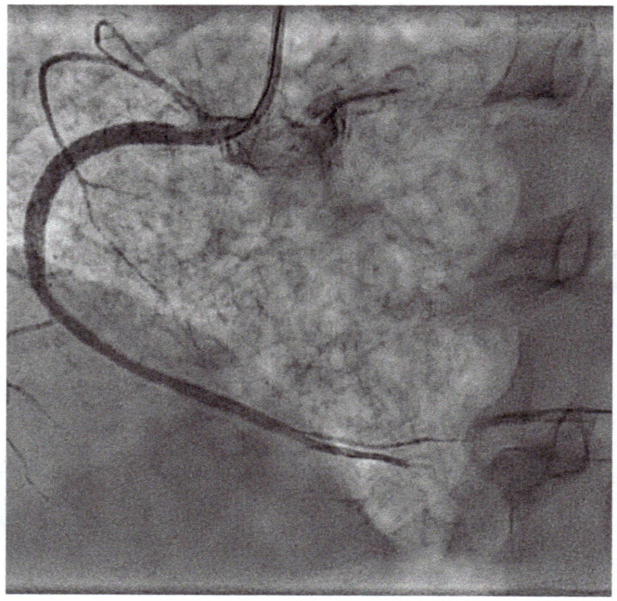

Figure 3: Right coronary artery (RCA) postpercutaneous intervention (PCI).

3. Discussion

Woven coronary artery anomaly is defined as a condition in which an epicardial vessel is divided into multiple thin vessel channels that share the same tunica proximally and converge into one lumen without any disruption of blood flow distally [1]. Beyond the intertwining or "woven" segment which averages at about 2.2 cm with a range of 1-5 cm, blood flow is TIMI-III in the involved vessel [2]. A limited number of cases have been published on this anomaly. The recent rise in WCAA reports may be due to the greater usage and advancement of intravascular imaging modalities that have made the anomaly easier to detect.

The first ever reported case of WCAA was in 1988. Sane and Vidaillet published a case report describing a 55-year-old female with rheumatic heart disease and valvular disorders. She presented with what were presumably symptoms of congestive heart failure with involvement of the mitral valve, but upon further evaluation, the proximal RCA was visualized and said to have a "figure 8" pattern on the arteriogram [3].

We have conducted a literature review that encompasses all published cases of WCAA from 1998 until June 2021, with a total of 37 cases. The demographic's information and the clinical details of these cases are in Tables 1 and 2. The mean age was found to be 53.2 ± 12.4 years, with the male gender being predominantly affected; out of the 37 patients, only 2 were female (male to female ratio of 17.5 : 1). All listed patients are adults, except for one case, a 9-month-old infant with Kawasaki disease [4].

The most common vessels involved in WCAA are RCA (70.2%), LAD (32.4%), and LCX (18.9%). WCAA malformation can affect more than one vessel at once and is more frequently found within a segmental artery [5]. The percentage of 2 or more vessels involved concurrently is 17.9%.

Table 1: A compiled list of case reports published in the literature and demographic's information.

#	Year	Author	# of cases	Age (year)	M/F	Risk factors				Past medical history
						Hypertension	Dyslipidemia	Smoking	IHD	
1	1988 [3]	Sane and Vidaillet	1	55	F	0	0	0	0	RHD, aortic valve replacement, and mitral valve commissurotomy
2	1990 [9]	Berman et al.	1	51	M	0	1	1	0	Family history of premature CAD
3	1995 [26]	Gregorini et al.	3 (3A)	60	NA	0	0	0	0	
			3 (3b)	62	M	0	0	0	0	
			3 (3c)	45	F	0	0	0	0	
4	2000 [27]	Martuscelli et al.	1	42	M	0	0	0	1	Angina and family history of hypercholesterolemia
5	2006 [28]	Kursaklioglu et al.	1	48	M	0	0	0	0	
6	2010 [4]	Yildirim et al.	1	0.75 (9 m)	M	0	0	0	0	
7	2010 [2]	Iyisoy et al.	1	58	M	0	0	1	0	
8	2012 [11]	Soylu et al.	1	48	M		1	0	0	
9	2012 [29]	Tasal et al.	1	60	M	1	0	1	0	
10	2013 [14]	Yuan	1	62	M	1	0	0	1	
11	2013 [30]	Akyuz et al.	1	45	M	1	1	1	0	Carotid artery occlusion
12	2013 [13]	Ayhan et al.	1	42	M	0	0	0	0	
13	2013 [17]	Bozkurt et al.	1	52	M	0	0	0	1	
14	2013 [31]	Oylumlu et al.	1	53	M	0	0	1	0	
15	2013 [19]	Uribarri et al.	1	73	M	0	0	0	0	
16	2013 [32]	Abaci et al.	1	46	M	0	0	0	0	
17	2014 [33]	Acar et al.	1	54	M	0	0	0	0	
18	2015 [34]	Alsancak et al.	1	54	M	0	0	0	0	
19	2015 [35]	Baysal et al.	1	61	M	1	1	0	0	
20	2015 [12]	Chikata et al.	1	75	M	0	1	0	0	Atrial flutter
21	2017 [10]	Val-Bernal et al.	1	39	M	0	0	0	0	
22	2017 [36]	Xing et al.	1	51	M	0	0	0	0	Mitral regurge
23	2018 [7]	Akcay and Soylu	1	41	M	0	0	0	0	
24	2019 [5]	Wang et al.	3(3A)	62	M	1	0	0	0	Atrial fibrillation
			3(3B)	61	M	1	0	0	1	
			3(3C)	66	M	1	0	1	0	

Table 1: Continued.

#	Year	Author	# of cases	Age (year)	M/F	Risk factors				Past medical history
						Hypertension	Dyslipidemia	Smoking	IHD	
25	2019 [21]	Bi et al.	1	59	M	0	0	0	0	
26	2019 [23]	Wen et al.	1	67	M	0	0	0	0	
27	2020 [1]	Wei et al.	1	67	M	0	0	1	0	
28	2020 [8]	Liu and Li	1	44	M	0	0	0	1	Atrial fibrillation, RHD, and severe mitral regurge
29	2020 [18]	Wang et al.	1	48	M	0	0	0	0	
30	2020 [20]	Uemura et al.	1	53	M	0	0	0	0	
31	2020 [37]	Li et al.	1	47	M	0	0	1	0	
32	2020 [24]	Vilalta et al.	1	59	M	1	0	1	1	
33	2021	Almasood et al.	1	57	M	0	0	1	0	Idiopathic pulmonary fibrosis

Risk factors: 1 = existant risk factor. 0 = non − existent risk factor.

Multiple theories have been proposed regarding the etiology of WCAA, despite the exact cause being unknown. In the literature, there have been 2 main proposed theories regarding pathology. Some believe that this disorder is congenital and more specifically sporadic as no reported cases are identifying a genetic predisposition or hereditary cause [1] [6]. Others believe that it is a consequence of spontaneous cardiac dissection or recanalized thrombus [1, 7]. The causes of WCAA can be vasculitic disorders such as spontaneous coronary artery dissection, recanalized thrombus, or Kawasaki disease, and it may be associated with long-term chronic conditions such as rheumatoid arthritis [1] [2] [3] [6, 8]. It is important to understand that WCAA can be due to spontaneous cardiac dissection or recanalized thrombus but can also mimic those pathological states. It is therefore advised to keep these similar pathologies in your list of differential diagnoses when considering a potential case of a woven coronary artery anomaly [9]. Despite an unknown pathophysiology, it has been postulated that certain growth factors involved in arteriogenesis and angiogenesis are key in the underlying pathophysiology of this disorder [1, 6]. Overall, the most commonly supported theory in the literature is that WCAA is of congenital origin [6, 10].

We believe that WCAA can be both congenital and acquired, provided that the typical characteristics of multiple thin vessels share the same tunica proximally and converge into one lumen distally without any disruption of blood flow. The presence of 3 distinct vessel wall layers indicates a congenital origin, while the preexistence of cardiac dissection or recanalized thrombus may hint at an acquired state of the anomaly.

Patients with the underlying woven anomaly of the coronary arteries tend to be asymptomatic for years and may even go undetected. This led to the anomaly being deemed as benign in the literature. However, there is now a rise in cases reported of patients presenting with acute coronary syndrome, ischemic stroke, myocardial infarction, or sudden cardiac death [7] [10–12]. Underlying risk factors may contribute to a malignant presentation of WCAA. The prevalence of predetermined risk factors in the patient population of woven coronary artery anomalies in the literature is as follows: 21.6% of patients have hypertension, 13.5% have dyslipidemia, 27% are smokers, and 16.2% have a preexisting history of ischemic heart disease.

The literature proposes WCAA as the culprit responsible for thrombus formation [11, 13]. The intertwining of the thin channels gives rise to an environment prone to thrombus formation [4]. A case report in 2018 strongly suggests that WCAA should be categorized under the umbrella of atherosclerotic disease, as complications of this disorder require similar treatment [7]. Up until 2012, reported cases of WCAA have not been associated with ischemia. The first reported case of WCAA causing ischemia was a 48-year-old man who presented with myocardial infarction due to the woven anomaly. This patient had a previous diagnosis of spontaneous coronary artery dissection 6 years before the MI, which may support the hypothesis that WCAA can be caused by coronary dissection [11]. Spontaneous dissection of the artery initially forms pseudolumens. It is theorized that over time, these pseudolumens join and form true lumens which spiral around each other in a woven formation, predisposing the patient to a thrombus [10, 11] Closer inspection and follow-up is required for such patients, to prevent adverse or life-threatening complications.

Coronary angiography is deemed as the gold standard method of identifying and diagnosing WCAA [2, 14]. Without familiarization of the disorder with imaging, woven anomaly may be missed [5]. WCAA can be viewed as a filling defect and as previously mentioned can appear similar to

Table 2: Outline of the clinical details of the woven anomaly case reports found in the literature.

#	Presenting symptom	ECG	Echocardiography	Ischemia assessment	OCT	IVUS	Woven anomaly vessel	Diseased artery	Treatment	Outcome or F/U
1	Shortness of breath				Not done	Not done	Proximal RCA			
2	Incidental			Exercise ECG: diffuse ST depression in anterolateral and inferior leads+thallium scan: inferoposterior defect	Not done	Not done	Middistal RCA	PDA		
3	ACS			Positive thallium scan	Not done	Not done	LAD, LCX, and OM			
	ACS				Not done	Not done	Proximal LCX	LAD, LCX	PTCA for mid LAD (percutaneous transluminal coronary angioplasty)	
	ACS				Not done	Not done	Distal LAD	LAD		
4	Chest pain				Not done	Not done	Middistal RCA	RCA		
5	Chest pain	Normal	Moderate aortic insufficiency	Stress ECG: ST depression in inferior leads	Not done	Not done	Mid LCX	RCA	PCI+aortic valve replacement	Unremarkable 5-year follow-up
6	Kawasaki disease	Prolonged PR interval			Not done	Not done	Proximal RCA		Aspirin and IV immunoglobulin for Kawasaki disease	Unremarkable 4-year follow-up
7	Chest pain		Normal LV wall motion, left ventricular EF: 60%	Stress ECG: ST depression in V1-V4+myocardial perfusion imaging: reversible ischemia in the anterior wall	Not done	Not done	Proximal RCA	LAD	PCI	Unremarkable 3-year follow-up on the woven artery. However, distal LAD developed 70% stenosis which required medical treatment
8	Atypical left arm pain	Old inferior infarction and T-wave inversion in V5-v6	Normal systolic function, inferior wall akinesis, and mild mitral regurge	Stress and rest Tc 99 m sestamibi scan: stress-induced myocardial ischemia in inferior and lateral leads	Not done	Not done	RCA	RCA	Medical treatment	Unremarkable 2-year follow-up
9	ACS	Normal	LV hypertrophy, mild diastolic dysfunction, and		Not done	Not done			PCI	Unremarkable 1-year follow-up

Table 2: Continued.

#	Presenting symptom	ECG	Echocardiography	Ischemia assessment	OCT	IVUS	Woven anomaly vessel	Diseased artery	Treatment	Outcome or F/U
			hypokinesia of the posterolateral wall with an ejection fraction of 55%				LAD, LCX, and OM2	LAD, LCX, and OM2		
10	ACS	ST depression in lead II, III, aVF, and V4-V6	LV hypokinesis, mild mitral insufficiency		Not done	Not done	Distal RCA	LM, LAD, LCX, and RCA	Medical treatment+CABG operation	Unremarkable postop
11	Chest pain	Normal	Normal wall motion, left ventricular EF: 65%	Stress ECG: ST-segment depression+thallium-201 myocardial perfusion imaging: no ischemia	Not done	Not done	LAD, LCX, RCA		Medical treatment+smoking cessation	
12	Chest pain	Sinus tachycardia, RBBB with marked ST-segment depression in precordial leads	Global hypokinesis, left ventricular EF: 30%		Not done	Not done	Proximal-distal RCA, proximal-mid LAD			
13	Incidental	Abnormal Q waves in leads V1–V6	Severe hypokinesia in the apical and anterior walls of the left ventricle, left ventricular EF: 45%	Infarction in the anterior and apical walls of the left ventricle, without any myocardial ischemia	Done	Not done	Proximal-mid LAD, proximal DI branch	LAD	Medical treatment	
14	ACS	Normal	Normal LV wall motion, left ventricular EF: 60%	Dobutamine stress echo: reversible ischemia in inferior wall	Not done	Not done	RCA	RCA due to stenosis before the woven segment	Medical treatment	
15	Chest pain			SPECT: stress-induced ischemia in the inferior wall of LV	Done	Not done	Mid-RCA	Distal RCA stenosis, CTO of PDA	CABG	
16	ACS				Not done	Not done	Proximal LAD, RCA, OM, and	LAD	CABG	Unremarkable postop

Table 2: Continued.

#	Presenting symptom	ECG	Echocardiography	Ischemia assessment	OCT	IVUS	Woven anomaly vessel	Diseased artery	Treatment	Outcome or F/U
17	Chest pain	Negative T waves in leads DII, DIII, and aVF	Normal LV wall motion, left ventricular EF: 65%	Myocardial perfusion imaging: no ischemia in the anterior wall	Not done	Not done	1st diagonal Distal LAD	LCX	Medical treatment	Unremarkable 1-year follow-up
18	Chest pain	Q waves and extrasystoles on D3 and aVF	Akinesia at inferior and posterior walls, left ventricular EF: 44%	Inferior wall ischemia was detected which approximately refers to 14% of the left ventricle	Not done	Not done	Mid-RCA	RCA	PCI	
19	Chest pain	Incomplete LBBB	Normal systolic function, LV hypertrophy	Myocardial perfusion imaging: reversible ischemia in inferior and posterior walls	Not done	Not done	RCA		Medical treatment	
20	Palpitations	Atrial flutter	Akinesia in the anterior and apical walls, severe hypokinesia in the other LV walls, and left ventricular EF: 22.5%	Stress-induced ischemia and a fixed low uptake in the anterior and apical walls	Not done	Done	Proximal-mid LAD		Cavotricuspid isthmus (CTI) ablation	
21	Sudden cardiac death	Asystole which could not be converted back to sinus rhythm					Mid RCA	RCA		Death
22	Exertional shortness of breath				Not done	Not done	LCX	LCX	CABG+mitral valve repair	Unremarkable 4-week follow-up
23	Incidental [symptoms of acute ischemic stroke of embolic origin]	Q waves in inferior leads	Akinesia in inferior and inferobasal walls, mild mitral regurgitation, and left ventricular EF: 40%	Myocardial perfusion scintigraphy: inferior wall fixed hypoperfusion, infarct, and mild peri-infarct ischemia	Not done	Not done	RCA	RCA	Medical treatment	Unremarkable 2-year follow-up
24	Congestive heart failure	Normal	Normal left ventricular EF		Done	Not done	LAD		Medical treatment	
	ACS		Regional inferior wall motion abnormality		Done	Not done	Distal RCA	RCA	PCI	
	Chest pain	Inverted T waves on precordial and inferior leads	NA		Done	Not done	Proximal RCA	LAD	PCI	Unremarkable 1-year follow-up

Table 2: Continued.

#	Presenting symptom	ECG	Echocardiography	Ischemia assessment	OCT	IVUS	Woven anomaly vessel	Diseased artery	Treatment	Outcome or F/U
25	ACS	ST-segment elevation in the inferior leads	Normal LV wall motion, left ventricular EF: 59%		Not done	Not done	Proximal-mid RCA	RCA	CABG	
26	Chest pain	Atrial fibrillation in rhythm and Q wave in the inferior leads	Left ventricular EF: 40%		Not done	Done	RCA	RCA	PCI	Unremarkable 9-month follow-up. LVEF improved by 4% (44%)
27	Chest pain				Done	Done	RCA			
28	Exertional shortness of breath		Rheumatic heart disease		Not done	Not done	Middistal RCA	LAD	CABG+mitral valve replacement	
29	ACS	ST-segment elevation in the anterior V1-V5 leads	Akinesia at anterior walls, left ventricular EF: 54%		Done	Not done	LAD	LAD	PCI	Unremarkable 4-year follow-up
30	ACS			Ischemia in the inferior wall	Done	Not done	RCA	RCA	PCI	
31	Chest pain				Not done	Not done	LAD, LCX, RCA	LAD	PCI	Unremarkable 3-year follow-up
32	ACS [referred]				Done	Not done	RCA	RCA	PCI	
33	Incidental	Normal	Normal LV systolic function, left ventricular EF: >55%, moderately severe pulmonary hypertension, and mild dilatation of the right atrium	Not performed	Done	Done	RCA	RCA	PCI	Unremarkable 3-month follow-up

spontaneous coronary dissection or recanalized thrombus, with the images being described as "honeycomb," "spiral" [8], "braid-like," or having a "figure 8" pattern [3, 8].

A published case series in 2020 argues that some of the case reports on woven anomalies are misdiagnosed and could be recanalized organized thrombi. It further states that merely doing an angiogram is not sufficient to determine the diagnosis as both these pathological states will present as a "braid-like lesion" [15].

Optical coherence tomography (OCT) and intravascular ultrasound (IVUS) [16] are intravascular imaging modalities that will provide a definitive diagnosis with a high-resolution illustration of the lumen of the vessel and the three layers of the vessel wall [5, 17].

Evidence supporting the theory that WCAA is of congenital origin can be supported by using OCT. In a woven anomaly, OCT findings will demonstrate intertwined thin segments separated by fibrous tissue with no cross-communication between those segments, undisrupted arterial wall integrity without dissection, and high signal intensity and low signal attenuation [5, 18, 19]. You may also visualize a thrombus formation in more malignant cases of woven anomaly [19]. Cross-communication is a key feature in distinguishing WCAA and recanalized thrombus. On OCT, the recanalized thrombus has been described as a "lotus-root" or "swiss-cheese" appearance due to the presence of multiple interconnected channels within the thrombus [20, 21]. This is unlike a congenital woven anomaly, which has no cross-communication between channels [22].

Because of the interchangeable usage of description terms, a key feature distinguishing these pathologies will help prevent any misdiagnosis. We believe OCT to be an essential tool for confirmation and avoidance of any undesirable operative complications due to misdiagnosis. OCT may not be suitable for all cases. In some instances, OCT wires may be difficult to penetrate through the complex structure of a woven anomaly associated with a thrombus or may simply be unavailable at the given facility. One case was able to overcome this by utilizing a patient's previous angiogram 3 years prior to deduce the location of the thrombus; the previously done angiogram revealed a hazy lesion followed by stenosis in the RCA, which was medically treated. Based on the assumption that the woven anomaly must have been caused by progression and recanalization of that thrombus, a PCI was performed afterward in addition to an IVUS [23].

Treatment modalities of WCAA vary from conservative percutaneous intervention to bypass surgery. Asymptomatic patients should be kept under observation especially if there is no evidence of ischemia. However, once symptoms such as angina are noted, patients must undergo further testing to confirm ischemia before deciding upon interventions such as surgical or percutaneous revascularization [21–23]. A method that can be helpful in deciding upon an intervention is the usage of fractional flow reserve (FFR) [24]. FFR determines the adequacy of coronary blood flow using a formula that takes the distal coronary pressure of a stenosed vessel and divides it by aortic pressure. In 2019, a study applied fluid dynamic principles to understand the variables affecting the pressure drop along a woven coronary artery. The number of channels and length of the diseased segment were found to have an inversely proportional relationship with pressure along the artery. The greater the length and the number of channels, the greater the pressure will drop. This supported their hypothesis that FFR is more effective in determining the adequacy of coronary blood flow as compared to coronary angiography [25].

Before ischemic WCAA was established in the literature, PCI was ruled as an ineffective treatment modality [11]. In our reported case, the decision was made to perform PCI on the RCA, based on clinical judgment and angiographic evaluation of TIMI flow I-II. Adequate blood supply was established in the RCA territory, with a TIMI-III grade flow.

4. Conclusion

WCAA is a rare braid-like pathology that can lead to a serious clinical sequela. We believe that it can arise in both an acquired and congenital form. Familiarization and proper identification of this anomaly are necessary with the use of coronary angiogram and more specifically OCT; visualization of the vessel wall layers and lumen will help distinguish a woven anomaly from similar pathologies such as spontaneous coronary artery dissection, recanalized thrombus, or bridging collaterals. Based on the ischemic assessment of the patient, treatment modalities can be chosen. Patients found to have an incidental benign woven anomaly must also be observed, as the anomaly can convert to a malignant variant and cause devastating medical consequences such as acute coronary syndrome or sudden cardiac death.

Abbreviations

WCAA: Woven coronary artery anomaly
RHD: Rheumatic heart disease
PCI: Percutaneous intervention
PTCA: Percutaneous coronary intervention
CABG: Coronary artery bypass graft
OCT: Optical coherence tomography
FFR: Functional flow reserve
IVUS: Intravenous ultrasound
TIMI: Thrombolysis in Myocardial Infarction
RCA: Right coronary artery
LAD: Left anterior descending
LCX: Left circumflex
IHD: Ischemic heart disease.

References

[1] W. Wei, Q. Zhang, and L.-M. Gao, "Woven coronary artery: a case report," *World Journal of Clinical Cases*, vol. 8, no. 20, pp. 4917–4921, 2020.

[2] A. Iyisoy, T. Celik, U. C. Yuksel, and E. Isik, "Woven right coronary artery: a case report and review of the literature," *Clinical Cardiology*, vol. 33, no. 7, pp. E43–E45, 2010.

[3] D. C. Sane and H. J. Vidaillet, ""Woven" right coronary artery: a previously undescribed congenital anomaly," *American Journal of Cardiology*, vol. 61, no. 13, p. 1158, 1988.

[4] A. Yıldırım, D. Oğuz, and R. Olguntürk, "Woven right and aneurysmatic left coronary artery associated with Kawasaki disease in a 9-month-old patient," *Cardiology in the Young*, vol. 20, no. 3, pp. 342–344, 2010.

[5] X. Wang, X.-Q. Cai, Q. Wang et al., "Optimizing woven coronary artery management by optical coherence tomography: three cases report," *Journal of Geriatric Cardiology : JGC*, vol. 16, no. 8, pp. 656–659, 2019.

[6] S. C. Joseph, A. V. D'antoni, R. S. Tubbs, J. Gielecki, and M. Loukas, "Woven coronary arteries: a detailed review," *Clinical Anatomy*, vol. 29, no. 4, pp. 502–507, 2016.

[7] M. Akcay and K. Soylu, "An unusual etiology of ischemic stroke: woven coronary artery anomaly," *Journal of the Saudi Heart Association*, vol. 30, no. 4, pp. 316–318, 2018.

[8] Z. Liu and Y. Li, "Rheumatic valvular heart disease combined with woven coronary artery: a case report," *Journal of Cardiothoracic Surgery*, vol. 15, no. 1, p. 124, 2020.

[9] A. D. Berman, D. Kim, and D. S. Baim, ""Woven" Right coronary artery: case report and therapeutic implications," *Catheterization and Cardiovascular Diagnosis*, vol. 21, no. 4, pp. 258-259, 1990.

[10] J. F. Val-Bernal, S. Malaxetxebarria, I. González-Rodilla, and M. Salas-García, "Woven coronary artery anomaly presenting as sudden cardiac death," *Cardiovascular Pathology*, vol. 26, pp. 7–11, 2017.

[11] K. Soylu, M. Meric, H. Zengin, S. Yüksel, and M. G. Kaya, "Woven right coronary artery," *Journal of Cardiac Surgery*, vol. 27, no. 3, pp. 345-346, 2012.

[12] A. Chikata, S. Sakagami, N. Kanamori et al., "Chronic ischemia induced by woven coronary artery anomaly with typical atrial flutter: insights from multiple imaging devices," *Internal Medicine*, vol. 54, no. 17, pp. 2185–2189, 2015.

[13] S. Ayhan, S. Ozturk, U. Y. Tekelioglu, and T. Ocak, "Woven coronary artery anomaly associated with acute Coronary Syndrome," *The International Journal of Angiology : Official Publication of the International College of Angiology, Inc*, vol. 22, no. 1, pp. 55–58, 2013.

[14] S.-M. Yuan, "Woven coronary artery: a case report and literature review," *Folia Morphologica*, vol. 72, no. 3, pp. 263–266, 2013.

[15] W.-X. Leng, H.-H. Wang, H. M. Liu et al., "Differential diagnosis, clinical characteristics, and interventions of braid-like coronary artery: case series analysis based on optical coherence tomography," *Journal of Interventional Cardiology*, vol. 2020, article 1031675, 11 pages, 2020.

[16] G. J. Tearney, E. Regar, T. Akasaka et al., "Consensus standards for acquisition, measurement, and reporting of intravascular optical coherence tomography studies: a report from the International Working Group for Intravascular Optical Coherence Tomography Standardization and Validation," *Journal of the American College of Cardiology*, vol. 59, no. 12, pp. 1058–1072, 2012.

[17] A. Bozkurt, O. Akkus, S. Demir, O. Kaypakli, and M. Demirtas, "A new diagnostic method for woven coronary artery," *Herz*, vol. 38, no. 4, pp. 435–438, 2013.

[18] F. Wang, J. Han, and L. Guo, "Optical coherence tomography and fractional flow reserve guided treatment of woven coronary artery anomaly presenting as acute myocardial infarction: a case report," *Medicine*, vol. 99, no. 7, p. e19163, 2020.

[19] A. Uribarri, R. Sanz-Ruiz, J. Elízaga, and F. Fernández-Avilés, "Pathological insights of a woven coronary artery with optical coherence tomography," *European Heart Journal*, vol. 34, no. 38, pp. 3005–3005, 2013.

[20] Y. Uemura, A. Tanaka, K. Takemoto, H. Ishii, T. Murohara, and M. Watarai, "Optical coherence tomography-guided stent implantation for woven coronary artery anomaly," *Circulation Journal*, vol. 84, no. 6, p. 1044, 2020.

[21] X. Bi, H. Yang, L. Liu, and Q. Wang, "Is every woven coronary artery benign? Case report," *Internal and Emergency Medicine*, vol. 14, no. 1, pp. 177-178, 2019.

[22] K. Toutouzas, A. Karanasos, K. Stathogiannis et al., "A honeycomb-like structure in the left anterior descending coronary artery: demonstration of Recanalized thrombus by optical coherence tomography," *JACC: Cardiovascular Interventions*, vol. 5, no. 6, pp. 688-689, 2012.

[23] W. Wen, H. Liu, J. Li, and Q. Zhang, "Woven-like change following intracoronary thrombosis recanalization: a case report," *BMC Cardiovascular Disorders*, vol. 19, no. 1, p. 317, 2019.

[24] V. Vilalta, O. Rodriguez-Leor, and O. Abdul-Jawad, "Physiology and imaging for woven disease management," *Revista Española de Cardiología (English Edition)*, vol. 73, no. 1, p. 85, 2020.

[25] S. Cito, R. Puri, J. Pallarès, O. Abdul-Jawad Altisent, and A. Bayes-Genis, "Woven Coronary Disease," *Circulation: Cardiovascular Interventions*, vol. 12, no. 9, p. e008087, 2019.

[26] L. Gregorini, R. Perondi, G. Pomidossi, A. Saino, I. M. Bossi, and A. Zanchetti, "Woven left coronary artery disease," *American Journal of Cardiology*, vol. 75, no. 4, pp. 311-312, 1995.

[27] E. Martuscelli, F. Romeo, M. Giovannini, and A. Nigri, "Woven coronary artery: differential diagnosis with diffuse intracoronary thrombosis," *Italian Heart Journal*, vol. 1, no. 4, pp. 306-307, 2000.

[28] H. Kursaklioglu, A. Iyisoy, and T. Celik, "Woven coronary artery: a case report and review of literature," *International Journal of Cardiology*, vol. 113, no. 1, pp. 121–123, 2006.

[29] A. Tasal, A. Bacaksiz, E. Erdogan, and Z. Küçükdurmaz, "Successful percutaneous management of occluded "woven" coronary artery: a case report," *Advances in Interventional Cardiology/Postępy w Kardiologii Interwencyjnej*, vol. 2, pp. 168–172, 2012.

[30] A. Akyuz, S. Alpsoy, and D. C. Akkoyun, "Spontaneous coronary artery dissection and woven coronary artery: three cases and a review of the literature," *Korean Circulation Journal*, vol. 43, no. 6, pp. 411–415, 2013.

[31] M. Oylumlu, A. Yıldız, H. Kaya, and F. Ertaş, "An impressive image of woven right coronary artery," *Türk Kardiyol Dern Arş-Arch Turk Soc Cardiol*, vol. 41, no. 8, pp. 736-737, 2013.

[32] A. Abaci, I. I. Gonul, S. Ozkan, M. Cemri, and A. Yener, "Pathological examination of the woven coronary anomaly," *European Heart Journal*, vol. 34, supplement 1, p. P5682, 2013.

[33] R. D. Acar, M. Bulut, Z. A. Uslu, S. Öztürk, M. Akçakoyun, and S. Pala, "Woven left anterior descending coronary artery imaging with computed tomography," *Herz*, vol. 39, no. 6, pp. 774-775, 2014.

[34] Y. Alsancak, B. Sezenoz, S. Turkoglu, and A. Abacı, "Woven coronary artery disease successfully managed with percutaneous coronary intervention: a new case report," *Case Reports in Cardiology*, vol. 2015, Article ID 516539, 3 pages, 2015.

[35] E. Baysal, B. Acar, and C. Burak, "Woven right coronary artery: a rare coronary anomaly," *Indian Heart Journal*, vol. 67, no. 6, pp. 611-612, 2015.

[36] Z. Xing, L. Tang, J. Huang, and X. Hu, "Woven coronary anomaly leading to silent myocardial infarction: a case report," *Medicine*, vol. 96, no. 44, p. e8302, 2017.

[37] Y. Li, H. Liu, Y. Deng, and Y. Han, "Intracoronary imaging-guided percutaneous coronary intervention for woven coronary artery disease with chronic total occlusion," *Canadian Journal of Cardiology*, vol. 36, pp. e9–1977.e11, 2020.

23

Pregnancy-Associated Chest Pain: A Case of Spontaneous Coronary Artery Dissection

Vidhushei Yogeswaran[1] **Satvik Ramakrishna**[1,2] **John S. MacGregor**[1,2] **Lucas Zier**[1,2] **and Nora Goldschlager**[1,2]

[1]*Department of Medicine, University of California, San Francisco, CA, USA*
[2]*Division of Cardiology, Zuckerberg San Francisco General Hospital, San Francisco, CA, USA*

Correspondence should be addressed to Vidhushei Yogeswaran; vidhushei.yogeswaran@ucsf.edu

Academic Editor: Assad Movahed

Spontaneous Coronary Artery Dissection (SCAD) is an important cause of myocardial infarction that typically affects women without traditional cardiovascular risk factors. It is the most common cause of myocardial infarction in pregnant and postpartum women. SCAD is often underdiagnosed due to the lack of clinician familiarity, and patients with pregnancy-associated SCAD often have more severe clinical presentations than those without. We present a case of SCAD in a multiparous woman who presented with acute chest pain in the postpartum period.

1. Introduction

SCAD is a rare but important cause of myocardial infarction (MI) and sudden cardiac death. SCAD is defined as an epicardial coronary dissection not associated with atherosclerosis, trauma, or iatrogenic injury and is the most common cause of pregnancy-associated and postpartum MI [1]. SCAD typically occurs in women without traditional atherosclerotic cardiovascular risk factors, and the mechanism of injury is thought to be coronary artery obstruction from an intramural hematoma or intimal disruption [2]. Risk factors for SCAD are fibromuscular dysplasia, connective tissue disease, physical stress, emotional stress, pregnancy, and multiparity. It is hypothesized that hormonal changes during pregnancy weaken the coronary arterial vessel walls; multiparous women can accumulate these changes over several pregnancies [2].

Patients with pregnancy-associated SCAD often have more acute presentations and high-risk features than patients with non-pregnancy-associated SCAD. Most cases of pregnancy-associated SCAD occur in the first month postpartum, with the majority in the first week following delivery [3]. It is important to recognize SCAD in clinical practice as the population affected, and management is different than other causes of MI.

2. Case Report

A 44-year-old gravida 6 para 4 postpartum woman presented to the emergency department (ED) complaining of substernal chest pain. That afternoon, she experienced sudden-onset severe left-sided chest pain radiating to her back and shoulder. She had been discharged four days prior after induction of labor for chronic hypertension with an uncomplicated vaginal birth. Her medical history was notable only for hypertension, for which she took metoprolol. She was maintained on metoprolol with good blood pressure control for the duration of her pregnancy and after induction. The day prior to admission she was under significant emotional distress after her infant was hospitalized with hyperbilirubinemia.

In the ED, the patient was afebrile, her blood pressure was 164/101 mm Hg, her heart rate was 60 beats per minute, and she was breathing 16 breaths per minute. Her cardiovascular examination was unremarkable with normal heart sounds with no murmurs, rubs, or gallops and no jugular

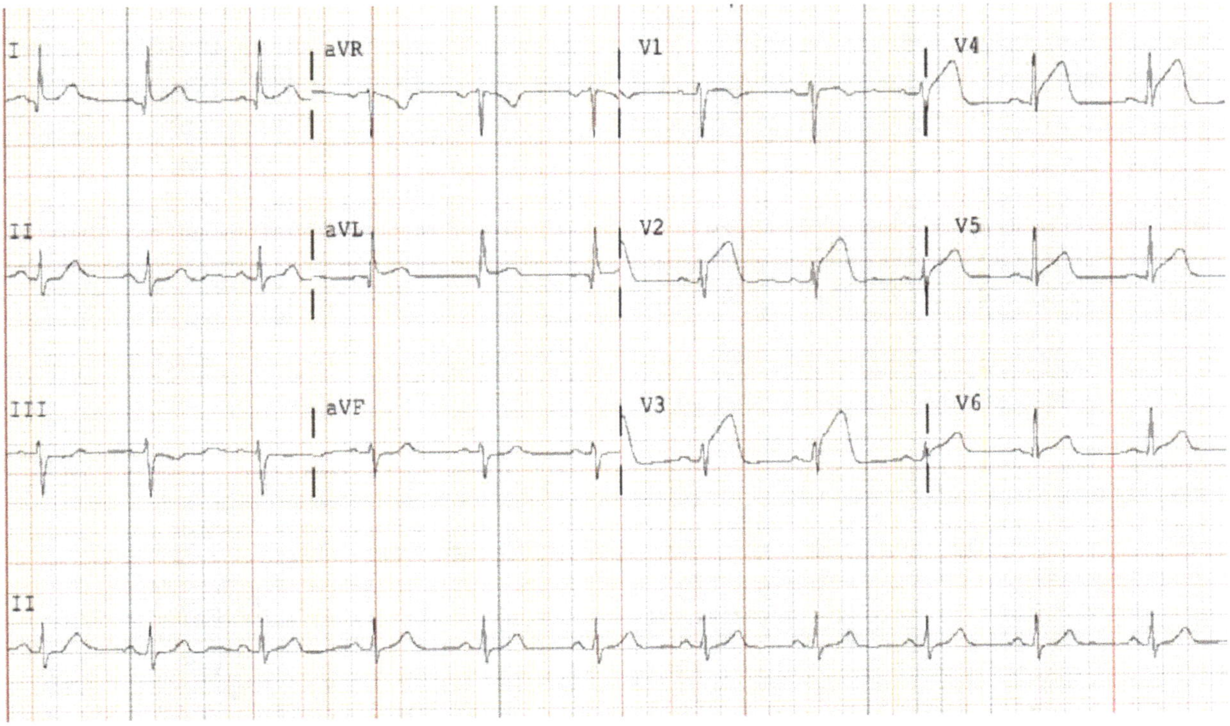

FIGURE 1: Patient's initial ECG showing ST-segment elevation in V2-V5, consistent with anterior STEMI.

venous distension. Her lungs were clear, her abdomen was soft, and she had no extremity edema. Her complete blood count and comprehensive metabolic panel results were within normal limits. Her initial troponin I was 0.41 ng/mL (reference range, <0.04 ng/mL), and her electrocardiogram (ECG) (Figure 1) was significant for ST elevation in leads V2-V5 consistent with an anterior ST-segment elevation myocardial infarction (STEMI). Her chest X-ray showed normal mediastinum, no signs of cardiomegaly, and clear lungs.

Given the concern for acute coronary syndrome (ACS), the patient was emergently taken to the cardiac catheterization lab. Her coronary angiogram showed haziness of the midleft anterior descending (LAD) artery followed by an abrupt change in arterial caliber extending to the distal LAD and diagonal branches (Figure 2(a)). There was no clear visualization of a dissection flap, but there was a visible long segment of diffuse vessel narrowing in the mid to distal LAD highly suspicious for coronary dissection. Contrast flow in the distal vessel was normal (TIMI 3), and there were no luminal changes with the administration of intracoronary nitroglycerin. There was no angiographic evidence of atherosclerotic disease in any of her coronary arteries, and no evidence of narrowing in the coronary arteries outside of the LAD. Her chest pain was resolved during the procedure, and her ECG showed normalization of her ST elevation. Given the patient's hemodynamic stability, normal blood flow in the distal LAD, resolution of chest pain, and suspicion for dissection, she was managed conservatively.

She was started on IV nitroglycerin for hypertension, metoprolol, and dual antiplatelet therapy with aspirin and clopidogrel and then transferred to the coronary care unit for close observation. Her transthoracic echocardiogram showed normal left ventricular function with an ejection fraction of 68% and hypokinetic septal and apical walls in the distribution of the LAD. Her repeat ECG (Figure 3) showed the expected evolution of her STEMI with QS waves and T-wave inversions seen in leads V2-V5. She was weaned off the nitroglycerin and transitioned to captopril and nifedipine for strict blood pressure control and safety with breastfeeding.

She remained chest-pain free during the course of the hospitalization and underwent a repeat angiogram to evaluate for the progression of disease given the diagnostic uncertainty. Her repeat angiogram on day 6 of hospitalization showed complete resolution of the LAD lesion (Figure 2(c)) consistent with dissection. Compared to the initial angiogram, the area of haziness was no longer present, and the vessel tapered appropriately towards the apical LAD. However, a new tubular narrowing with abrupt vessel caliber change (Figure 2(d)) was noted in the midposterior descending artery (PDA), compared to her initial angiogram (Figure 2(b)) with normal flow and no clear dissection flap. This event was concerning for a new dissection event. The patient was asymptomatic throughout her hospitalization and was discharged home with close obstetric, primary care, and cardiology outpatient follow-up.

3. Discussion

In this postpartum woman presenting with a STEMI with angiographic findings suggestive of coronary dissection and no evidence of atherosclerotic disease, a diagnosis of SCAD was made. SCAD commonly presents as ACS with ST-

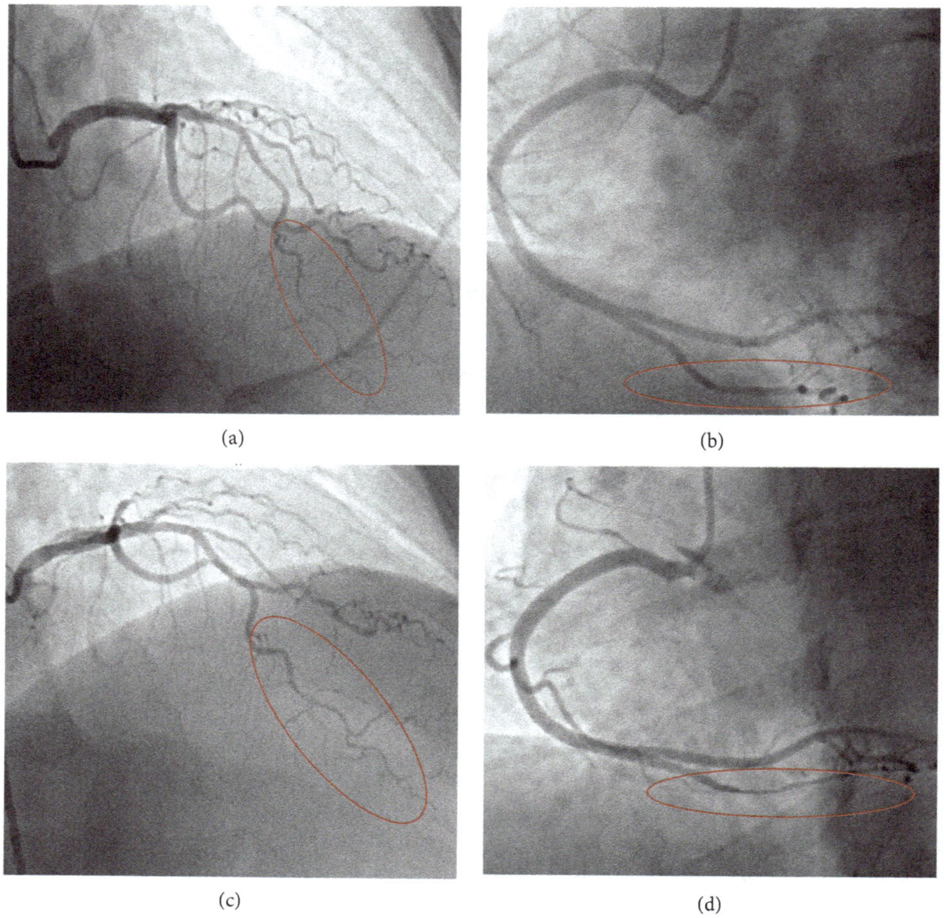

FIGURE 2: Frame A: initial angiogram showing Type 2 SCAD, with a long segment of diffuse vessel narrowing in the mid to distal LAD. Frame B: initial angiogram showing the PDA with no angiographic disease or narrowing. Frame C: repeat angiogram on hospital day 6 showing healing of initial SCAD lesion after medical therapy. Frame D: repeat angiogram showing new Type 2 SCAD lesion in the mid-PDA.

segment changes, and early angiography should be performed to confirm the diagnosis, assess the coronary anatomy, and facilitate revascularization when necessary [2–4]. SCAD is often misdiagnosed and a research group recently published a flowchart to aid in the diagnosis [5]. Angiographically, SCAD has three main classifications: Type 1 is identified by contrast staining showing multiple lumens, Type 2 is an abrupt change in vessel caliber with diffuse tubular stenoses of varying length, and Type 3 is a focal stenosis that mimics atherosclerosis and intracoronary imaging using intravascular ultrasound or optical coherence tomography is often required to confirm the diagnosis. The angiographic appearance of Type 2 is often missed and shorter lengths, such as 20-30 mm, may require repeat angiography or intracoronary imaging to make the diagnosis [4, 6]. The patient in this case had a Type 2 SCAD lesion with suggestive features on the initial angiogram that was confirmed with a repeat angiogram showing healing of her lesion. The LAD is the most common artery affected in both pregnancy-associated and non-pregnancy-associated SCAD [2, 3]. Patients with pregnancy-associated SCAD often have more severe clinical presentations than non-pregnancy-related SCAD with multivessel dissections and acute heart failure [3].

Once a diagnosis is made, SCAD consensus guidelines recommend a conservative approach in patients who are hemodynamically stable and without active ischemia [2, 4, 6]. Invasive management in SCAD is associated with a high incidence of iatrogenic coronary dissection. Patients should be initiated on aspirin, beta-blockade, and additional antiplatelet therapy with clopidogrel for up to 12 months after the initial event. The role of antiplatelet therapy in SCAD is unclear but is extrapolated from its evidence in acute coronary syndrome and may be beneficial with prothrombotic intimal tears. Beta-blockade is thought to reduce arterial shear stress and may be beneficial through mechanisms similar to that of the treatment of aortic dissection [6]. The majority of SCAD patients (70-90%) managed conservatively have spontaneous healing of their dissection. However, patients with hemodynamic instability, electrical instability, ongoing/recurrent ischemia, abnormal blood flow (TIMI 0-1), and/or left-main coronary artery dissection should be considered for urgent revascularization [2].

Due to the risk of early dissection recurrence or extension, SCAD patients should be observed inpatient for 2-4 days until asymptomatic and clinically stable [4, 6]. Patients with pregnancy-associated SCAD have been found to have

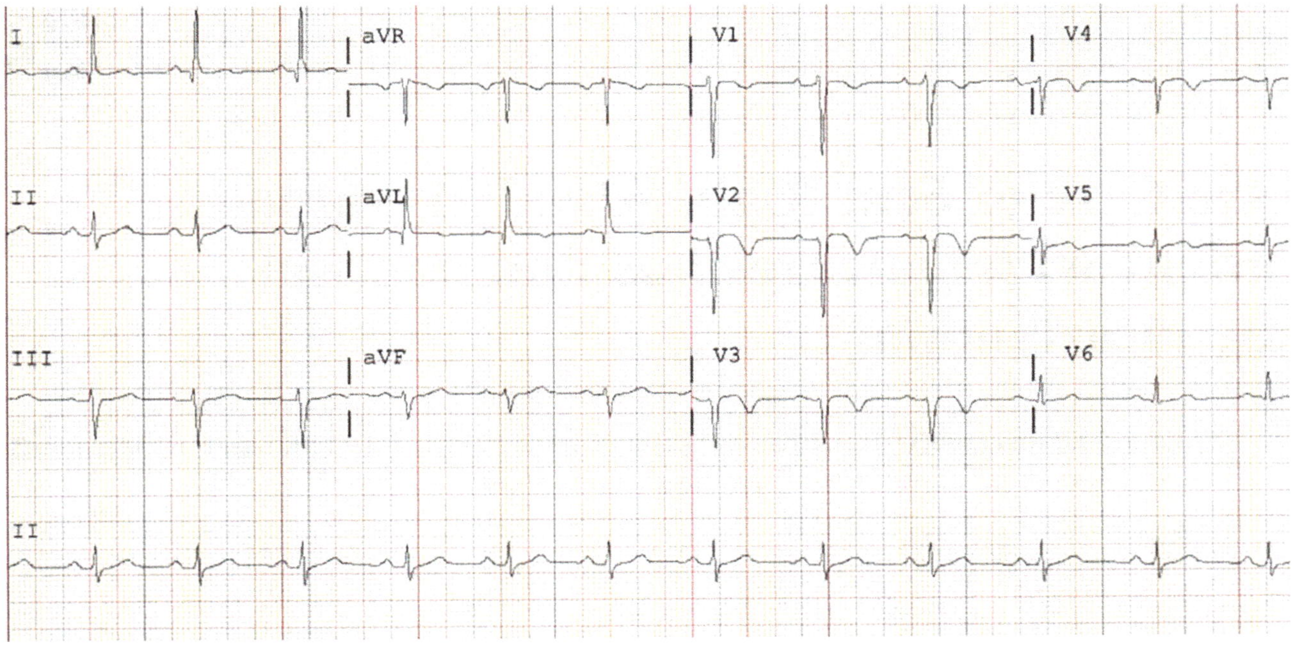

FIGURE 3: Repeat ECG on day 2 of hospitalization showing the expected evolution of anterior STEMI with QS waves and T-wave inversions seen in V2-V5.

a higher prevalence of multivessel dissection events [3]. The patient had a new dissection event on her repeat coronary angiogram but remained chest-pain free without any new evidence of ischemia. There is growing evidence into the role that pregnancy and future pregnancy play with SCAD recurrence and the rates of recurrence have been reported to be as high as 30 percent [7]. This creates a relevant ethical question, and a recent experience-based survey reported that the majority of responders discourage future pregnancy after SCAD [8]. Patients who decide to proceed with pregnancy should have dedicated care with cardiologists and obstetric specialists [7].

4. Conclusion

SCAD is an important and underdiagnosed cause of MI associated with pregnancy. Clinicians should maintain high suspicion in women presenting with chest pain in the postpartum period. The diagnosis of SCAD should be made with early angiography, and a conservative approach with medical management is recommended if possible. All patients with SCAD should be followed closely outpatient as researchers learn more information on the factors associated with recurrence.

Authors' Contributions

All authors had a role in writing and reviewing this case report.

References

[1] U. Elkayam, S. Jalnapurkar, M. N. Barakkat et al., "Pregnancy-associated acute myocardial infarction: a review of contemporary experience in 150 cases between 2006 and 2011," *Circulation*, vol. 129, no. 16, pp. 1695–1702, 2014.

[2] S. N. Hayes, E. S. H. Kim, J. Saw et al., "Spontaneous coronary artery dissection: current state of the science: a scientific statement from the American Heart Association," *Circulation*, vol. 137, no. 19, pp. e523–e557, 2018.

[3] M. S. Tweet, S. N. Hayes, E. Codsi, R. Gulati, C. H. Rose, and P. J. M. Best, "Spontaneous coronary artery dissection associated with pregnancy," *Journal of the American College of Cardiology*, vol. 70, no. 4, pp. 426–435, 2017.

[4] J. Saw, E. Aymong, T. Sedlak et al., "Spontaneous coronary artery dissection: association with predisposing arteriopathies and precipitating stressors and cardiovascular outcomes," *Circulation Cardiovascular Interventions*, vol. 7, no. 5, pp. 645–655, 2014.

[5] D. Buccheri, D. Piraino, and G. Andolina, "Sistema de puntuacion para el enfoque diagnostico y terapeutico de la diseccion coronaria espontanea," *Revista Espa de Cardiologia (English Edition)*, vol. 69, no. 9, pp. 878-879, 2016.

[6] A. Yip and J. Saw, "Spontaneous coronary artery dissection—a review," *Cardiovascular Diagnosis and Therapy*, vol. 5, no. 1, pp. 37–48, 2015.

[7] M. S. Tweet, S. N. Hayes, R. Gulati, C. H. Rose, and P. J. Best, "Pregnancy after spontaneous coronary artery dissection: a case series," *Annals of Internal Medicine*, vol. 162, no. 8, pp. 598–600, 2015.

[8] D. Buccheri, G. Zambelli, F. Alfonso, and B. Cortese, "Pulse on spontaneous coronary artery dissections: experience-based survey," *JACC: Cardiovascular Interventions*, vol. 10, no. 14, pp. 1469–1471, 2017.

Rare Case of 6cm Right Atrial Myxoma in Patient with Synchronous Endometrial Adenocarcinoma

Mohammad Altujjar,[1] Feras Zaiem,[2] Erin Sheehan,[3] Willy Gan,[4] Mohammed Mhanna,[4] Waleed Khokher,[4] Ikram Ullah,[1] and Mohammad Tokir Mujtaba[1]

[1]*Dartmouth Hitchcock Medical Center, Lebanon, USA*
[2]*Wayne State University, Detroit, USA*
[3]*Indiana University, Indianapolis, Indiana, USA*
[4]*University of Toledo, Toledo, USA*

Correspondence should be addressed to Mohammad Altujjar; tujjarmd@hotmail.com

Academic Editor: Francesco Nappi

Primary cardiac tumors are extremely rare. Cardiac myxomas most frequently appear in the left atrium. In this article, we present a case of an asymptomatic 6 cm right atrial mass in a patient undergoing staging for endometrial cancer. The mass was resected, and final pathology was consistent with cardiac myxoma.

1. Case Presentation

1.1. History of Presentation. A 55-year-old female presented to the hospital with vaginal bleeding. Diagnostic hysteroscopy with dilation and curettage showed endometrioid endometrial adenocarcinoma. During staging, a CT chest revealed a 6 cm right heart atrial mass. The patient denied chest pain, shortness of breath, or palpation. Physical exam and auscultation of the heart and lung were unremarkable. Complete blood count and basic metabolic profile were within normal limits.

Past medical history: essential hypertension and hyperthyroidism

Differential diagnosis: benign cardiac tumor, malignant cardiac tumor, intracardiac thrombus, valvular vegetation, and pericardial cyst

1.2. Investigations. A transthoracic echocardiogram (TTE) confirmed the presence of a large round echogenic right atrial mass with a possible stalk (Figure 1). Transesophageal echocardiogram (TEE) measured the echogenic mass at 5.5 × 4.6 cm, originating from a tiny stalk over the right atrium appendage (Figure 2). The patient underwent right and left heart catheterization to assess for possible coronary artery disease and was found to have no significant coronary artery disease. Right atrial angiogram demonstrated a large and immobile-appearing mass attached to the wall of the right atrium.

1.3. Management. The patient underwent surgery and excision of the mass. The resected mass measured 6 × 6 × 3.5 with a small lobulated stalk measuring 2 × 2 cm (Figure 3). Intraoperative section was consistent with a benign lesion (Figures 4(a) and 4(b)). The permanent histology section (Figures 4(c) and 4(d)) and immunostains (Figure 4(f)) showed finding consistent with cardiac myxoma.

2. Discussion

Primary cardiac tumors are extremely rare with an estimated incidence rate of 0.1%. In certain studies, benign cardiac tumors are estimated to represent more than 90% of cardiac tumors [1].

Myxomas account for more than half of all benign cardiac tumors and most frequently appear in the left atrium (up to 75%) [2]. Other benign cardiac tumors include

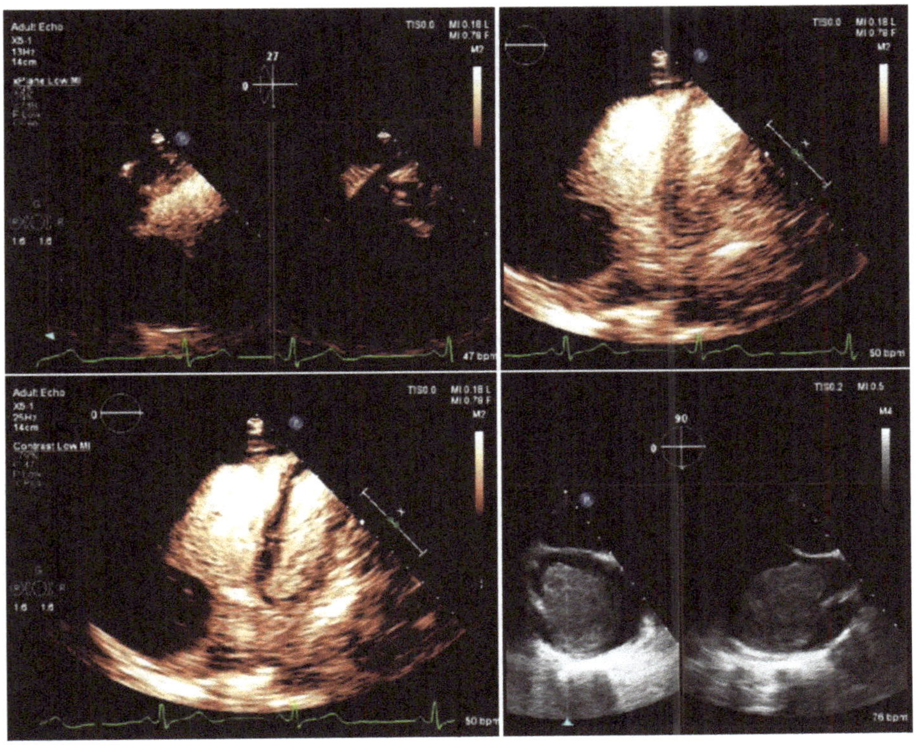

Figure 1: Transesophageal echocardiography showing echogenic right atrial mass with a possible noted stalk.

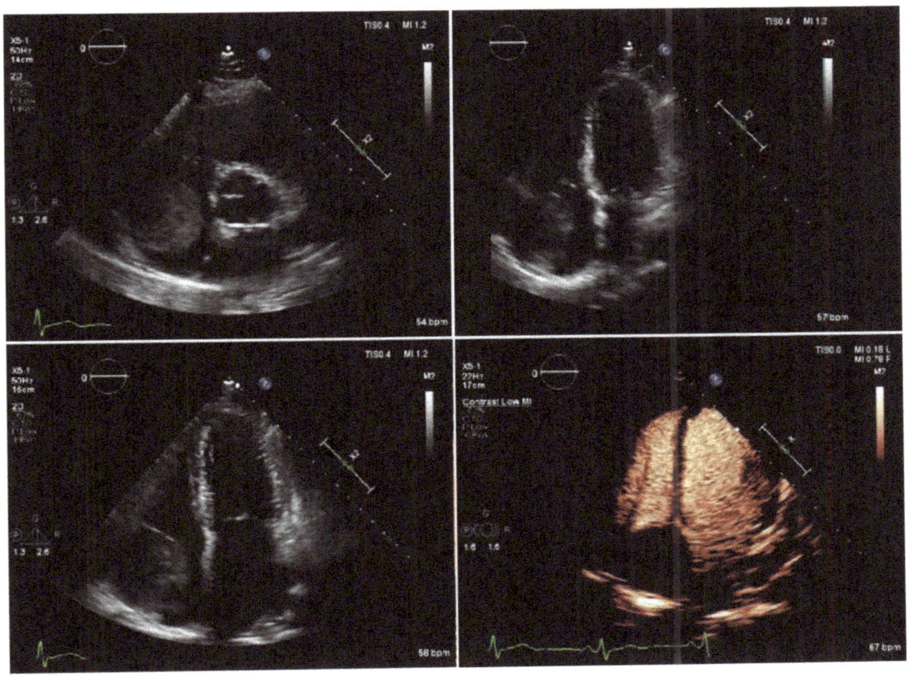

Figure 2: Transthoracic echocardiogram (TEE) view of the mass. Myocardial contrast echo findings suggest minimal to no vascularity within the mass.

pericardial cysts (6.5%), papillomas (4%), fibromas (2.5%), rhabdomyosarcomas (2.5%), hematic cysts (1.5%), teratomas (1.5%), hemangiomas (0.8%), celotheliomas (0.8%), and lipomas (0.8%).

The most common malignant cardiac tumors are mesothelioma and myosarcoma (each 2.5%), followed by angiosarcoma (1.5%), fibrosarcoma (1.5%), and leiomyosarcoma (1.5%) [3]. The rate of incidence of metastatic cardiac

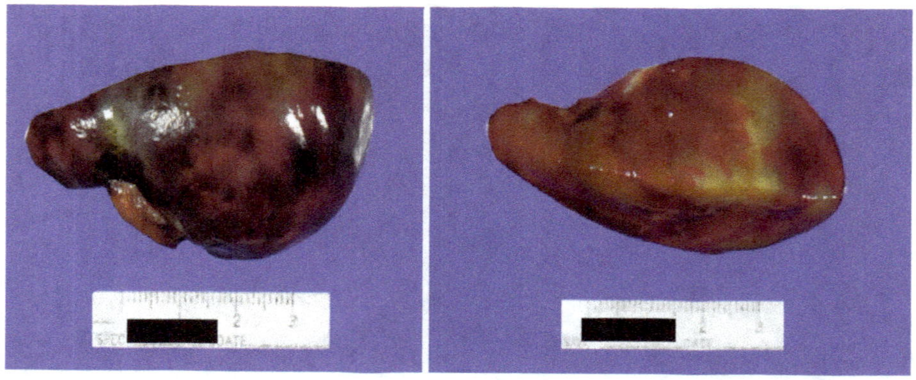

FIGURE 3: The resected tumor showed a $6 \times 6 \times 3.5$ cm oval-shaped mass with a small lobulated stalk.

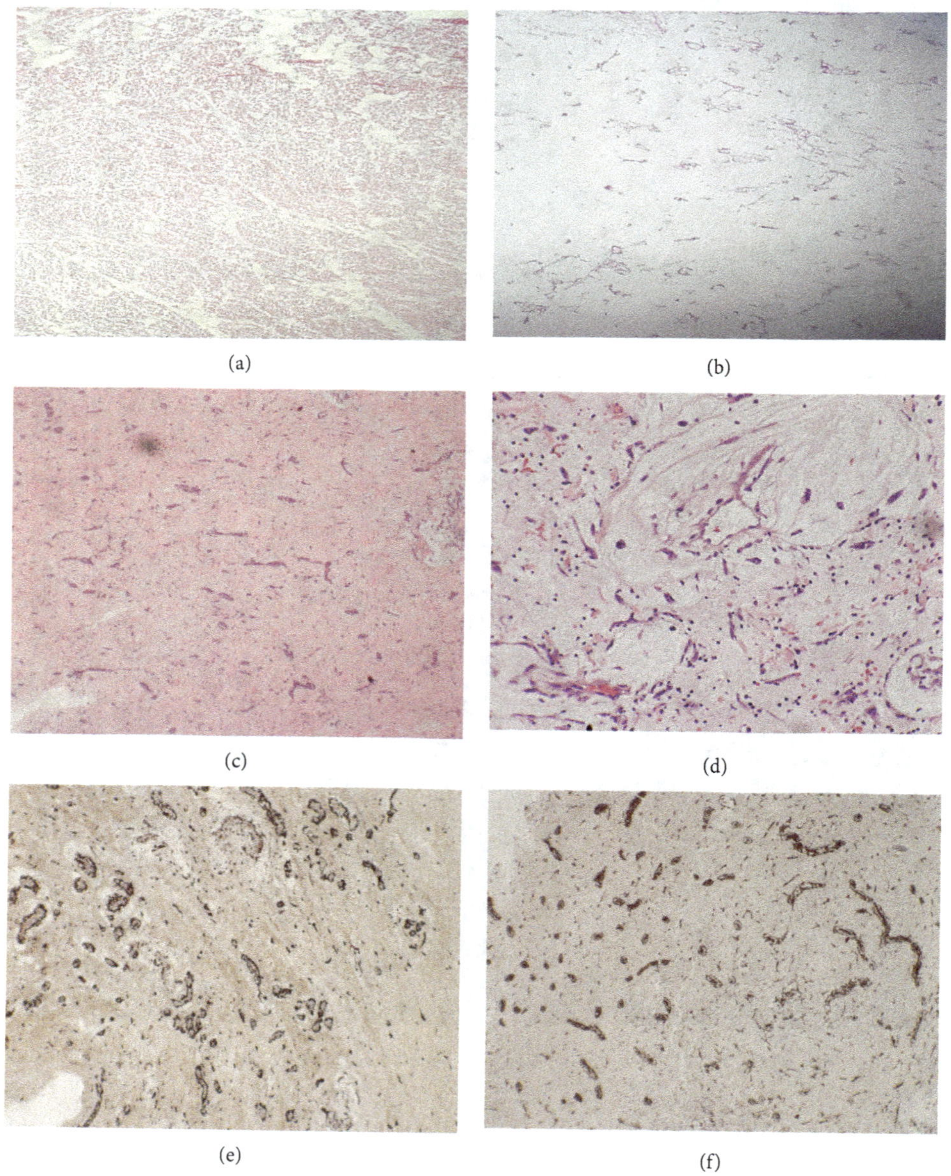

FIGURE 4: The intraoperative frozen section showed unremarkable skeletal heart muscle with abundant myxoid stroma (a, b). The hematoxylin and eosin histology sections (c, d) showed no cytologic atypia or necrosis. The lesional cells are immunoreactive for calretinin (e) and CD34 immunostains (f).

tumors is not precisely known; however, one study reported 8% cardiac involvement in patients who died from metastatic cancer. [4]

Presentation of cardiac tumors, including myxomas, can be variable and mainly depends on the tumor location, size, and mobility. Asymptomatic cardiac myxoma cases have been reported in 10% in some studies [5]. Symptomatic cardiac myxomas can present with constitutional, obstructive, or embolic symptoms. Constitutional symptoms were reported in as high as 90% of the cases; however, these symptoms are nonspecific. Obstructive symptoms may manifest as progressive heart failure, syncope, valvular abnormalities variable with position, or sudden cardiac death. Arterial blood supply can also be affected by left atrial myxomas, with systemic emboli reported in 10-45% of cases; embolization to cerebral, coronary, renal, splenic, ocular, and cutaneous arteries have been reported [5].

In contrast to left atrial myxomas, right-sided atrial myxomas tend to be asymptomatic until relatively late in their development. One study demonstrated that right atrial myxomas are only symptomatic when 7 cm or greater, corresponding to around twice the size of when left atrial myxomas become symptomatic [6]. A right atrial tumor can obstruct the flow of blood through the tricuspid valve, leading to tricuspid stenosis and right heart failure. There is also a chance the tumor may break off and embolize to the lungs, causing pulmonary embolism [7], or cause systemic embolism if a patent foramen ovale or atrial septal defect is present. Villous surface of the mass increases the risk of embolization [7].

Physical exam findings are mainly auscultative. The pathognomonic "tumor plop" is a protodiastolic heart sound with low frequency and heard after the second heart sound. It can be confused with the third heart sound. An association between auscultative findings and symptomatic presentations has been reported [5].

The rarity of primary cardiac tumors, including intracardiac myxomas, makes them a challenge to diagnose. Many cardiac myxomas are found incidentally via imaging studies. Two-dimensional echocardiography is the gold-standard in diagnosis of intracardiac myxomas, with a transesophageal approach being superior to the transthoracic approach in its ability to visualize and define these tumors. Diagnosis can be adequately made with echocardiography alone by identifying the typical appearance of an atrial myxoma as a mobile mass attached by a visible stalk to the surface of the endocardium, commonly from the fossa ovalis [2]. Echocardiogram is also useful to assess hemodynamics and degree of obstruction. If this is not visible, typically, cardiac CT or MRI is required to better characterize the tumor and attempt to distinguish it from the appearance of mural thrombi. It also can help mapping coronary and cardiac anatomy for planning of a cardiothoracic surgery [8].

To our knowledge, there have been no documented cases of a right atrial myxoma concurrent with an endometrial adenocarcinoma. In the management of synchronous tumors, the most life-threatening condition should be treated first [9]. Another case of a left atrial myxoma and endometrial adenocarcinoma being managed concurrently has been reported in a 77-year-old female; surgeons elected to respect her pelvic mass to address her malignancy and left her asymptomatic cardiac tumor in place [10]. In our case, the patient underwent cardiac surgery to resect the mass, and the endometrial cancer was managed subsequently.

2.1. Follow-Up. The patient recovered well after the heart surgery. She underwent total laparoscopic hysterectomy and bilateral salpingo-oophorectomy for the endometrial cancer. Final pathology diagnosis was stage IIIC1 endometrioid endometrial adenocarcinoma. She was started on chemotherapy and continues to be followed. A follow-up TEE was significant for mild tricuspid regurgitation and showed a preserved ejection fraction of 60-65%.

3. Conclusion

Primary cardiac tumors are rare compared to metastatic tumors. These tumors can present with embolic or obstructive symptoms; it can also be asymptomatic even with larger sizes depending on its location. Multiple imaging modalities including echocardiography, cardiac CT, and MRI can be utilized to diagnose the tumors. Surgical resection is the treatment of choice for cardiac myxomas. Although no known available medical treatment for cardiac myxomas, it can still be used to manage tumor complications.

Abbreviations

CD4: Cluster differentiation 4
TEE: Transesophageal echocardiogram
CT: Computerized tomography.

Additional Points

Learning Objectives. (1) To be able to approach intracardiac masses and make a differential diagnosis. (2) To understand the possible different presentations of cardiac myxomas.

References

[1] A. Cresti, M. Chiavarelli, M. Glauber et al., "Incidence rate of primary cardiac tumors: a 14-year population study," *Journal of Cardiovascular Medicine*, vol. 17, no. 1, pp. 37–43, 2016.

[2] G. Ma, D. Wang, Y. He, R. Zhang, Y. Zhou, and K. Ying, "Pulmonary embolism as the initial manifestation of right atrial myxoma: a case report and review of the literature," *Medicine*, vol. 98, no. 51, article e18386, 2019.

[3] C. Basso, M. Valente, A. Poletti, D. Casarotto, and G. Thiene, "Surgical pathology of primary cardiac and pericardial tumors," *European Journal of Cardio-Thoracic Surgery*, vol. 12, no. 5, pp. 730–738, 1997.

[4] R. Bussani, M. Castrichini, L. Restivo et al., "Cardiac tumors: diagnosis, prognosis, and treatment," *Current Cardiology Reports*, vol. 22, no. 12, p. 169, 2020.

[5] L. Pinede, P. Duhaut, and R. Loire, "Clinical presentation of left atrial cardiac myxoma. A series of 112 consecutive cases," *Medicine*, vol. 80, no. 3, pp. 159–172, 2001.

[6] G. K. Munirathinam, B. Kumar, and H. Singh, "Right atrial myxoma with pulmonary artery hypertension: role of transesophageal echocardiography in detection of cause and perioperative management," *Journal of Cardiothoracic and Vascular Anesthesia*, vol. 32, no. 2, pp. 801–806, 2018.

[7] E. Kuon, M. Kreplin, W. Weiss, and J. B. Dahm, "The challenge presented by right atrial myxoma," *Herz*, vol. 29, no. 7, pp. 702–709, 2004.

[8] K. Haji and A. Nasis, "Radiological characteristics of atrial myxoma in cardiac computed tomography," *Journal of Cardiovascular Computed Tomography*, vol. 11, no. 3, pp. 234–236, 2017.

[9] I. N. Nuño, Kang TY 4th, H. Arroyo, and V. A. Starnes, "Synchronous cardiac myxoma and colorectal cancer: a case report," *Texas Heart Institute Journal*, vol. 28, no. 3, pp. 215–217, 2001.

[10] L. N. Abaid, H. D. Epstein, M. Chang, R. Kankus, and B. H. Goldstein, "Endometrial adenocarcinoma with concomitant left atrial myxoma," *Case Reports in Oncology*, vol. 2, no. 2, pp. 150–156, 2009.

25

Plaque Rupture-Induced Myocardial Infarction and Mechanical Circulatory Support in Alpha-Gal Allergy

Sohab S. Radwan,[1] **Gauravpal Gill**,[1] **Amre Ghazzal**,[1] **Awais Malik**,[2] **and Christopher Barnett**[1]

[1]*MedStar Washington Hospital Center, Washington, DC, USA*
[2]*MedStar Georgetown University Hospital, Washington, DC, USA*

Correspondence should be addressed to Sohab S. Radwan; sohab_radwan@hotmail.com

Academic Editor: Kathleen Ngu

Alpha-gal (AG) allergy is an IgE-mediated allergic reaction to galactose-alpha-1,3-galactose found in mammalian meat. Heparin, being derived from porcine intestinal tissue, may have a degree of cross-reactivity with AG antigen and thus place patients at risk for allergic and even anaphylactic reactions. This is especially important in patients with myocardial infarction (MI) and mechanical circulatory support, such as a left ventricular assist device (LVAD), since anticoagulation is immediately required. Therefore, individualized assessment and preoperative planning is needed regarding the use of heparin vs. nonheparinoid products in such a population.

1. Introduction

AG allergy, also known as AG syndrome or red meat allergy, is an IgE-mediated allergic reaction to galactose-alpha-1,3-galactose carbohydrate found in mammalian meat such as pork and beef. It usually occurs following a tick bite, with the lone star tick being the most predominant cause in the US [1]. The prevalence of AG allergy is steadily increasing with an estimated 10% of certain populations, especially in southeastern US, reported to have elevated antibody titers against AG antigen [2]. The severity of the reaction varies, but it usually manifests as a late yet powerful anaphylactic reaction 3-6 hours after ingestion, rather than a simple allergic one, and is therefore important to recognize [3]. Heparin products, either unfractionated or low-molecular weight, are derived from porcine intestinal tissue. Although data on the degree of heparin cross-reactivity with AG antigen is still lacking, it is highly likely that such patients will react to heparin [4]. Intolerance to heparin products poses challenges for anticoagulation in patients with MI and postoperatively, in those with mechanical circulatory support devices such as LVAD.

2. Case Presentation

A 56-year-old male with a past medical history of coronary artery disease (status post percutaneous coronary intervention (PCI) to the distal left anterior descending artery (LAD) in 2011), ischemic cardiomyopathy (ejection fraction of 20-25%), type 2 diabetes mellitus, hypertension, hyperlipidemia, and AG allergy presented with chest pain and dyspnea on exertion of one-day duration. On initial presentation, he was hemodynamically stable. Electrocardiogram revealed 3 mm ST segment elevation in leads V2-V4 and reciprocal 1 mm ST segment depression in leads I and aVL, consistent with a diagnosis of anterior wall ST segment elevation MI. The patient was taken immediately to the catheterization lab, where he underwent left heart catheterization, which revealed 50% stenosis of the proximal LAD, 100% occluded mid LAD with thrombus in place, and 30% in-stent restenosis in the distal LAD. He underwent PCI with successful drug-eluting stent placement in the mid LAD. He was anticoagulated with bivalirudin given his AG allergy. His hospital course was complicated by cardiogenic shock approximately 48 hours following PCI requiring intravenous diuresis and inotrope support. His hemodynamics subsequently deteriorated, and a refractory requirement for progressively increasing doses of inotropes leads to evaluation for advanced heart failure therapies. He underwent an exhaustive evaluation and planning for LVAD placement with periprocedural anticoagulation using bivalirudin. He was eventually discharged to a cardiac rehabilitation center. The patient is currently doing well and follows up periodically in the advanced heart failure clinic at our hospital.

3. Discussion

This article describes a case of anterior wall ST segment elevation MI leading to shock requiring inotrope therapy and eventually mechanical circulatory support. A history of ischemic cardiomyopathy with poor functional reserve at an ejection fraction of 20-25% at baseline, along with new acute coronary plaque rupture, leads to cardiogenic shock in our patient which did not resolve with revascularization and diuresis. An important consideration on the differential was a separate entity of acute coronary syndrome, previously described in the literature, called Kounis syndrome. Also known as allergic angina or allergic acute coronary syndrome, Kounis syndrome is usually precipitated by an acute allergic reaction triggering the release of several inflammatory mediators [5]. Pathogenesis involves mast cell activation and degranulation, which can ultimately lead to coronary artery vasospasm and atheromatous plaque erosion, rupture, and thrombus formation [5, 6]. It is diagnosed infrequently; however, it is common in individuals with an allergic background [5]. Despite having a significant allergic history, anaphylaxis is a less likely etiology for shock in this patient without exposure to known allergens and stable hemodynamics on presentation. Therefore, while managing this patient, serum tryptase levels, which reflect mast cell burden and help in determining the presence of anaphylaxis, were not measured [7].

There are no available standardized desensitization protocols that could have facilitated the use of heparin in this patient. Moreover, the amount of heparin required to trigger an allergic reaction is unclear, since a nonstandardized amount of AG antigen is present in each lot of heparin [4]. However, there have been reported cases of patients with AG allergy who received heparin products during cardiac surgery after being preoperatively treated with steroids and antihistamines, with acceptable outcomes. Interestingly, heparin has also been shown to induce anaphylaxis in individuals without AG allergy [8]. This mainly occurs as part of the heparin-induced thrombocytopenia syndrome as well as through the contact system-activating effects of unknown contaminants within heparin lots [9]. Given the risk for cross-reactivity between heparin and AG antigen, proposed alternative options for anticoagulation include bivalirudin and direct oral anticoagulants, specifically apixaban or rivaroxaban [10]. However, the lack of experience with those drugs and varied duration of action in this setting as compared to heparin presents a challenge as well.

Furthermore, stents themselves may act as antigenic stimuli and induce hypersensitivity reactions [11]. Culprit components include the polymer coating, metallic platform, and the released drugs, which are thought to result in chronic and repetitive hypersensitivity irritation to the coronary intima [11]. This eventually results in attracting several proteins, mainly fibrinogen and complement, leading to complement system activation [11]. As such, this constitutes a variant of allergic acute coronary syndrome, manifesting as stent thrombosis, which is unlikely in our patient given the sequence of events. The current emphasis in research revolves around the use of biodegradable stent technology in an effort to reduce the trigger for persistent inflammation within the coronary intima [12]. With such technology, all stent components (drug, polymer, or scaffold) are absorbed and none is left behind [13]. Although the evidence on such technology is promising, it is still limited [14].

4. Conclusion

Further research regarding AG cross-reactivity with heparin in acute coronary syndrome as well as perioperative anticoagulation alternatives in mechanical circulatory support is necessary. Moreover, hypersensitivity reactions to implanted materials within stent structures must be emphasized on. Lastly, establishing standardized heparin desensitization protocols in patients with AG allergy is crucial.

References

[1] J. W. Steinke, T. A. Platts-Mills, and S. P. Commins, "The alpha-gal story: lessons learned from connecting the dots," *The Journal of Allergy and Clinical Immunology*, vol. 135, no. 3, pp. 589–96; quiz 597, 2015.

[2] S. P. Commins, S. M. Satinover, J. Hosen et al., "Delayed anaphylaxis, angioedema, or urticaria after consumption of red meat in patients with IgE antibodies specific for galactose-alpha-1,3-galactose," *The Journal of Allergy and Clinical Immunology*, vol. 123, no. 2, pp. 426–433, 2009.

[3] W. L. Jackson, "Mammalian meat allergy following a tick bite: a case report," *Oxford Medical Case Reports*, vol. 2018, no. 2, article omx098, 2018.

[4] K. A. Sell-Dottin, M. Sola, and T. G. Caranasos, "Impact of newly emerging alpha-gal allergies on cardiac surgery: a case series," *Clinics in Surgery*, vol. 2, article 1477, 2017.

[5] H. Adachi, M. Ihara, Y. Nojima, T. Kurimoto, and S. Nanto, "Kounis syndrome caused by anaphylaxis without skin manifestations after cefazolin administration," *The Journal of Allergy and Clinical Immunology: In Practice*, vol. 7, no. 1, pp. 317–319, 2019.

[6] N. G. Kounis and G. M. Zavras, "Histamine-induced coronary artery spasm: the concept of allergic angina," *The British Journal of Clinical Practice*, vol. 45, no. 2, pp. 121–128, 1991.

[7] M. C. Carter, K. N. Ruiz-Esteves, L. Workman, P. Lieberman, T. A. E. Platts-Mills, and D. D. Metcalfe, "Identification of alpha-gal sensitivity in patients with a diagnosis of idiopathic anaphylaxis," *Allergy*, vol. 73, no. 5, pp. 1131–1134, 2018.

[8] S. Despotopoulos, A. Roumeliotis, N. G. Kounis, G. Tsigkas, G. Hahalis, and P. Davlouros, "Severe allergic reaction during angioplasty culminating to fatal acute stent thrombosis: an

association with Kounis syndrome," *Heart Lung*, vol. 48, no. 2, pp. 138–140, 2019.

[9] T. K. Kishimoto, K. Viswanathan, T. Ganguly et al., "Contaminated heparin associated with adverse clinical events and activation of the contact system," *The New England Journal of Medicine*, vol. 358, no. 23, pp. 2457–2467, 2008.

[10] V. Parikh, U. Parikh, A. M. Ramirez et al., "Novel oral anticoagulants in patients with continuous flow left ventricular assist devices," *The Journal of Heart and Lung Transplantation*, vol. 38, no. 4, article S425, 2019.

[11] N. G. Kounis, I. Koniari, A. Roumeliotis et al., "Thrombotic responses to coronary stents, bioresorbable scaffolds and the Kounis hypersensitivity-associated acute thrombotic syndrome," *Journal of Thoracic Disease*, vol. 9, no. 4, pp. 1155–1164, 2017.

[12] J. Bil and R. J. Gil, "Bioresorbable vascular scaffolds-what does the future bring?," *Journal of Thoracic Disease*, vol. 8, no. 8, pp. E741–E745, 2016.

[13] D. J. Kereiakes, Y. Onuma, P. W. Serruys, and G. W. Stone, "Bioresorbable vascular scaffolds for coronary revascularization," *Circulation*, vol. 134, no. 2, pp. 168–182, 2016.

[14] F. Alfonso, J. Cuesta, T. Bastante et al., "Bioresorbable vascular scaffolds in patients with acute myocardial infarction: a new step forward to optimized reperfusion?," *Journal of Thoracic Disease*, vol. 8, no. 6, pp. E417–E423, 2016.

26

Ventricular Tachycardia or Fibrillation Storm in Coronavirus Disease

Muhammad H. Khan,[1] Obadah Aqtash,[2] David M. Harris,[2] Alexandru I. Costea,[2] and Myron C. Gerson[2]

[1]*Department of Internal Medicine, University of Cincinnati, USA*
[2]*Department of Cardiovascular Medicine, University of Cincinnati, USA*

Correspondence should be addressed to Myron C. Gerson; myron.gerson@uc.edu

Academic Editor: Kathleen Ngu

Ventricular tachycardia (VT) or ventricular fibrillation (VF) storm associated with severe acute respiratory syndrome coronavirus 2 infection is a potentially fatal complication; the correlation of these 2 disorders, however, has not been well studied. This retrospective case series examined outcomes of 2 patients who were admitted for repeated implantable cardioverter-defibrillator shocks with or without syncope and observed to have VT/VF storms with COVID-19. Mechanisms of VT/VF storms in COVID-19 are multifactorial including myocarditis, systemic inflammation, hyperadrenergic state, hemodynamic instability, hypoxia, acidosis, and proarrhythmic drugs. A higher incidence of VT/VF storm is observed in patients with comorbidities and those requiring critical care, with some studies reporting increased mortality. In our cohort, 1 of the 2 patients succumbed to the complications from COVID-19, and the other patient was discharged to home in stable condition. Monitoring of life-threatening arrhythmias in the setting of COVID-19 may need to be adopted to prevent morbidity and mortality.

1. Introduction

The coronavirus disease (COVID-19) pandemic caused by the severe acute respiratory syndrome coronavirus 2 (SARS-CoV-2) began in December 2019 and continues to spread globally. The virus primarily causes pulmonary infections; however, major cardiovascular complications are commonly reported in higher risk patients with diabetes, hypertension, and hyperlipidemia [1]. Additionally, a higher reported incidence of ST elevation myocardial infarction in COVID-19 indicates a different pathophysiological mechanism promoting an acute overthrombotic status favoring intracoronary vessel thrombosis and ST elevation myocardial infarction [2]. Myocardial injury from SARS-CoV-2 infection can lead to multiple complications, including cardiomyopathies with heart failure or cardiogenic shock, venous thromboembolism, and increased incidence of cardiac arrhythmias. Our study is aimed at highlighting the importance of recognizing malignant ventricular tachyarrhythmia (VT) or ventricular fibrillation (VF) in the acute or convalescent phase of the infection.

2. Materials and Methods

This is a single-center, observational case-series study of ventricular arrhythmia in 2 COVID-19 survivors previously treated with automatic implantable cardioverter-defibrillator (AICD). We retrospectively identified patients between the period of 01/2021 and 03/2020, who were admitted to the cardiovascular ICU with VT storm and a confirmed positive COVID-19 based on reverse transcription polymerase chain reaction testing.

3. Case Presentation

3.1. Case 1. A 53-year-old woman presented with a history of repaired ventricular septal defect, atrial fibrillation, tricuspid valve endocarditis with tricuspid valvuloplasty and replacement, coronary artery disease, and biventricular heart failure with reduced left ventricular ejection fraction (40–45%) with biventricular AICD placement. Prior to her hospital visit, she complained of lightheadedness, palpitations, and experienced 1 episode of syncope. She additionally noted that her biventricular ICD had fired approximately 5 times in the past 24 hours which prompted her to present to the hospital for evaluation. Soon after being admitted, she once again lost consciousness and was noted to have VT and VF storm and received 26 shocks. Reverse transcription polymerase chain reaction testing revealed positive SARS-CoV-2. She additionally complained of mild dyspnea and denied any other COVID-19-related symptoms like fevers, chills, diarrhea, headache, or muscle aches. Initial laboratory tests were significant for hypokalemia and low-normal magnesium levels. Transthoracic echocardiography revealed reduced left ventricular ejection fraction (25–30%) with severe diffuse hypokinesis, abnormal left ventricular relaxation, and increased left ventricular filling pressures. Left ventricular size and wall thickness were normal. The bioprosthetic tricuspid valve was functioning normally. She already had coronary angiography performed 4 years ago which was unremarkable other than minor luminal irregularities in the left anterior descending artery. Electrocardiogram on admission illustrated biventricular paced rhythm with a corrected QT interval of 546 ms. AICD interrogation revealed polymorphic VF with 26 appropriate and effective shocks that terminated the arrhythmia (see Figure 1).

Her laboratory data revealed electrolyte imbalance that required replacing potassium and magnesium. She was not on any antiarrhythmic drug at home; however, she used ciprofloxacin (for spontaneous bacterial peritonitis prophylaxis) which was discontinued. She was treated with 150 mg intravenous bolus of amiodarone and then started on infusion at 1 mg/min for 6 hours which resolved her VT. Throughout her hospital course, she was treated with low molecular weight heparin. She briefly required 1-2 liters of oxygen via nasal cannula for dyspnea associated with mild COVID-19 pneumonia, which was successfully treated with a one-time dose of bamlanivimab 700 mg intravenous infusion. Prior to discharge, her QT interval had improved to 385 ms, and she was discharged in stable condition on 200 mg of oral amiodarone daily and 5 mg of Eliquis twice a day.

3.2. Case 2. An 82-year-old man with a medical history significant for coronary artery disease, coronary artery bypass grafting in 1997 complicated by VT with AICD implantation, atrial fibrillation, and atrial flutter with ablation and watchman procedure in 2016 was admitted to the hospital for complaints of exertional angina. He tested positive for SARS-CoV-2, after he underwent RT-PCR testing due to high clinical suspicion. Additionally, he complained of shortness of breath requiring 2-3 liters of supplemental oxygen via nasal cannula. He underwent left heart catheterization which revealed a severe 3 vessel disease with complete occlusion of RCA, no intervention was performed, and a decision was made to pursue medical management given high surgical risk. During his hospitalization, he developed VT storm and received 38 AICD shocks. AICD interrogation revealed 38 episodes of polymorphic ventricular tachycardia, which were not resolved with antitachycardia pacing and were then followed by 38 effective ICD shocks. Transthoracic echocardiogram was performed which revealed a moderately dilated left ventricle with 35–40% systolic function. Severe wall motion abnormality was observed predominantly in the basal to mid inferolateral and basal to mid inferoseptal segments with no evidence of intracardiac thrombus. Pacemaker leads were present in the right atrium and right ventricle (see Figure 2).

During hospitalization, he was treated with multiple intravenous antiarrhythmic agents including lidocaine, amiodarone, and esmolol. He responded well to amiodarone infusion and was subsequently switched to 400 mg twice a day of oral amiodarone with the resolution of VTs on the third day of hospitalization. His AICD settings were adjusted to lower VT detection threshold. His device settings were changed to DDD 60, and the atrioventricular delay was reduced to 180 ms. For afterload reduction, he was treated with Isordil 20 mg every 8 hours and hydralazine 50 mg every 8 hours. Electrocardiogram subsequently revealed an AV dual-paced rhythm at 60 beats per minute. A transesophageal echocardiogram was later obtained which revealed a normal left ventricular systolic function with no signs of valvular vegetations.

Cardiac magnetic resonance and VT ablation were initially considered but later canceled due to worsening of his medical condition with development of septic shock, acute renal failure, and respiratory failure from COVID-19 pneumonia. He required broad-spectrum antibiotics including vancomycin and vasopressors (vasopressin, norepinephrine, and dobutamine) for the treatment of septic shock. Due to worsening of respiratory function, he was intubated, put on mechanical ventilation, and treated with dexamethasone and remdesivir for acute respiratory distress syndrome secondary to COVID-19 pneumonia. He was managed in the cardiovascular intensive care unit during his treatment but eventually succumbed to sepsis and multiorgan failure.

4. Discussion

4.1. Potential Mechanisms of Ventricular Tachycardia/Ventricular Fibrillation Storm in COVID-19. SARS-CoV-2 infection predominantly affects the respiratory system but has been causally linked to acute myocardial injury manifesting as elevated cardiac markers, namely, troponin I and T [3, 4]. Several factors can cause myocardial injury following SARS-CoV-2 infection, including type 1 myocardial infarction due to plaque rupture, type 2 myocardial infarction due to increased oxygen demand or reduced supply, myocarditis due to direct viral cytopathic effects, or indirect effects of systemic infection or cytokine storm in a hyperinflammatory state resulting in stress cardiomyopathy [1, 2, 5, 6]. Additionally, patients with hyperglycemia are noted to

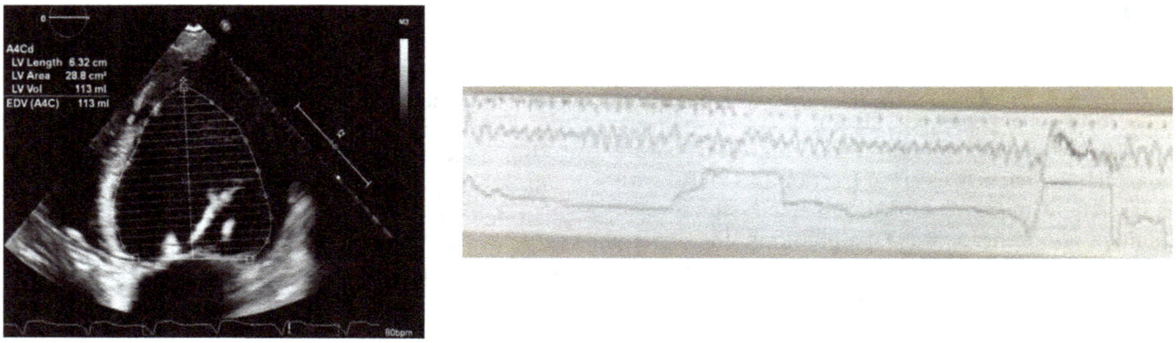

Figure 1: Case 1. Apical four-chamber view of left ventricle with Simpson disk summation method showing increased left ventricular end diastolic volume and diameter. Telemetry strip showing polymorphic ventricular fibrillation rhythm.

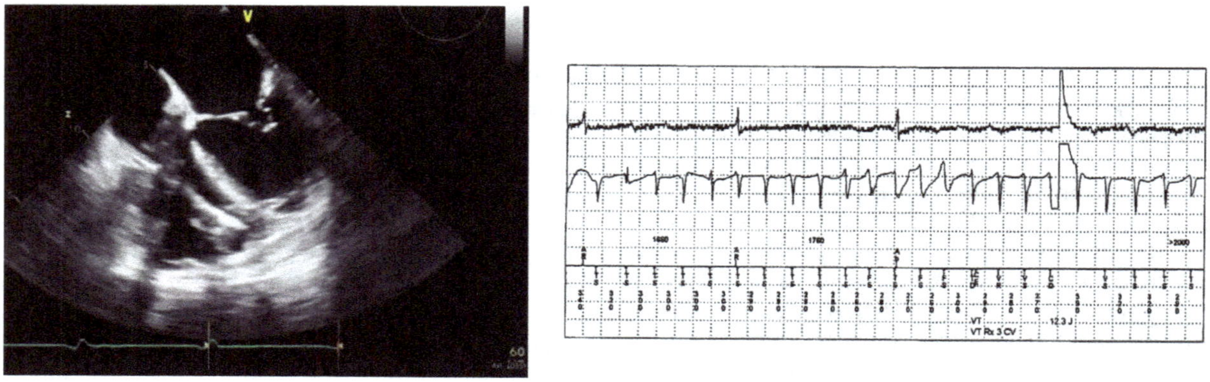

Figure 2: Case 2. Left atrium and moderately dilated left ventricle shown. Pacemaker leads present in the right ventricle. Telemetry strip showing ventricular tachycardia storm.

have a significantly higher levels of inflammatory cytokines that blunt the effects of anti-inflammatory therapy [7]. The predominant mechanisms suspected to be involved in inducing VT/VF storm in the 2 cases reported are myocarditis, systemic inflammation, hemodynamic instability and hyperadrenergic state, hypoxia and acidosis, and use of proarrhythmic drugs. The demographic data and pertinent medical history are shown in Table 1. Mechanisms responsible for the VT/VF storm pertaining to the 2 cases are discussed below (Figure 3).

4.1.1. Myocarditis. Myocarditis is the predominant mechanism of VT/VF storm in this patient cohort, which is marked by elevated cardiac high-sensitivity troponin levels as noted in both the cases described. Myocarditis due to SARS-CoV-2 infection is not generally associated with pathognomonic findings on an electrocardiogram, and often times, the common presenting symptoms of fever, chest pain, and palpitations maybe absent or obscured thus making clinical diagnosis difficult. Two large scale studies have reported acute myocarditis as the cause of SARS-CoV-2-induced myocardial injury. A cardiac autopsy study of 39 confirmed COVID-19 cases proved cardiac infection by documenting the viral genome in myocardial tissue of 60% of patients [8]. Another study identified the SARS-CoV-2 genome in 5 out of 104 endomyocardial biopsy samples with histological assessment revealing myocarditis, necrosis, and granulation tissue [9]. COVID-19-related myocarditis has been documented in several other studies; however, only few studies have demonstrated association between myocarditis and VT/VF storm in the setting of COVID-19-related myocarditis [10–14]. Tachyarrhythmias particularly nonsustained VT have been documented to be related to severity of acute illness and level of troponin elevation and found to be an independent factor of in-hospital mortality [15]. Additionally, SARS-CoV-2-related fulminant myocarditis is now a major consideration in patients who present with chest

Table 1: Demographic data and relevant comorbidities of patients presenting with ventricular tachycardia.

	Patient 1	Patient 2
Age (years)	53	82
Sex	F	M
Hx of VT	—	+
Hx of AF/AFL	+	+
Hx of CAD	+	+
LVEF (%)	40–45%	35–40%

AF: atrial fibrillation; AFL: atrial flutter; CAD: coronary artery disease; Hx: history; LVEF: left ventricular ejection fraction; VT: ventricular tachycardia.

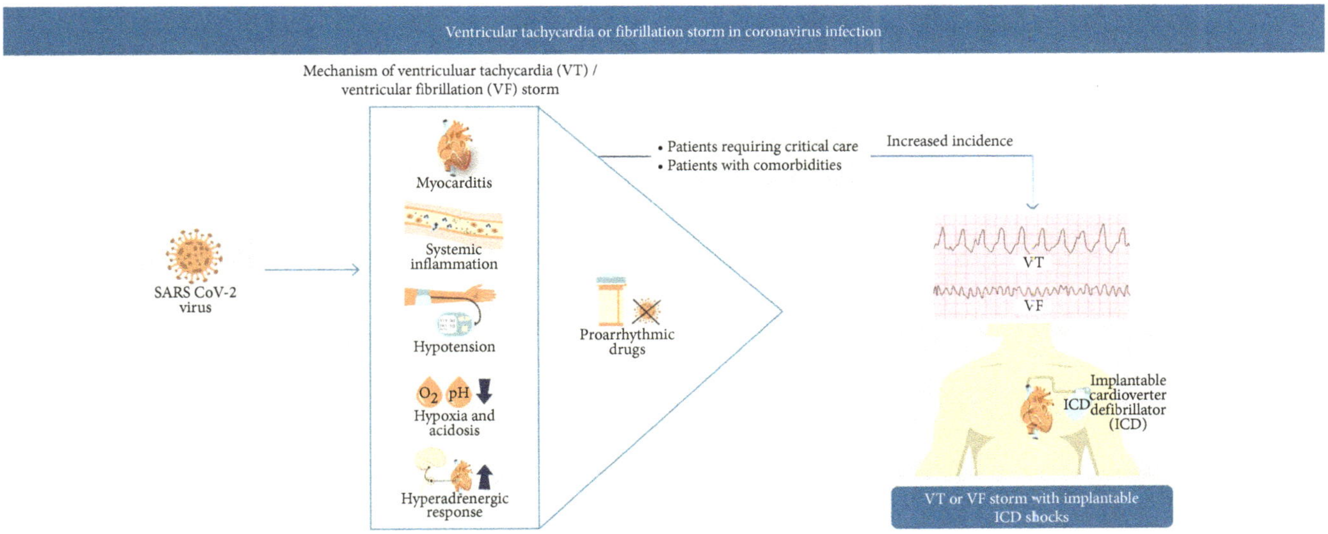

Figure 3: Potential mechanisms of VT/VF storm in COVID-19. Complications resulting from SARS-CoV-2 infection can lead to myocarditis, systemic inflammation, hypotension, hypoxia and acidosis, and a hyperadrenergic response. These along with the use of proarrhythmic drugs can lead to VT/VF storm which are more commonly observed in patients with multiple comorbidities who are critically ill. Abbreviations: COVID-19: coronavirus disease; ICD: implantable cardioverter-defibrillator; SARS-CoV-2: severe acute respiratory syndrome coronavirus 2; VF: ventricular fibrillation; VT: ventricular tachycardia.

Table 2: Diagnostic test results in patients with COVID-19 and ventricular tachycardia.

	Patient 1	Patient 2
HS troponin (ng/L)	*24*	*3,767*
QTc (ms)	*546*	*596*
BNP (pg/mL)	*232*	*435*
Serum potassium (mmol/L)	**3.1**	3.8
Serum magnesium (mmol/L)	**1.5**	2.5
Venous O_2 saturation (mmHg)	40	29
Lactic acid (mmol/L)	0.8	2.2
Sepsis	—	+
ARDS	—	+
AKI	+	+
D-dimer (μg/mL)	*6.67*	*>20.0*
Lymphocytes (%)	*11.9*	*10.2*
Ferritin (ng/mL)	*411.5*	223.4
CRP (mg/L)	6	*158.4*

Italics: above normal limit. Bold: below normal limit. AKI: acute kidney injury; ARDS: acute respiratory distress syndrome; BNP: brain natriuretic peptide; CRP: C-reactive protein; HS: high sensitivity.

pain, elevated cardiac troponins and arrhythmias with hemodynamic instability, and left ventricular dysfunction on imaging [16]. These findings suggest early measurement of cardiac biomarkers in COVID-19 may help identify patients at risk of poor clinical outcome as reflected by the mortality of case 2 in our cohort (Table 2) [16].

4.1.2. Systemic Inflammation. Another possible mechanism responsible for ventricular arrhythmia in our patient cohort is cytokine-mediated myocardial dysfunction, which can promote VT/VF storm in severe COVID-19 cases. The presence of inflammatory cytokines, i.e., interleukin-1, interleukin-6, and high-sensitivity C-reactive protein, has been associated with electrical storm in ICD implanted patients in previous studies [17]. Additionally, numerous case studies have documented an association between VT/VF storm and increased inflammatory markers like C-reactive protein in COVID-19 patients, which resolved with the resolution of inflammatory status [18, 19]. The mechanism by which inflammatory cytokines like tumor necrosis factor, interleukin-1, and interleukin-6 propagate arrhythmia involves altering function of cardiac ion channels also known as inflammatory cardiac channelopathy. These cytokines specifically alter the function of gap junctions, outward K^+ currents, and L-type Ca^{2+} channels in the atrial and ventricular myocytes leading to prolongation of action potential duration and/or QT interval which is associated with malignant arrhythmias [20]. In patients with rheumatoid arthritis, elevated inflammatory markers like IL-6 and CRP are known to be associated with QTc prolongation. Interestingly, both cases in our cohort presented with QTc prolongation > 500 ms and elevated inflammatory markers as shown in Table 2 [21]. This suggests that therapeutic interventions targeting inflammatory cytokines can help in ameliorating the effects of systemic inflammation to reduce acute cardiovascular complications including VT/VF storms while promoting recovery from multiorgan dysfunction.

4.1.3. Hemodynamic Instability and Hyperadrenergic State. Severe SARS-CoV-2 infection can cause sepsis with hemodynamic instability and shock. This can lead to organ level cardiac ischemia resulting in scarring or fibrosis. Functional electrical pathways can form in the scar tissue, creating reentrant circuits that cause ventricular arrhythmias [22].

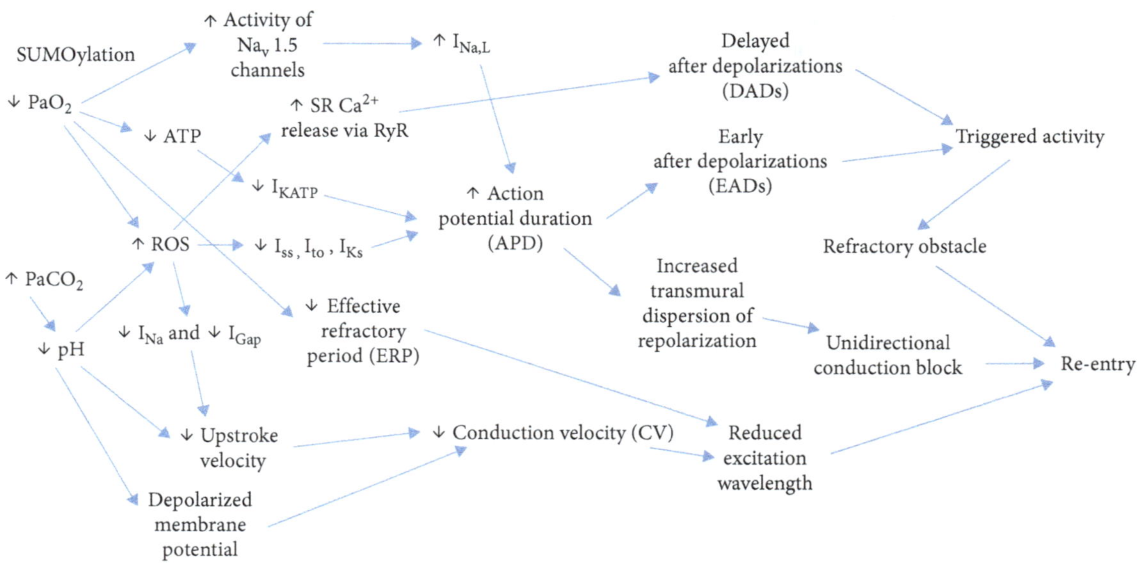

FIGURE 4: Electrophysiological mechanisms underlying ventricular arrhythmias from hypoxia and hypercapnia [23]. Decreased partial pressure of oxygen, increased partial pressure of carbon dioxide, and decreased pH lead to reduced ATP, reduced upstroke velocity, and increased ROS. These electrophysiological changes with interplay of additional variables promote arrhythmia via non-reentrant and reentrant mechanisms. Source: Lee et al. [25]. Reproduced with permission. Abbreviations: ATP: adenosine triphosphate; $PaCO_2$: partial pressure of carbon dioxide; PaO_2: partial pressure of oxygen; ROS: reactive oxygen species; RyR: ryanodine receptors; SR: sarcoplasmic reticulum.

Although scars are commonly caused by ischemic events, replacement fibrosis can also occur in nonischemic cardiomyopathies. Unfortunately, antiarrhythmic drugs tend to have poor efficacy in VAs due to scars [22].

Alternatively, as a response to cardiac injury, there may be a compensatory response with neurohumoral system activation, leading to sympathetic hyperactivity (hyperadrenergic state) and reduced vagal tone, which helps maintain cardiac output. However, if the cardiac sympathovagal imbalance continues, it creates a maladaptive environment of continued sympathetic activity resulting in cardiac tissue remodeling and ultimately paving pathways for fatal malignant arrhythmias, including electrical storm [23].

4.1.4. Hypoxia and Acidosis. Multiple studies have reported acute respiratory distress syndrome and pulmonary embolism as common complications of severe COVID-19 [24]. Resultant hypoxia can predispose patients to tachycardia which further increases oxygen demand of the cardiomyocytes. Decreased oxygen in the cardiomyocytes alters the function of multiple ion channels, including the L-type Ca^{2+} ion channel, voltage-gated sodium channels, and outward potassium currents, inducing increased oxidative stress through the generation of reactive oxygen species [25]. Additionally, acidosis secondary to hypercapnia in respiratory failure settings can cause persistent membrane depolarization and reduced phase 0 slope of the cardiac action potential in the ventricular fibers [26]. These changes act as triggers for prolonged action potential, early afterdepolarization, and delayed afterdepolarization [27]. These electrophysiological abnormalities together promote ventricular arrhythmias via both non-reentrant and reentrant mechanisms [27]. Figure 4 summarizes the mechanisms via which hypoxia and hypercapnia can lead to ventricular arrhythmias [25].

4.1.5. Proarrhythmic Drugs. It is crucial to be aware of the proarrhythmic effects of some of the drugs commonly used in the treatment of COVID-19. In the context of systemic inflammation, hemodynamic, and/or metabolic instability, proarrhythmic drugs used in the treatment of COVID-19 should be targeted to reduce the burden of arrhythmias. Case 1 received a one-time dose of bamlanivimab, and case 2 was treated with a 5-day course of dexamethasone and remdesivir in combination. Other than systemic steroids, no other anti-inflammatory drugs were used in the two reported cases.

One group of drugs that has been extensively researched during the COVID-19 pandemic is chloroquine and hydroxychloroquine (HCQ). They are mainly used for their antimalarial properties; however, these drugs received emergency use authorization during the early days of the pandemic based on limited-quality and nonrandomized data. Multiple studies have now concluded that chloroquine or HCQ does not improve outcomes in SARS-CoV-2 infected individuals or act as a prophylaxis to prevent symptomatic infection [28]. Notably, the RECOVERY trial confirmed this analysis by reporting no significant improvement in 28-day mortality with the use of chloroquine or HCQ [29]. Additionally, the chronic use of chloroquine or HCQ is associated with QTc prolongation by binding to and inhibiting the hERG-potassium channel, thereby blocking the delayed rectifier potassium current leading to prolonged ventricular repolarization. Delayed ventricular repolarization enables early afterdepolarizations, which can trigger torsades de pointes and other ventricular arrhythmias [30].

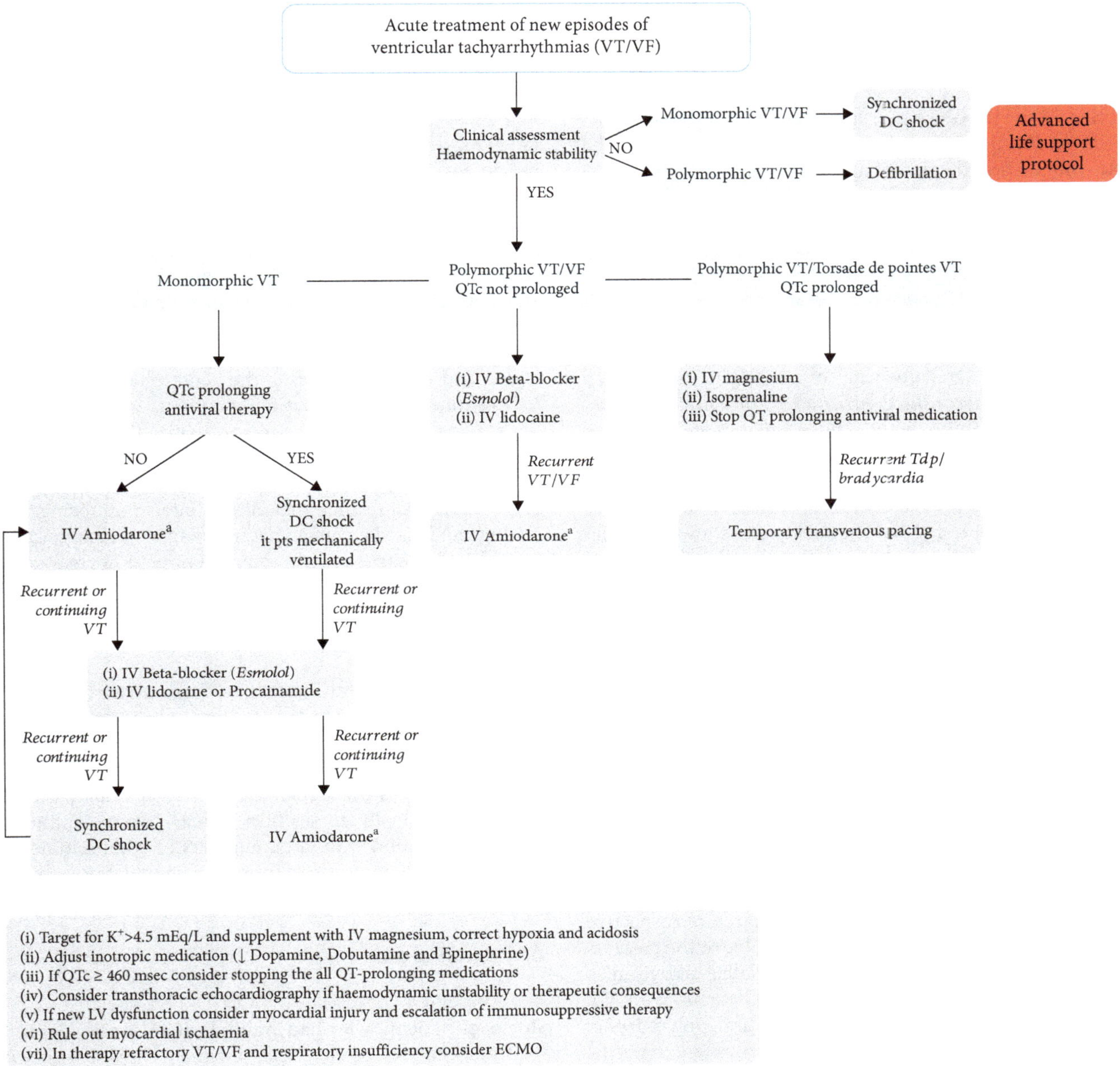

FIGURE 5: Acute treatment of new episodes of ventricular tachyarrhythmias (VT/VF) [40]. Recommendations for treatment of monomorphic and polymorphic ventricular arrhythmias based on clinical assessment and hemodynamic stability. The benefit of IV amiodarone treatment should be balanced against the polymorphic risk in patients taking QR-prolonging antiviral therapy. Reproduced from https://www.escardio.org/Education/COVID-19-and-Cardiology/ESC-COVID-19-Guidance with permission from The European Society of Cardiology 2021. Abbreviations: DC: direct current; ECMO: extracorporeal membrane oxygenation; IV: intravenous; LV: left ventricle; Pts: patients; TdP: torsade de pointes; VF: ventricular fibrillation; VT: ventricular tachycardia.

Use of chloroquine or HCQ was initially combined with azithromycin which is used to treat gram-positive and atypical bacterial respiratory infections. Additionally, azithromycin has an anti-inflammatory effect via the down-regulation of inflammatory cytokines. Numerous studies at the start of the pandemic reported that patients treated with azithromycin in addition to HCQ had a reduction in detectable viral load, which led to widespread use of the HCQ-azithromycin combination in COVID-19 patients [31]. However, randomized trials have now demonstrated more adverse events, including QTc prolongation in patients who received the HCQ-azithromycin combination [32]. In addition to QTc prolongation, sustained and non-sustained monomorphic ventricular tachycardias have also been reported with the combination of these drugs [33]. Therefore, the CDC recommends against the use of HCQ and azithromycin in hospitalized or nonhospitalized patients as the cardiac risk imposed by the concurrent use of these medications increases the risk of serious cardiac arrhythmias.

Based on anecdotal evidence, protease inhibitors like lopinavir and ritonavir (KALETRA) have also been considered for the treatment of SARS-CoV-2 infection. However, results of 2 large control trials, RECOVERY and SOLIDARITY, have reported failure to reduce mortality, need for mechanical ventilation, or duration of hospitalization [29, 34]. A study on the triple combination therapy of azithromycin, lopinavir/ritonavir, and chloroquine or HCQ resulted in extreme QTC prolongation in 23% of hospitalized COVID-19 patients, with a TdP incidence in 1.14% of study population [35]. Studies have documented association of remdesivir with sinus bradycardia but no such association has been reported with hemodynamic instability or ventricular arrhythmias [36].

4.2. Risk and Consequences of COVID-19-Associated Ventricular Tachycardia/Ventricular Fibrillation Storm. Cardiac viral infection with a high inflammatory burden predisposes patients to arrhythmias, especially if other metabolic dysfunctions are present. According to the American College of Cardiology, the overall incidence of arrhythmias due to COVID-19 is 16.7%. The incidence is lower in mild infection (8.9%) and increases to 44.4% in severe illnesses [6]. Supraventricular tachycardia is the most common type of arrhythmia noted in COVID-19 patients [37]. A study reported that sinus tachycardia resulting from hypoxia, hypovolemia, and fever was the most common supraventricular tachycardia, followed by atrial fibrillation [37]. Other supraventricular tachycardias such as atrioventricular nodal reentry tachycardia and conduction blocks continue to be reported but are not well documented due to the benign nature of these arrhythmias [38].

Numerous studies have documented increased proportions of patients developing ventricular arrhythmias in COVID-19. A study by Guo et al. reported VT/VF in 5.9% of COVID-19 patients, with the majority of the cases in patients with myocardial injury [4]. In a large retrospective survey of 827 patients from 12 countries, 21% of the patients admitted for COVID-19 developed ventricular arrhythmias defined as VT, nonsustained VT, or VF. Patients with VT had equal proportions of monomorphic and polymorphic VT (4% each), and 3.4% had VF [39]. Ventricular arrhythmias were associated with significant mortality when compared to atrial arrhythmias, and only 38% of these patients survived to hospital discharge. Other than isolated case reports, observational studies documenting the prevalence of VT/VF storm observed in COVID-19 patients are still lacking [18, 19, 40]. Collectively, these studies suggest that malignant ventricular arrhythmias including VT/VF storm in the context of COVID-19 are more commonly observed in patients with comorbidities and those requiring intensive care unit admission.

4.3. Treatment, Prevention, and Monitoring. COVID-19-related VAs in acute settings should be treated with intravenous amiodarone (American College of Cardiology/American Heart Association–Class of Recommendation 1 and Level of Evidence A). For cases of new malignant VAs unrelated to QT prolongation, imaging via transthoracic echocardiography is warranted to assess ventricular function. Cardiac magnetic resonance imaging should also be considered for myocardial involvement. According to European Society of Cardiology guidelines, intravenous lidocaine is a less effective alternative to amiodarone but may be used, especially if underlying ischemia is suspected (Figure 5) [41]. Temporary pacemaker implantation for overdrive termination or antitachycardia pacing is an option for emergency cases. Following recovery from acute SARS-CoV-2 infection, the need for prevention with either catheter ablation or ICD implantation for secondary prophylaxis should be considered [41]. Additionally, a personalized approach for ICD programming is required to balance unnecessary ICD shocks vs. detecting potential life-threatening VAs.

The general consensus among experts is that patients who developed overt cardiac disease should be closely monitored and reassessed during the acute phase of the SARS-CoV-2 infection. Risk stratifying patients is important during recovery. Some have proposed that patients at high risk should receive repeat transthoracic echocardiography and an electrocardiogram 2–6 months after COVID-19 diagnosis [42]. Additional testing, including Holter monitoring, stress testing, and cardiac magnetic resonance imaging, can be considered in some cases to guide return to normal activity or aerobic exercise, including competitive sports.

5. Study Limitations

This study has several limitations. First, given the observational nature of the study, the association between ICD shocks for COVID-19 induced VT/VF storm cannot be interpreted as causal. Second, in patients with a history of arrhythmias, numerous factors other than COVID-19 may play a role in ICD shocks. Finally, this cohort of ICD patients is a unique patient population with large numbers of comorbidities that may not be representative of the general population and hence reduces generalizability of these findings.

6. Conclusions

We presented 2 cases of COVID-19-associated VT/VF storm in patients who had multiple ICD shocks delivered. The mechanisms of electrical storm in COVID-19 can be attributed to multiple mechanisms as detailed above. Other than previously published isolated case reports, this is the first case-series study that details the possible mechanisms, risks, and complications of VT/VF storm as a complication of COVID-19. The true burden of electrical storm in COVID-19 may not be fully appreciated due to the incomplete understanding of virus-induced injury to the myocardial conduction system and a large proportion of out-of-hospital mortality. Future investigations of COVID-19-related malignant ventricular arrhythmias are needed to risk-stratify and adopt an effective long-term monitoring and treatment plan in this population.

Consent

Due to the retrospective nature of the study, institutional review board of the University of Cincinnati waived the need for informed consent in both cases.

References

[1] N. D'Onofrio, L. Scisciola, C. Sardu et al., "Glycated ACE2 receptor in diabetes: open door for SARS-COV-2 entry in cardiomyocyte," *Cardiovascular Diabetology*, vol. 20, no. 1, p. 99, 2021.

[2] R. Marfella, P. Paolisso, C. Sardu et al., "SARS-COV-2 colonizes coronary thrombus and impairs heart microcirculation bed in asymptomatic SARS-CoV-2 positive subjects with acute myocardial infarction," *Critical Care / the Society of Critical Care Medicine*, vol. 25, no. 1, p. 217, 2021.

[3] C. Huang, Y. Wang, X. Li et al., "Clinical features of patients infected with 2019 novel coronavirus in Wuhan, China," *In The Lancet*, vol. 395, no. 10223, pp. 497–506, 2020.

[4] T. Guo, Y. Fan, M. Chen et al., "Cardiovascular implications of fatal outcomes of patients with coronavirus disease 2019 (COVID-19)," *JAMA Cardiology*, vol. 5, no. 7, pp. 811–818, 2020.

[5] A. A. F. de Vries, "SARS-CoV-2/COVID-19: a primer for cardiologists," *Netherlands Heart Journal: Monthly Journal of the Netherlands Society of Cardiology and the Netherlands Heart Foundation*, vol. 28, no. 7-8, pp. 366–383, 2020.

[6] M. Imazio, "COVID-19 as a possible cause of myocarditis and pericarditis. American College of Cardiology," June, 2021 https://www.acc.org/latest-in-cardiology/articles/2021/02/05/19/37/covid-19-as-a-possible-cause-of-myocarditis-and-pericarditis.

[7] R. Marfella, P. Paolisso, C. Sardu et al., "Negative impact of hyperglycaemia on tocilizumab therapy in Covid-19 patients," *Diabetes & Metabolism*, vol. 46, no. 5, pp. 403–405, 2020.

[8] D. Lindner, A. Fitzek, H. Bräuninger et al., "Association of cardiac infection with SARS-CoV-2 in confirmed COVID-19 autopsy cases," *JAMA Cardiology*, vol. 5, no. 11, pp. 1281–1285, 2020.

[9] F. Escher, H. Pietsch, G. Aleshcheva et al., "Detection of viral SARS-CoV-2 genomes and histopathological changes in endomyocardial biopsies," *ESC Heart Failure*, vol. 7, no. 5, pp. 2440–2447, 2020.

[10] S. Sala, G. Peretto, M. Gramegna et al., "Acute myocarditis presenting as a reverse Tako-Tsubo syndrome in a patient with SARS-CoV-2 respiratory infection," *European Heart Journal*, vol. 41, no. 19, pp. 1861-1862, 2020.

[11] J.-H. Zeng, Y.-X. Liu, J. Yuan et al., "First case of COVID-19 complicated with fulminant myocarditis: a case report and insights," *Infection*, vol. 48, no. 5, pp. 773–777, 2020.

[12] A. Beri and K. Kotak, "Cardiac injury, arrhythmia, and sudden death in a COVID-19 patient," *HeartRhythm Case Reports*, vol. 6, no. 7, pp. 367–369, 2020.

[13] H. Hu, F. Ma, X. Wei, and Y. Fang, "Coronavirus fulminant myocarditis treated with glucocorticoid and human immunoglobulin," *European Heart Journal*, vol. 42, no. 2, p. 206, 2021.

[14] G. Tavazzi, C. Pellegrini, M. Maurelli et al., "Myocardial localization of coronavirus in COVID-19 cardiogenic shock," *European Journal of Heart Failure*, vol. 22, no. 5, pp. 911–915, 2020.

[15] V. Russo, M. Di Maio, F. F. Mottola et al., "Clinical characteristics and prognosis of hospitalized COVID-19 patients with incident sustained tachyarrhythmias: a multicenter observational study," *European Journal of Clinical Investigation*, vol. 50, no. 12, article e13387, 2020.

[16] V. Russo, R. Bottino, A. Carbone et al., "COVID-19 and heart: from clinical features to pharmacological implications," *Journal of Clinical Medicine Research*, vol. 9, no. 6, p. 1944, 2020.

[17] F. Streitner, J. Kuschyk, C. Veltmann et al., "Role of proinflammatory markers and NT-proBNP in patients with an implantable cardioverter-defibrillator and an electrical storm," *Cytokine*, vol. 47, no. 3, pp. 166–172, 2009.

[18] G. Mitacchione, M. Schiavone, A. Gasperetti, and G. B. Forleo, "Ventricular tachycardia storm management in a COVID-19 patient: a case report," *European Heart Journal. Case Reports*, vol. 4, no. FI1, pp. 1–6, 2020.

[19] O. Elsaid, P. A. McCullough, K. M. Tecson, R. S. Williams, and A. Yoon, "Ventricular fibrillation storm in coronavirus 2019," *The American Journal of Cardiology*, vol. 135, pp. 177–180, 2020.

[20] P. E. Lazzerini, F. Laghi-Pasini, M. Boutjdir, and P. L. Capecchi, "Cardioimmunology of arrhythmias: the role of autoimmune and inflammatory cardiac channelopathies," *Nature Reviews. Immunology*, vol. 19, no. 1, pp. 63-64, 2019.

[21] P. E. Lazzerini, M. Acampa, P. L. Capecchi et al., "Antiarrhythmic potential of anticytokine therapy in rheumatoid arthritis: tocilizumab reduces corrected QT interval by controlling systemic inflammation," *Arthritis Care & Research*, vol. 67, no. 3, pp. 332–339, 2015.

[22] W. G. Stevenson, "Ventricular scars and ventricular tachycardia," *Transactions of the American Clinical and Climatological Association*, vol. 120, pp. 403–412, 2009.

[23] M. Kalla, N. Herring, and D. J. Paterson, "Cardiac sympatho-vagal balance and ventricular arrhythmia," *Autonomic Neuroscience: Basic & Clinical*, vol. 199, pp. 29–37, 2016.

[24] A. Garcia-Ortega, G. Oscullo, F. Calvillo et al., "Incidence, risk factors, and thrombotic load of pulmonary embolism in patients hospitalized for COVID-19 infection," *The Journal of Infection*, vol. 82, no. 2, pp. 261–269, 2021.

[25] S. Lee, G. Li, T. Liu, and G. Tse, "COVID-19: electrophysiological mechanisms underlying sudden cardiac death during exercise with facemasks," *Medical Hypotheses*, vol. 144, article 110177, 2020.

[26] Y. Kagiyama, J. L. Hill, and L. S. Gettes, "Interaction of acidosis and increased extracellular potassium on action potential characteristics and conduction in guinea pig ventricular muscle," *Circulation Research*, vol. 51, no. 5, pp. 614–623, 1982.

[27] G. Tse, "Mechanisms of cardiac arrhythmias," *Journal of Arrhythmia*, vol. 32, no. 2, pp. 75–81, 2016.

[28] J. Geleris, Y. Sun, J. Platt et al., "Observational study of hydroxychloroquine in hospitalized patients with Covid-19," *The New England Journal of Medicine*, vol. 382, no. 25, pp. 2411–2418, 2020.

[29] RECOVERY Collaborative Group, "Dexamethasone in hospitalized patients with Covid-19," *The New England Journal of Medicine*, vol. 384, no. 8, pp. 693–704, 2021.

[30] L. Jankelson, G. Karam, M. L. Becker, L. A. Chinitz, and M.-C. Tsai, "QT prolongation, torsades de pointes, and sudden death with short courses of chloroquine or hydroxychloroquine as used in COVID-19: a systematic review," *Heart Rhythm: The Official Journal of the Heart Rhythm Society*, vol. 17, no. 9, pp. 1472–1479, 2020.

[31] P. Gautret, J.-C. Lagier, P. Parola et al., "Hydroxychloroquine and azithromycin as a treatment of COVID-19: results of an

open-label non-randomized clinical trial," *International Journal of Antimicrobial Agents*, vol. 56, no. 1, article 105949, 2020.

[32] A. B. Cavalcanti, F. G. Zampieri, R. G. Rosa et al., "Hydroxychloroquine with or without azithromycin in mild-to-moderate Covid-19," *The New England Journal of Medicine*, vol. 383, no. 21, pp. 2041–2052, 2020.

[33] M. Saleh, J. Gabriels, D. Chang et al., "Effect of chloroquine, hydroxychloroquine, and azithromycin on the corrected QT interval in patients with SARS-CoV-2 infection," *Circulation. Arrhythmia and Electrophysiology*, vol. 13, no. 6, article e008662, 2020.

[34] WHO Solidarity Trial Consortium, H. Pan, R. Peto et al., "Repurposed antiviral drugs for Covid-19 - interim WHO solidarity trial results," *The New England Journal of Medicine*, vol. 384, no. 6, pp. 497–511, 2021.

[35] V. Russo, A. Carbone, F. F. Mottola et al., "Effect of triple combination therapy with lopinavir-ritonavir, azithromycin, and hydroxychloroquine on QT interval and arrhythmic risk in hospitalized COVID-19 patients," *Frontiers in Pharmacology*, vol. 11, p. 582348.h, 2020.

[36] E. Attena, S. Albani, A. E. Maraolo et al., "Remdesivir-induced bradycardia in COVID-19: a single center prospective study," *Circulation. Arrhythmia and Electrophysiology*, vol. 14, no. 7, article e009811, 2021.

[37] Y. Wang, L. Chen, J. Wang et al., "Electrocardiogram analysis of patients with different types of COVID-19," *Annals of Noninvasive Electrocardiology: The Official Journal of the International Society for Holter and Noninvasive Electrocardiology, Inc*, vol. 25, no. 6, article e12806, 2020.

[38] B. Long, W. J. Brady, R. E. Bridwell et al., "Electrocardiographic manifestations of COVID-19," *The American Journal of Emergency Medicine*, vol. 41, pp. 96–103, 2021.

[39] E. J. Coromilas, S. Kochav, I. Goldenthal et al., "Worldwide survey of COVID-19-associated arrhythmias," *Circulation. Arrhythmia and Electrophysiology*, vol. 14, no. 3, article e009458, 2021.

[40] F. Vetta, L. Marinaccio, G. Vetta, and D. Marchese, "Electrical storm in a patient with COVID-19 treated with hydroxychloroquine: a case report," *SAGE Open Medical Case Reports*, vol. 8, p. 2050313X2097421, 2020.

[41] ESC guidance for the diagnosis and management of CV disease during the COVID-19 pandemic(n.d.). Retrieved September 11, 2021, from https://www.escardio.org/Education/COVID-19-and-Cardiology/ESC-COVID-19-Guidance.

[42] R. D. Mitrani, N. Dabas, and J. J. Goldberger, "COVID-19 cardiac injury: implications for long-term surveillance and outcomes in survivors," *Heart Rhythm: The Official Journal of the Heart Rhythm Society*, vol. 17, no. 11, pp. 1984–1990, 2020.

Subaortic Membrane Papillary Fibroelastoma

Robyn Bryde,[1] **Kevin Landolfo**,[2] **Jordan C. Ray**,[3] **Pragnesh Parikh**,[3] **Qihui "Jim" Zhai**,[4] **and Carolyn Landolfo**[3]

[1]*Department of Internal Medicine, Mayo Clinic Florida, 4500 San Pablo Road South, Jacksonville, Florida 32224, USA*
[2]*Department of Cardiothoracic Surgery, Mayo Clinic Florida, 4500 San Pablo Road South, Jacksonville, Florida 32224, USA*
[3]*Department of Cardiovascular Disease, Mayo Clinic Florida, 4500 San Pablo Road South, Jacksonville, Florida 32224, USA*
[4]*Department of Pathology, Mayo Clinic Florida, 4500 San Pablo Road South, Jacksonville, Florida 32224, USA*

Correspondence should be addressed to Robyn Bryde; bryde.robyn@mayo.edu

Academic Editor: Ertugrul Ercan

A 61-year-old male presented for an annual exam and received a transthoracic echocardiogram (TTE) which revealed a mobile mass arising from a subaortic membrane. Further investigations with a transesophageal echocardiogram (TEE) and cardiac computerized tomography angiography (CTA) confirmed the presence of a mobile 9 mm × 3 mm mass on a subaortic membrane. Cardiothoracic surgery was performed with an open operation removing the mass and subaortic membrane. Upon visual inspection, the mass was likened to a sea anemone and immunohistochemical staining performed pathologically confirmed the diagnosis of cardiac papillary fibroelastoma. This case represents the first reported example of a cardiac papillary fibroelastoma (PFE) arising from a subaortic membrane. Although PFEs are benign cardiac tumors, proper identification and consideration for excision of these lesions may be indicated to prevent thromboembolic complications.

1. Introduction

Cardiac papillary fibroelastomas (PFEs) ensue as the second most common form of primary cardiac tumors in the adult population and are frequently found incidentally during cardiac imaging [1, 2]. Approximately 85% of PFEs are isolated to valvular surfaces in the following order of frequency: aortic, mitral, tricuspid, and pulmonary valves [1]. The remaining 15% of tumors involve nonvalvular sites, typically left-sided endocardial surfaces. We present a rare case of a PFE arising from a subaortic membrane, which has not been reported previously. The tumor and subaortic membrane were surgically resected without complications.

2. Case Report

A 61-year-old gentleman presented for a health maintenance examination. His medical history was significant for diabetes mellitus type 2, hypertension, hyperlipidemia, and IgM monoclonal gammopathy of unknown significance. He reported no symptoms and maintained an active lifestyle by exercising several times per week. Physical exam findings revealed a BP of 139/81 and heart rate of 70 beats per minute with a regular rate and rhythm and no murmurs or gallop. Other systems were unremarkable, including the absence of systemic symptoms. The patient's baseline ECG showed minor abnormalities. In the setting of chronic hypertension and ECG abnormalities, a TTE was obtained and showed normal left ventricular size and function, but incidentally revealed a subaortic membrane in addition to a highly mobile mass arising from the membrane (Figure 1(a)). Differential diagnosis of the mass included endocardial tumor, thrombus, or endocarditis. Due to the highly mobile nature of the mass, endocardial thrombus was less likely. Additionally, in the absence of clinical evidence of infection, endocarditis was ruled out. The patient was referred to cardiovascular medicine for further investigation of the cardiac mass.

TEE confirmed the presence of a mobile 9 mm × 3 mm mass on the subaortic membrane within the LVOT suspicious for a PFE (Figure 1(b)) (video file 1). No Doppler evidence of

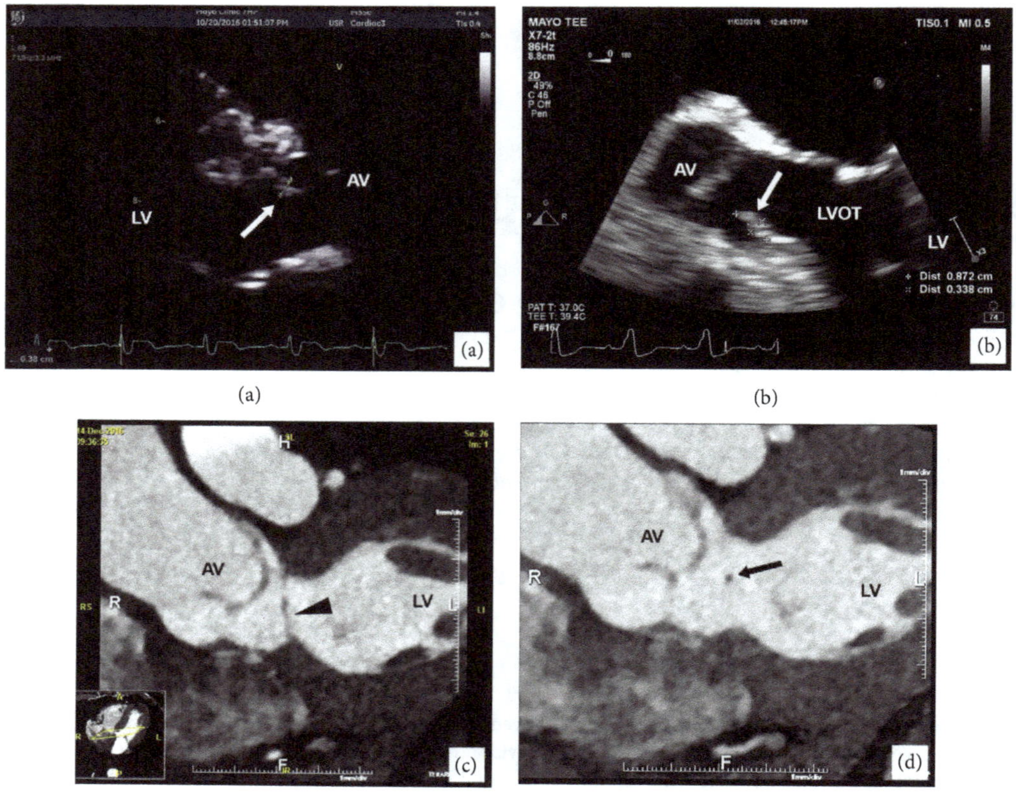

Figure 1: (a) TTE imaging of a subaortic membrane and mass (arrow) on the anterior wall of the LVOT. (b) TEE imaging showing the mass (arrow) in close proximity to the aortic valve. (c) CTA showing a subaortic membrane (arrowhead) with an area of extension, likely representing a mass (arrow) in (d).

significant left ventricular outflow tract (LVOT) obstruction was present; however, due to the size, mobility, and location of the mass, cardiothoracic surgery was consulted for surgical removal of the mass.

In preparation for surgery, the patient received a preoperative cardiac CTA which showed an insignificant coronary atherosclerotic plaque and confirmed the presence of the mass on a nonobstructive subaortic membrane 11 mm from the aortic valve (Figures 1(c) and 1(d)).

The operation was performed through a median sternotomy, and the patient was placed on cardiopulmonary bypass. Inspection of the LVOT revealed a multifaceted mass extending from a partial subaortic membrane, the appearance of which was consistent with a papillary fibroelastoma. The mass was excised and the subaortic membrane was dissected to the muscular portion of the septum (Figure 2(a)). The specimen was submerged in water revealing the frond-like appearance which can be likened to a sea anemone (Figure 2(b)). The patient had an uneventful postoperative course.

Histologically, hematoxylin and eosin (H&E) stain of the specimen revealed branching papillae (Figure 2(c)) which were avascular and rich in collagen (Figure 2(d)). CD34 stain highlighted the surface composed of a single layer of endothelial cells (Figure 2(e)). The pathologic examination confirmed the diagnosis of PFE.

3. Discussion

PFEs are the second most common primary cardiac tumor after myxomas, accounting for approximately 5% to 15% of all cardiac tumors [1]. Additionally, they are the most common type of valvular tumor and usually arise from the mid portion of the valve [1, 3]. PFEs preferentially involve the aortic, mitral, tricuspid, and least commonly the pulmonary valve. These lesions can be rarely found on endocardial surfaces.

The pathogenesis of PFEs remains controversial with origins related to reactive, hamartomatous, thrombotic, viral, or neoplastic processes [4]. Differential diagnosis includes other cardiac tumors (myxoma, fibroma, and rhabdomyoma), thrombi, vegetations (sterile or septic), calcifications, and Lambl's excrescences. Location, mobility, and patient demographics can be used to further characterize PFEs from other cardiac masses.

After surgical excision, submerging the specimen in water will remove adherent clot and reveal the unique appearance which can be likened to a sea anemone with frond-like arms arising from a pedunculated stalk. Diagnosis is confirmed by immunohistochemical staining with Alcian blue, CD34, and elastin revealing mucopolysaccharide, endothelial, and elastic composition, respectively [2].

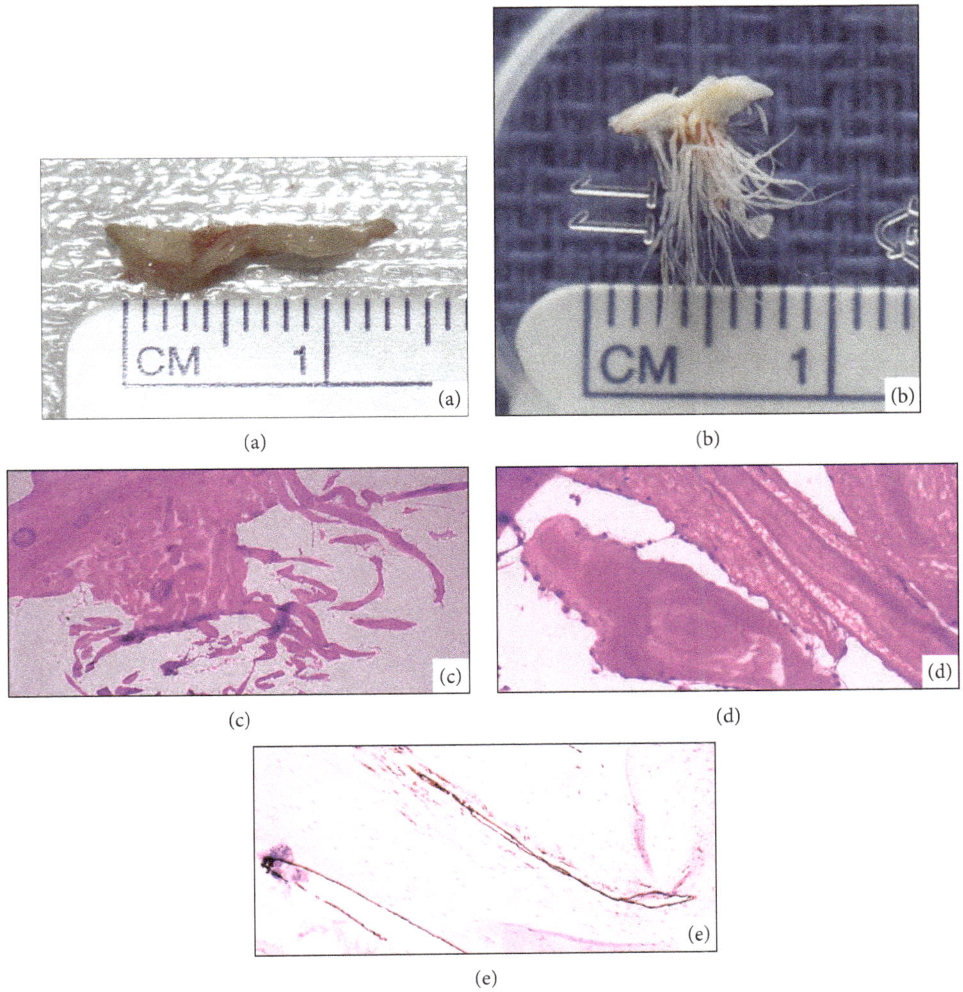

FIGURE 2: Gross specimens of the resected subaortic membrane (a) and mass (b) which has the classic frond-like appearance after being submerged in water. Histopathology with H&E stain revealing multiple papillae (c) which are avascular and rich in collagen (d) and CD34 staining highlighting the dark single layer of epithelial cells lining the mass.

Most cases are found in asymptomatic patients as incidental findings during cardiac imaging. Symptomatic patients usually present with complications related to thromboembolic events such as transient ischemic attacks, stroke, chest pain, myocardial infarction, syncope, and blindness. Embolism occurs from either the tumor itself which is soft and flimsy or from adherent clot localized within the fronds. Because PFEs more commonly arise from the higher pressure ventricular surface of valves, they have a higher rate of thromboembolism (34%) in comparison to tumors arising from the lower pressure atrial chambers such as myxomas (24%) [3].

There is general agreement that symptomatic patients be treated with surgical intervention. In asymptomatic patients, surgical intervention should be considered for mobile tumors and/or size > 1 cm [5].

4. Conclusion

Cardiac papillary fibroelastomas are rare and benign cardiac tumors with the majority occurring on left-sided cardiac valves. This case presents a novel example of a PFE emanating from a subaortic membrane. Although PFEs typically present as asymptomatic incidental findings on imaging, proper identification is important to prevent thromboembolic events. Treatment with surgical resection tends to be curative and with low risk of recurrence [1].

Abbreviations

AV: Aortic valve
CTA: Computerized tomography angiography
LV: Left ventricle
LVOT: Left ventricular outflow tract
PFE: Papillary fibroelastoma
TTE: Transthoracic echocardiogram
TEE: Transesophageal echocardiogram.

References

[1] R. M. Gowda, I. A. Khan, C. K. Nair, N. J. Mehta, B. C. Vasavada, and T. J. Sacchi, "Cardiac papillary fibroelastoma: a comprehensive analysis of 725 cases," *American Heart Journal*, vol. 146, no. 3, pp. 404–410, 2003.

[2] J. F. Val-Bernal, M. Mayorga, M. F. Garijo, D. Val, and J. F. Nistal, "Cardiac papillary fibroelastoma: retrospective clinicopathologic study of 17 tumors with resection at a single institution and literature review," *Pathology - Research and Practice*, vol. 209, no. 4, pp. 208–214, 2013.

[3] A. W. ElBardissi, J. A. Dearani, R. C. Daly et al., "Survival after resection of primary cardiac tumors: a 48-year experience," *Circulation*, vol. 118, 14_Supplement_1, pp. S7–S15, 2008.

[4] A. N. Kurup, H. D. Tazelaar, W. D. Edwards et al., "Iatrogenic cardiac papillary fibroelastoma: a study of 12 cases (1990 to 2000)," *Human Pathology*, vol. 33, no. 12, pp. 1165–1169, 2002.

[5] G. Mariscalco, V. D. Bruno, P. Borsani, C. Dominici, and A. Sala, "Papillary fibroelastoma: insight to a primary cardiac valve tumor," *Journal of Cardiac Surgery*, vol. 25, no. 2, pp. 198–205, 2010.

Wedged Sensor in Distress? Lessons Learned from Troubleshooting Dampened Transmitted PA Waveforms of CardioMEMS Device

Robby Singh,[1] **Santo Scarfone**,[2] **and Marcel Zughaib**[1]

[1]*Providence Hospital, Michigan State University, USA*
[2]*Georgetown University, USA*

Correspondence should be addressed to Robby Singh; robby9697@gmail.com

Academic Editor: Hajime Kataoka

Introduction. Cardiovascular disease is a leading cause of morbidity and mortality with heart failure constituting a large portion of this spectrum. Heart failure patients have 90-day readmission rates of nearly 41% associated with a high expense. Numerous strategies to reduce readmissions have been attempted with the CardioMEMS pulmonary artery pressure monitoring system as one of the more successful ones. As this device becomes used more frequently, it is important to recognize procedural complications. We present of a rare complication where a patient underwent successful device placement and was subsequently found to have dampened waveforms which were due to device migration. *Case Report.* A 79-year-old male underwent successful CardioMEMS placement due to recurrent heart failure hospitalizations. 6 months later, the transmitted waveforms appeared dampened, and repeat angiography revealed a device that had migrated. Rather than abandoning the device, it was recalibrated and continued to transmit data and helped manage the patient's heart failure. *Conclusion.* CardioMEMS is a cost-effective tool to help reduce heart failure hospitalizations. Device migration is a rare complication and can lead to inaccurate data. However, as seen in this case, the device can be successfully recalibrated and can continue to be utilized to help reduce heart failure admissions.

1. Introduction

Cardiovascular disease (CVD) is a leading cause of morbidity and mortality worldwide and in the US and encompasses a wide variety of diseases. Heart failure constitutes a large portion of this spectrum with close to 6 million adults affected in the US [1]. That number is expected to increase over the next 15 years with CVD-related costs projected to reach up to $1.1 trillion, a large portion of which can be attributed to heart failure (HF) rehospitalizations [2]. Clinical trials have shown that HF patients have 90-day readmission rates of nearly 41% with a mean per-patient expense of $16,000 [2]. Further, the average lifetime expense of each HF patient is roughly $83,980, 80% of which is thought to be accumulated during these hospitalizations [2]. During the final two years of life of HF patients, costs are estimated to be $156,000 [3]. Chronic HF cases are expected to reach 8 million by 2030 and HF management costs to increase two- to threefold [3]; patients and healthcare providers alike face a significant financial burden that has been attempted to be addressed by multiple novel strategies.

While guideline-directed medical therapy with regular outpatient follow-up has long been a cornerstone of heart failure treatment, the CHAMPION trial found a significant reduction in heart failure hospitalizations in patients who underwent a CardioMEMS device placement [4, 5]. This pulmonary artery pressure (PAP) remote monitoring device has proven to be an effective tool for treating HF. The PAP sensor system is comprised of a "... coil and a pressure-sensitive capacitor encased in a hermetically sealed capsule covered by silicone" [6]. The CardioMEMS device is placed in the distal pulmonary artery (PA) branch, and the coil and capacitor create an electrical circuit which monitors the pressure fluctuation in the PA as frequencies in the form of wavelengths

[6]. This information is paramount in treating heart failure patients with physicians able to make dynamic adjustments of treatment regimens and being able to see nearly real-time changes in patients which help reduce heart failure-related hospitalizations.

Although the CardioMEMS system is a relatively safe device, it can rarely be associated with adverse events, with less than 3% of patients experiencing an adverse event [7]. Pulmonary injury or hemoptysis is the most common complication, roughly 18% of all complications but overall procedure complication incidence of only 2% [6]. Since FDA approval in 2014, thousands of CardioMEMS devices have been implanted worldwide, and there have been only 46 instances of sensor failure, migration, or malfunction, "... of which 35 required recalibrations, 13 reimplantations, and 11 hospitalizations" [7]. We herein present such a case where a patient underwent CardioMEMS device placement and was subsequently found to have dampened waveforms which were found to be a result of device migration.

2. Case Report

A 79-year-old male with past medical history of coronary artery disease and prior coronary artery bypass graft surgery, multiple myeloma on long-term immunotherapy, hypertension, diabetes, and cardiomyopathy presented with worsening dyspnea on exertion, peripheral edema, and scrotal edema. The patient had had a heart failure-related hospitalization in the previous year and the presenting NYHA II-III symptoms prompted CardioMEMS device placement. A right heart catheterization with angiography was performed on July 2018 that revealed suitable target vessels for device placement (Figure 1). A CardioMEMS device was successfully deployed (Figure 2), and good quality waveforms were transmitted and recorded (Figure 3). The patient tolerated the procedure well and was discharged safely without complications. For the next 6 months, the patient did not have any heart failure hospitalizations and transmitted daily readings from the CardioMEMS device that revealed a well-controlled PA diastolic pressure.

However, 6 months later, the patient's CardioMEMS transmissions were noted to have a dampened waveform (Figure 4). While the patient remained asymptomatic, a possible thrombus was hypothesized as the etiology of the dampening, leading to decreased blood flow in the vessel. The decision was made reevaluate the device by right heart catheterization. Angiography revealed a device that had migrated distally compared to the original implantation site and wedged at the vessel bifurcation (Figure 5). No evidence of thrombus was seen. The device was then recalibrated using the pulmonary artery catheter, but because of the dampening of the waveform, only the PA mean could be recalibrated. The patient was then discharged in stable condition and continued to follow up as an outpatient. 6 months after the recalibration and 1 year after device implantation, the CardioMEMS device continued to transmit data (Figure 6) and the mean PA values helped manage the patient's heart failure and help reduce the risk of repeat heart failure hospitalizations.

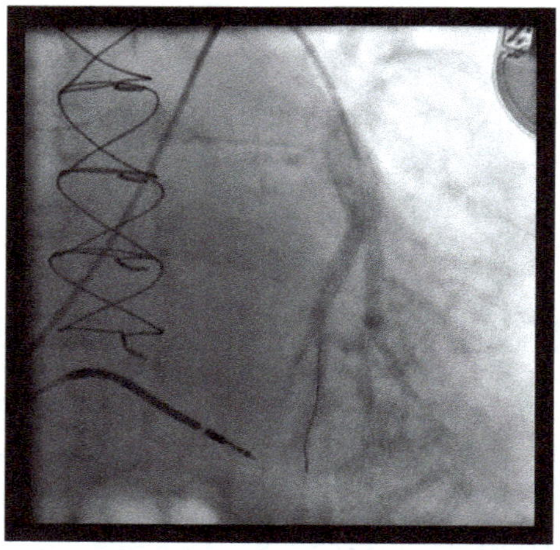

FIGURE 1: Left pulmonary artery vasculature on angiography revealed suitable vessels for CardioMEMS device placement.

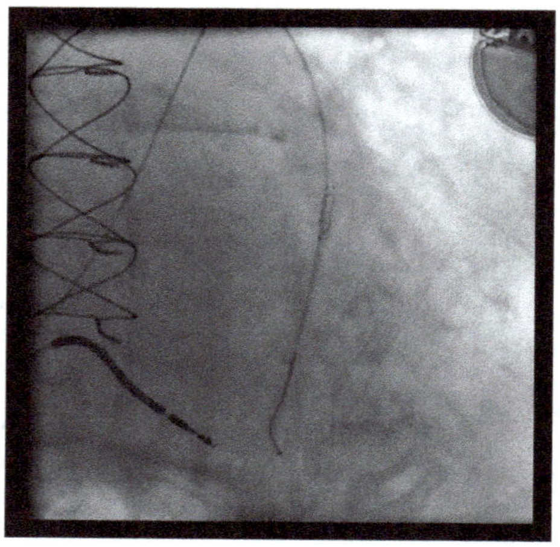

FIGURE 2: CardioMEMS device successfully deployed.

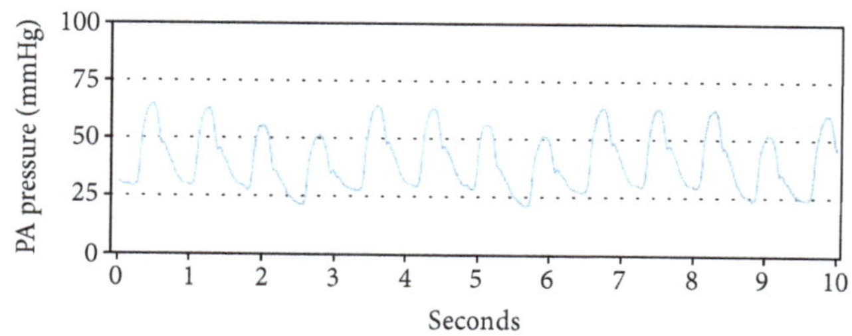

FIGURE 3: CardioMEMS transmission on the day of implantation showing a good quality waveform.

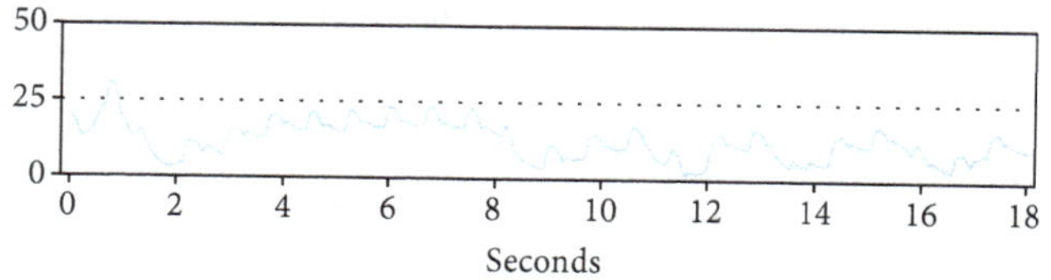

FIGURE 4: CardioMEMS transmissions 6 months postprocedure showed a dampened waveform compared to baseline.

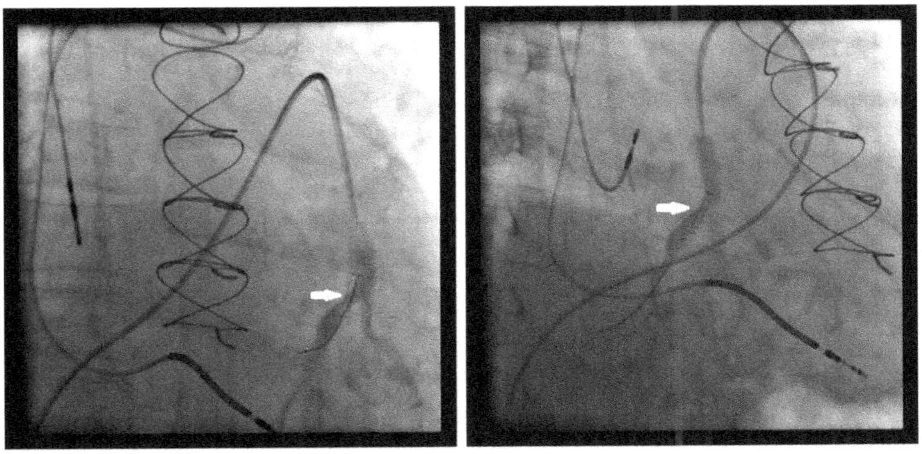

FIGURE 5: Repeat angiography revealed a migrated CardioMEMS device (arrow) compared to baseline.

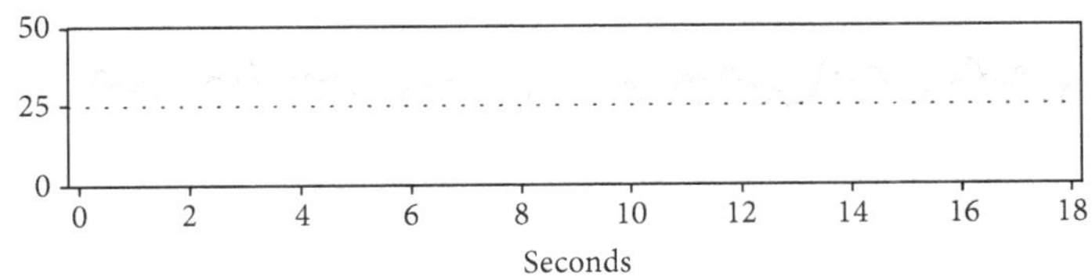

FIGURE 6: CardioMEMS continued transmission 6 months after recalibration and helped guide heart failure treatment and prevented rehospitalization.

3. Discussion

Heart failure remains a common cause of cardiovascular morbidity and mortality that places a tremendous burden on healthcare expenditure. The traditional approaches of close outpatient follow-up and guideline-directed medical therapy remain cornerstones of heart failure treatments, but newer technologies have allowed for more dynamic monitoring and, as a result, treatment of the disease. Chief among these, the CardioMEMS remote pulmonary artery pressure monitoring device has been shown to reduce heart failure hospitalizations by 37% in the CHAMPION trial [4, 5]. The recent CardioMEMS postapproval study showed an even greater decrease of 58% in heart failure hospitalizations at 1-year postimplantation [8] while a recent single-center study showed nearly an 80% reduction in heart failure admission and an almost 70% reduction in overall admissions [9].

Consequently, CardioMEMS has become an economically efficient technology, with the cost of device implantation being under $20,000 [1]. In contrast, using the 5-year observational period following the CHAMPION trial, heart failure treatment costs total nearly $170,000 which include future hospitalizations, monthly monitoring, and routine care and "... all costs are weighted based on the assumption that 75% of patients are covered by Medicare and 25% have commercial coverage" [1]. As the technology becomes more widespread, it is important for providers to be aware of the adverse events associated with the device.

Although pulmonary artery injury is the most common complication of the procedure, sensor malfunction is also a possibility, albeit very rare. A thrombus can lead to decreased blood flow and subsequently a dampened waveform. In our patient, we found that the device had likely embolized and wedged at a vessel bifurcation. To help avoid migration of the sensor, it is recommended to implant the device in a vessel with a diameter > 7 mm. However, despite implanting the device in such a location, as was done in our case, it may still not be enough to prevent migration. Using data from a right cardiac catheterization, the device was able to be calibrated and remained a viable tool to manage the patient's heart failure treatment. Conversely, it is also possible to recalibrate the device using noninvasive methods. With echocardiography, a pulmonary regurgitation jet can be used to obtain a mean PA pressure and diastolic PA pressure, which can then be used to calculate a PA systolic pressure. A tricuspid regurgitation jet can also be used to calculate the right ventricle systolic pressure which can substitute for a PA systolic pressure if there is no pulmonic stenosis. All this data can then be used to recalibrate the device, though this less-invasive approach is limited by the ability to acquire good echocardiographic windows. In addition, another possible but unlikely etiology of the dampened waveform may have been partial endothelialization of the device, and the resulting tissue growing over it may have triggered a drift-like process which resulted in inaccurate data. This was supported by cineangiography which showed that the proximal end of the device was free and the distal end was "jammed" in the vessel.

Interestingly, on detailed review of the waveforms after device implantation, a gradual change was noted instead of a sudden dampening. While sensor drift occurs with nearly all implanted sensors, the CardioMEMS device is very stable and only has a reported drift of.1 mm per year [10]. Therefore, the dampened pressures may have been misinterpreted as a well-controlled volume status of the patient and not a device migration. While the PA diastolic pressure is typically used to guide heart failure therapy, monitoring the PA systolic pressure may have alerted the physicians to the gradual decline of the pressure. Once a dampened waveform was identified, it is important to confirm the readings with a right cardiac catheterization. Though in some cases the data may not be useable, there is still an opportunity to recalibrate and utilize the device instead of implanting a new one.

4. Conclusion

CardioMEMS remote pulmonary artery pressure monitoring is a cost-effective tool to help reduce heart failure hospitalizations. As the technology gains more widespread acceptance and usage, physicians must be aware of possible adverse events associated with the device. Sensor malfunction is a possible issue that can lead to inaccurate data. We presented such a case where the CardioMEMS device developed a dampened waveform due to device migration and/or partial endothelialization. Despite this, the device can be recalibrated with a right cardiac catheterization and, as seen in our patient, can remain a suitable tool in monitoring and treating heart failure.

References

[1] J. K. Schmier, K. L. Ong, and G. C. Fonarow, "Cost-effectiveness of remote cardiac monitoring with the CardioMEMS heart failure system," *Clinical Cardiology*, vol. 40, no. 7, pp. 430–436, 2017.

[2] M. Kilgore, H. K. Patel, A. Kielhorn, J. F. Maya, and P. Sharma, "Economic burden of hospitalizations of Medicare beneficiaries with heart failure," *Risk Management and Healthcare Policy*, vol. 10, pp. 63–70, 2017.

[3] P. Ayyadurai, H. Alkhawam, M. Saad et al., "An update on the CardioMEMS pulmonary artery pressure sensor," *Therapeutic Advances in Cardiovascular Disease*, vol. 13, 2019.

[4] P. B. Adamson, W. T. Abraham, M. Aaron et al., "CHAMPION* Trial Rationale and Design: The Long-Term Safety and Clinical Efficacy of a Wireless Pulmonary Artery Pressure Monitoring System," *Journal of Cardiac Failure*, vol. 17, no. 1, pp. 3–10, 2011.

[5] W. T. Abraham, L. W. Stevenson, R. C. Bourge, J. A. Lindenfeld, J. G. Bauman, and P. B. Adamson, "Sustained efficacy of pulmonary artery pressure to guide adjustment of chronic heart failure therapy: complete follow-up results from the CHAMPION randomised trial," *The Lancet*, vol. 387, no. 10017, pp. 453–461, 2016.

[6] P. B. Adamson and E. D'Elia, "Implantable hemodynamic monitoring," *Heart Failure Management: The Neural Pathways*, A. Costea, E. Gronda, and E. Vanoli, Eds., pp. 91–95, Springer, 2016.

[7] M. Vaduganathan, E. M. DeFilippis, G. C. Fonarow, J. Butler, and M. R. Mehra, "Postmarketing adverse events related to the CardioMEMS HF system," *JAMA Cardiology*, vol. 2, no. 11, pp. 1277–1279, 2017.

[8] https://www.acc.org/~/media/Clinical/PDF-Files/Approved-PDFs/2019/03/15/ACC19_Slides/Mar17_Sun/1145amET_CardioMEMS-PAS-acc-2019.pdf.

[9] M. Assaad, S. Sarsam, A. Naqvi, and M. Zughaib, "CardioMems® device implantation reduces repeat hospitalizations in heart failure patients: a single center experience," *JRSM Cardiovascular Disease*, vol. 8, 2019.

[10] https://www.healio.com/cardiology/intervention/news/print/cardiology-today-intervention/%7B1f4f8554-c5e8-48fa-bfe2-f7ebdc73b20e%7D/cardiomems-experts-in-intervention-hf-provide-their-take-on-the-fda-approval.

Pericardial Tamponade and Elevated Serum CA-125 Level in Inadequately Treated Hypothyroidism

Moaaz Baghal, Viralkumar Amrutiya, Bhoomi Patel, Rutwik Patel, Jonathan Hernandez, Mohamed Ahmed, Abraham Lo, and Mark Gabelman

Hackensack Meridian Health Palisades Medical Center, Department of Internal Medicine, USA

Correspondence should be addressed to Moaaz Baghal; moaaz.baghal@gmail.com

Academic Editor: Assad Movahed

Cardiac tamponade is a medical emergency and must be managed promptly, and reaching a diagnosis is imperative to prevent recurrence. Herein, we present a case of a young female patient that presented with progressive shortness of breath and abdominal distension and was found to have cardiac tamponade with the finding of elevation of a blood tumor marker, CA-125, in the setting of nonadherence to thyroid replacement therapy. She was managed by surgical pericardial window and abdominal paracentesis, with replacement of thyroid hormones leading to resolution of the tamponade and ascites. CA-125 elevation associated with cardiac tamponade and myxedema ascites due to hypothyroidism is very rare, and we aim to shed light on the importance of having a broad differential when approaching cardiac tamponade and understand the association between CA-125 and hypothyroidism.

1. Introduction

Primary hypothyroidism is prevalent in 4.6% of the US population, with a higher prevalence in women. According to the American Thyroid Association, reportedly one in eight women will develop a thyroid disorder [1]. The disease is usually life-long but can be well controlled with adherence to medical management. However, poor medical care or nonadherence can put the patient at risk for complications, which can range from mild to life-threatening, the latter of which can include the accumulation of fluids in the body cavities presenting as cardiac tamponade and myxedema ascites, which occur in 4% of mild cases, and can go up to 30-80% in severe cases [1, 2]. Cardiac tamponade secondary to hypothyroidism is rare as the fluid accumulates slowly, gradually progressing to pericardial sac distension [2]. Herein, we report a case of a young female patient with uncontrolled postthyroidectomy hypothyroidism in the setting of medication nonadherence who presented with elevated CA-125 levels, cardiac tamponade, and ascites, all of which were secondary to severe hypothyroidism.

1.1. Patient Information. A 31-year-old female with hypothyroidism secondary to total thyroidectomy for papillary thyroid carcinoma, with chronic medication nonadherence, presented with abdominal distension that had been progressing over the 3 months prior to admission. She also complained of worsening dyspnea which progressed to inability to finish her sentence, along with back pain radiating to her shoulder that started one hour prior to admission.

The patient had a history of papillary thyroid carcinoma status postthyroidectomy one year prior to admission, with the patient reporting a several-month history of medication nonadherence. The patient had no personal or family cardiac history.

1.2. Clinical Findings. Upon presentation, her blood pressure was 103/90 mmHg, heart rate ranged from 75 to 89 beats/min, respiration was 16 breaths/min, SpO_2 was 98% on room air, and she was afebrile. Cardiovascular examination revealed a jugular venous pressure of 15 cm H_2O, distant heart sounds, and no murmurs, and Kussmaul's sign was not present. However, pulsus paradoxus was not appreciated, and peripheral

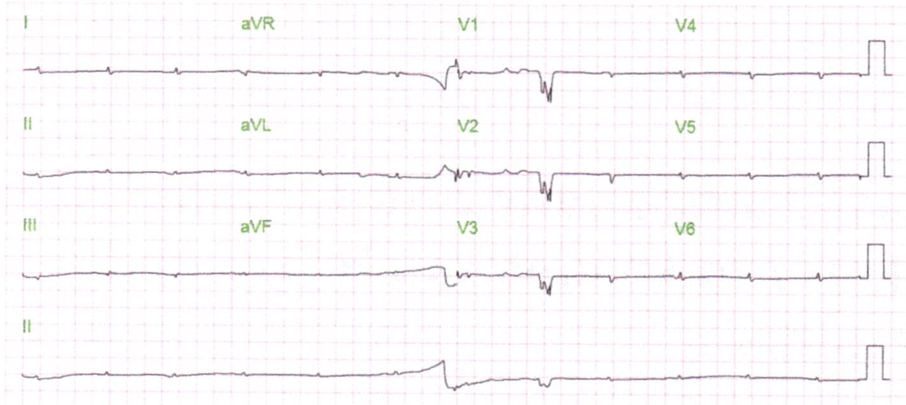

Figure 1: Electrocardiogram at presentation showing a sinus rhythm with a heart rate around 90 bpm and diffuse low voltage in both precordial and limb leads.

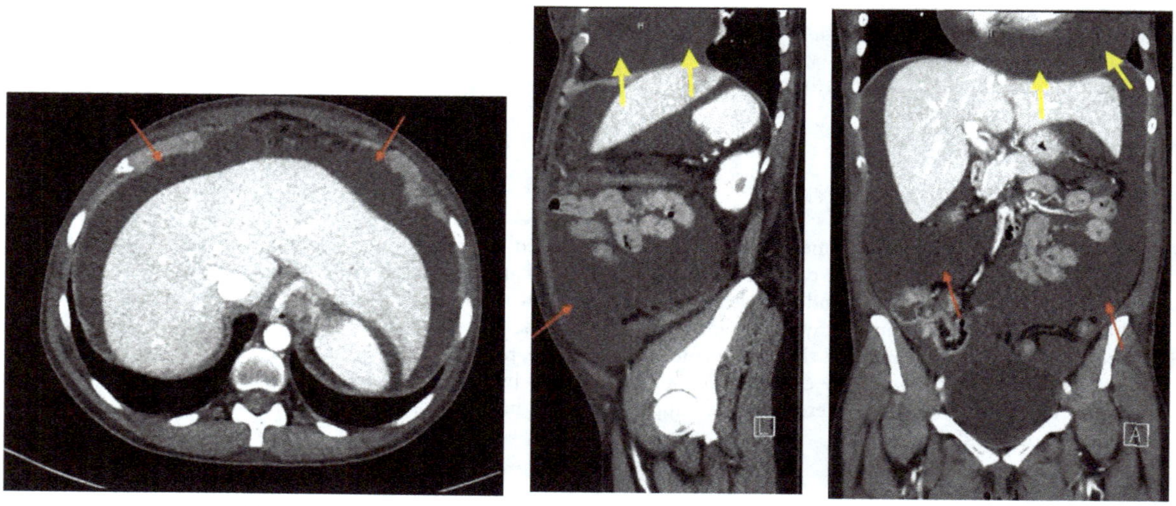

(a) (b) (c)

Figure 2: CT of the abdomen and pelvis with IV contrast on day 1. Mild bilateral basilar foci of atelectasis. Large pericardial effusion (yellow arrows in (b) and (c)). Large amounts of ascitic fluid (red arrows in (a)–(c)). Mild stranding of the peritoneum anteriorly.

edema was absent. There was a well-healed horizontal neck scar from a previous total thyroidectomy, also known as a Kocher incision. She was noted to have mild facial swelling, mild generalized hypopigmentation over her skin, and enlarged nontender abdominal girth.

1.3. Diagnostic Assessment. Laboratory analysis revealed serum TSH level > 100 mIU/L and elevated levels of CA-125 of 230.1 U/mL. A diffuse low voltage electrocardiogram (EKG) (Figure 1) raised a suspicion for pericardial effusion, which was confirmed on initial enhanced computed tomography (CT) of the abdomen and pelvis, showing large pericardial effusion and peritoneal fluid collection (Figure 2). An urgent transthoracic echocardiogram (TTE) confirmed the very large pericardial effusion with a swinging heart, right ventricular collapse, and marked mitral inflow respiratory variation (Figure 3), for which the patient was taken for an emergent pericardial window with removal of 1.5 liters of serous fluid and pericardial drain placement. Pericardial fluid analysis and pericardial tissue demonstrated exudative effusion with reactive mesothelial cells, which were positive for calretinin and negative for tumor marker results such as MOC31, BerEp4, TTF1, and mucin. Pericardial effusion also had negative cultures and cytology.

It was initially difficult to reconcile such a profound presentation of fluid overload with a unifying diagnosis. Pregnancy was first ruled out. Along with hypothyroidism, a highly elevated CA-125 led to considering peritoneal and gynecologic malignancies at the top of the differential diagnosis. Autoimmune (e.g., SLE and rheumatoid arthritis); bacterial, fungal, and viral infections; and postviral complications were considered, along with congenital disorders (e.g., Wilson's disease).

1.4. Investigations. A follow-up TTE (Figure 4) demonstrated a small pericardial effusion, a thickened and echogenic right ventricular (RV) free wall, and diffuse mild hypokinesis of the left ventricle (LV) with an Ejection Fraction (EF) of 45-

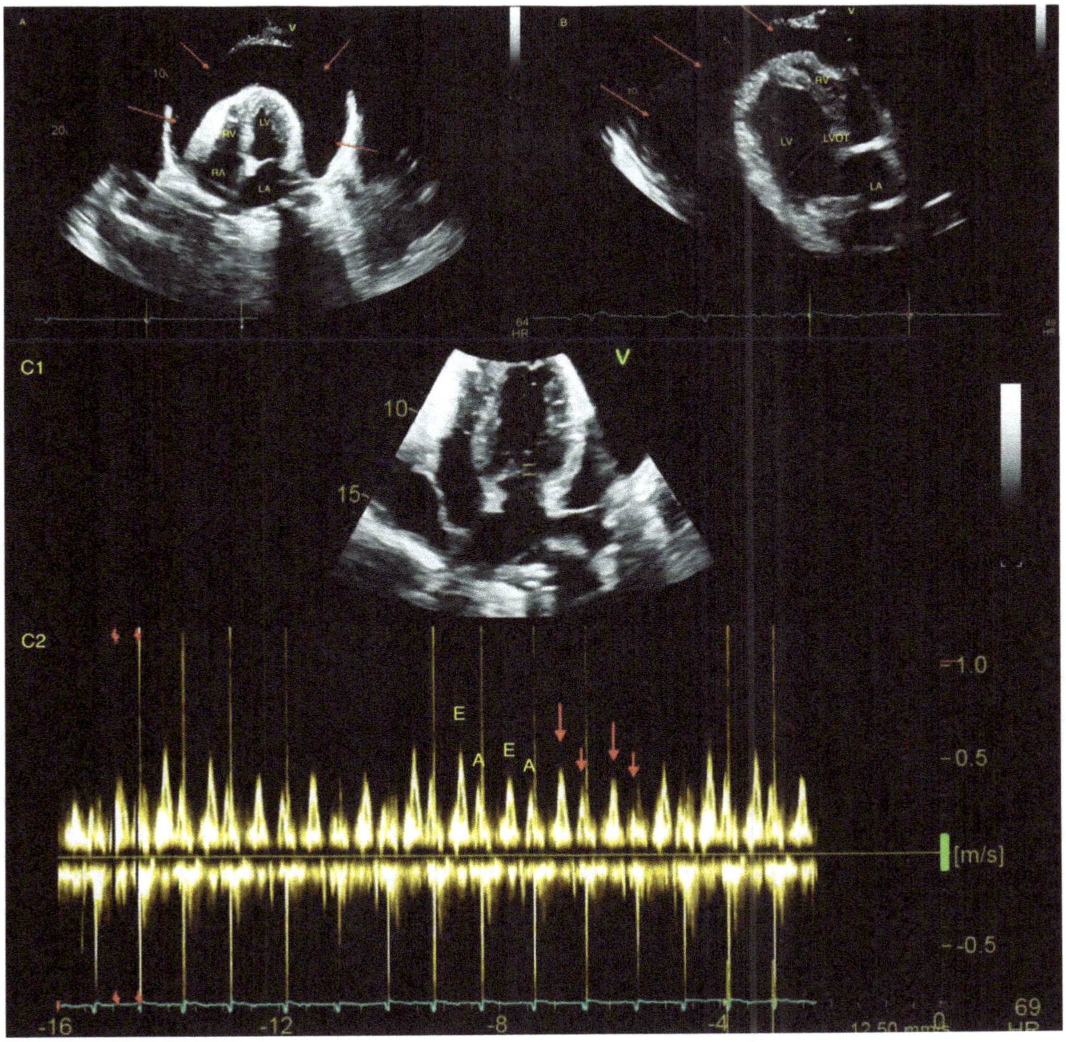

FIGURE 3: Transthoracic echocardiogram on day 0. Very large pericardial effusion with a swinging heart (red arrows in (a) and (b)), RV diastolic collapse, and marked mitral inflow respiratory variation (red arrows in (c)) consistent with significant tamponade. (a) Apical 4-chamber view; (b) parasternal long-axis view; (c) apical 4-chamber view showing the position of the Doppler pulse wave vector to obtain the mitral inflow waveform; (d) mitral inflow waveform.

50%. Serum lactic acid was normal, and serum lipase was unremarkable. The iron profile showed low iron levels 47 μg/dL with normal ferritin levels. B-Type Natriuretic Peptide (BNP) was 15 pg/mL. Initial serum troponin I levels were normal. Multiple serum tumor markers were tested; Carbohydrate Antigen (CA) 19-9 was 13 U/mL, CEA was 4.3 ng/mL, and Cancer Antigen (CA) 125 was 230.1 U/mL (reference: <35 U/mL). A SARS-CoV-2 rapid test was negative. Pericardial fluid analysis revealed a negative fungal culture, no mycobacterial species were isolated after 6 weeks of incubation, and bacterial culture was negative. Pericardial biopsy showed dense fibrosis and mesothelial cell changes, negative for malignancy. Peritoneal fluid analysis showed a SAAG of < 1.1/dL, and the rest of the peritoneal fluid studies were unremarkable. Serum lactate dehydrogenase was 162 U/L. Serum TSH levels were >100 μIU/mL (reference: 0.34-5.6 μIU/mL), serum free thyroxine level was <0.20 ng/dL (reference: 0.58-1.64 ng/dL), and total T3 level was <0.2 ng/mL (reference: 0.7-2.1 ng/mL). Serum thyroglobulin level was less than 0.4 ng/mL. Serum anti-thyroglobulin antibody level was 6 IU/mL (reference < 1). Pelvic vaginal ultrasound did not reveal any signs of ovarian mass or uterine pathology. The serum rheumatoid factor was negative. Serum ANA was negative. Serum ceruloplasmin and serum copper levels were normal. Epstein-Barr virus IgM and IgG were negative. Coombs' test was negative.

1.5. Therapeutic Intervention. Postprocedure, the size of the pericardial effusion remained stable. The condition was complicated by left-sided pneumothorax, which was considered a postprocedure complication, and required chest tube placement and admission to the critical care unit, where she was monitored. For hypothyroidism, the patient was started on thyroid replacement therapy. On day 1, a paracentesis was performed with removal of 3 liters of fluid from the abdomen. The patient was closely monitored, and she

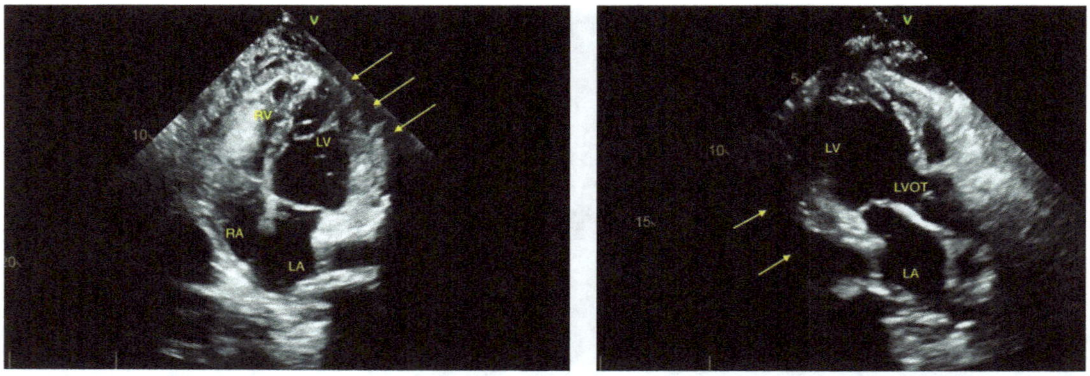

(a) (b)

Figure 4: Transthoracic echocardiogram on day 1. The left ventricle has normal size. There is diffuse mild hypokinesis, LVEF is 45-50%. The right ventricular free wall appears thickened and echogenic. There is a small pericardial effusion. (a) Apical 4-chamber view and (b) parasternal long-axis view.

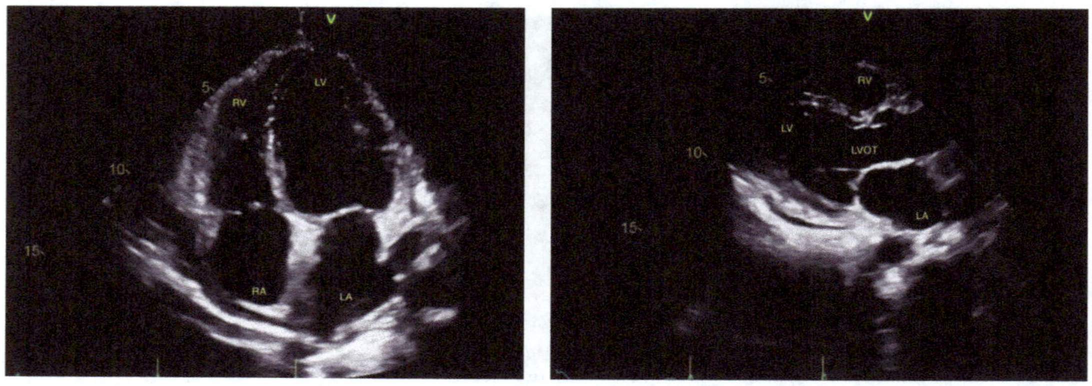

(a) (b)

Figure 5: Transthoracic echocardiogram 4 weeks since admission. The left ventricle has normal size. LVEF is 55-60%. LV strain is -19%. The right ventricle free wall is thick, and mitral valve leaflets are thickened. Small-to-moderate circumferential pericardial effusion. There is no evidence of tamponade. (a) Apical 4-chamber view and (b) parasternal long-axis view.

Table 1: Timeline.

Day 0	Patient undergoes surgical pericardial window, complicated postoperatively by left-sided pneumothorax that required chest tube placement. Thyroid replacement therapy started
Day 1	Paracentesis performed, with removal of 3 liters of fluid
Day 2	Resolution of pneumothorax with removal of the chest tube
Day 5	Discharged home on strict instructions to adhere to thyroid medication and follow-up with cardiology, obstetrics and gynecology, and endocrinology
Day 37	Outpatient follow-up showed downtrending of CA-125 levels. Follow-up echocardiogram revealed no recurrence of pericardial effusion. Thyroid hormone levels were within the normal range

remained hemodynamically stable on day 2; the pneumothorax was resolved with subsequent removal of the chest tube, and the patient was downgraded to medical floor for further medical care. The patient was later discharged home on levothyroxine with strict recommendations on the importance of adherence and outpatient follow-up.

1.6. Follow-Up and Outcomes. A close follow-up of our patient in the outpatient setting showed normal levels of TSH with no signs of recurrent malignancy on follow-up ultrasound of the neck. Follow-up transthoracic echocardiogram 4 weeks later showed improved LV and RV systolic function with improved LVEF with mild pericardial effusion and no evidence of pericardial effusion (Figure 5). Her CA-125 levels were trending down to 124.8 U/mL, and the patient reported no further symptoms on adherence to thyroid replacement therapy. An outpatient PET scan with the oncology workup returned negative (Table 1).

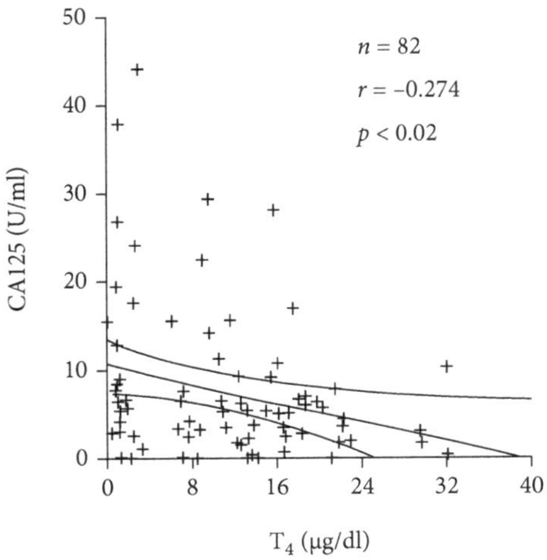

FIGURE 6: Graph showing the correlation between CA-125 and T4 concentrations in patients with altered thyroid states, demonstrated by Hashimoto et al. in their published article. Changes in tumor marker concentration in female patients with hyper-, eu-, and hypothyroidism [9].

2. Discussion

Depending on the severity of hypothyroidism, cardiac function can be impacted caused by changes in the cardiovascular system due to low T3 levels, leading to decreased cardiac output, increased diastolic blood pressure, narrowing of the pulse pressure, and bradycardia; in severe hypothyroidism, it can lead to pericardial effusion [2].

The mechanism of hypothyroidism-induced pericardial effusion is unclear, but it is believed to be associated with increased capillary permeability and reduced lymphatic drainage from the pericardial space [2]. It is hypothesized that the low synthesis of albumin, which usually occurs 2 to 3 months after a hypothyroid state, with increased interstitial pressure plays a major role [3]. In addition, it is believed that the increased extravascular accumulation of protein is a result of increased outward transcapillary transport rate of albumin and poor compensatory increased lymphatic flow with slow protein return rate to the intravascular space. Only in 4 percent of cases, extravascular plasma protein accumulation occurred in the heart, liver, kidneys, and spleen [4]. Pericardial effusion and cardiac tamponade are acutely managed by pericardiocentesis; in some cases, a prolonged pericardial drainage and a pericardial window are reverted in case of reaccumulation and signs of loculation, or biopsy material is required, as per the latest ESC 2015 guidelines. In our patient's case, the diagnosis of pericardial effusion in the setting of malignancy was suspected, and it was the cardiothoracic surgeon's decision to perform a pericardial window with pericardial drainage and collect the pericardial fluid and sac for pathological and cytological testing [3].

Noncardiac manifestations, such as ascites as in our patient's case, have had the same pathophysiological hypothesis as pericardial effusion. The ascitic fluid analysis showed a SAAG of 1.0 g/dL, indicating that the cause is not due to portal hypertension. As ascites is not considered a common complication of hypothyroidism, the suspicion for hypothyroidism was low and other causes needed to be excluded. Our patient's condition coupled with elevated levels of CA-125 warranted a workup for ovarian cancer as hypothyroidism has also been rarely associated with elevated CA-125 levels, with one case reported in Japan in 2007 [5].

CA-125 was first described in 1981 by Bast et al. as a glycoprotein raised in 90% of advanced ovarian tumors and has since been used prospectively as a marker for therapeutic efficacy and disease monitoring among ovarian cancer patients but has not been used for screening for ovarian cancer due to inadequate sensitivities, as proven by previous studies [6]. It is rare for hypothyroidism to be correlated with elevated levels of CA-125 [4], with the exact mechanism not being identified yet. One hypothesis explains that the elevation of CA-125 occurs in cases of stretching of the peritoneum with ascitic fluid accumulation, and elevated CA-125 can reach levels comparable to those in ovarian carcinoma; such correlations have been seen in nephritic syndrome and liver cirrhosis, as described by Castro et al. [7]. Another hypothesis is the elevation of CA-125 due to pericardial effusion with delayed clearance of CA-125 in hypothyroid states, with the possibility of CA-125 being related to the severity of hypothyroidism-associated pericardial effusion. A study done by Hashimoto et al. in 1989 showed an inverse relationship between the levels of T4 concentration in abnormal thyroid states and CA-125 (Figure 6) [8, 9].

Typical features of myxedema ascites include long duration of hypothyroidism and rapid resolution of ascites following thyroid hormone replacement therapy. In cases of ascites, the diagnostic workup includes paracentesis to analyze the ascitic fluid and to narrow the differential diagnosis, which can be divided into high protein ascites, which usually includes peritoneal malignancies, tuberculous peritonitis, pyogenic peritonitis, and pancreatic ascites, and low protein ascites, which is correlated with liver cirrhosis and congestive heart failure [10].

Peritoneal malignancy must be suspected when the composition of ascitic fluid and ultrasonography are not consistent with portal hypertension. Although in our case, we detected an elevated CA-125, workup for peritoneal malignancy and ovarian carcinoma was done while restarting thyroid hormone replacement therapy, performing a pericardial window for cardiac tamponade and paracentesis for ascites with a positive response noted in the patient's condition. When the initial workup for malignancy came back negative, the definitive answer would come in the outpatient follow-up setting, where close follow-up and patient adherence to her thyroid medication led to complete resolution of her presentation with no recurrence, and no evidence of peritoneal malignancy was found as well as excluding all other causes.

Early diagnosis of the causes of ascites and cardiac tamponade would prevent the inappropriate use of other management modalities such as frequent paracentesis, liver biopsies, and in cases of failure of diagnosis an exploratory laparotomy [5]. However, not all cases of hypothyroidism-associated ascites present with a SAAG < 1.1, as Oey et al. [4] presented in their study review that the patient can also present with a SAAG > 1.1. Therefore, levels of SAAG are variable, and neither high nor low SAAG has shown to be a constant feature of myxedema ascites.

Adequate history, physical examination, and guideline-directed management are essential for the early diagnosis of cardiac tamponade and myxedema ascites. Although the condition is rare, it is easily reversible and avoidable with thyroid hormone replacement therapy.

We report our experience to shed light on the importance to exercise caution when analyzing elevated tumor markers in patients with abnormal thyroid hormone levels and to consider the thyroid to be correlated with elevated CA-125 and fluid overload when other devastating causes have been ruled out without having to perform unnecessary invasive procedures. More studies are still needed to understand the mechanisms of pericardial effusion and elevated CA-125 in hypothyroidism.

Additional Points

Patient Perspective. The patient was contacted and declined to share her perspective on the case.

Consent

Verbal informed consent was obtained from the patient for her anonymized information to be published in this article.

Acknowledgments

The authors gratefully acknowledge and thank our patient for her kind support.

References

[1] https://www.thyroid.org/media-main/press-room/.

[2] https://seer.cancer.gov/statfacts/html/thyro.html.

[3] M. Imazio and Y. Adler, "Management of pericardial effusion," *European Heart Journal*, vol. 34, no. 16, pp. 1186–1197, 2013.

[4] R. C. Oey, H. R. van Buuren, and R. A. de Man, "The diagnostic work-up in patients with ascites: current guidelines and future prospects," *The Netherlands Journal of Medicine*, vol. 74, no. 8, pp. 330–335, 2016.

[5] N. Takahashi, T. Shimada, Y. Ishibashi, N. Oyake, and Y. Murakami, "Transient elevation of serum tumor markers in a patient with hypothyroidism," *The American Journal of the Medical Sciences*, vol. 333, no. 6, pp. 387–389, 2007.

[6] D. Gupta and C. G. Lis, "Role of CA125 in predicting ovarian cancer survival - a review of the epidemiological literature," *Journal of Ovarian Research*, vol. 2, no. 1, p. 13, 2009.

[7] F. de Castro, M. Bonacini, J. M. Walden, and T. T. Schubert, "Myxedema ascites. Report of two cases and review of the literature," *Journal of Clinical Gastroenterology*, vol. 13, no. 4, pp. 411–414, 1991.

[8] H. H. Parving, J. M. Hansen, S. L. Nielsen, N. Rossing, O. Munck, and N. A. Lassen, "Mechanisms of edema formation in myxedema–increased protein extravasation and relatively slow lymphatic drainage," *Journal of Postgraduate Medicine*, vol. 301, no. 9, pp. 460–465, 1979.

[9] T. Hashimoto and F. Matsubara, "Changes in the tumor marker concentration in female patients with hyper-, eu-, and hypothyroidism," *Endocrinologia Japonica*, vol. 36, no. 6, pp. 873–879, 1989.

[10] A. Jabbar, A. Pingitore, S. H. Pearce, A. Zaman, G. Iervasi, and S. Razvi, "Thyroid hormones and cardiovascular disease," *Nature Reviews Cardiology*, vol. 14, no. 1, pp. 39–55, 2017.

An Unusual Cause of Hypoxia: Ventricular Septal Defect, Pulmonary Artery Atresia and Major Aortopulmonary Collaterals Diagnosed in the Adult Cardiac Catheterization Lab

Katia Bravo-Jaimes, Brian Walton, Poyee Tung, and Richard W. Smalling

Division of Cardiology, University of Texas Health Science Center at Houston, Houston, Texas, USA

Correspondence should be addressed to Brian Walton; brian.walton@uth.tmc.edu

Academic Editor: Ertugrul Ercan

The association of pulmonary atresia, ventricular septal defect (VSD) and major aortopulmonary collaterals (MAPCA) is an extreme form of tetralogy of Fallot (TOF). It carries a high mortality risk if not intervened on during infancy with only 20% of unoperated patients surviving into adulthood. We present the case of a 40-year-old man who presented for evaluation prior to retinal surgery and was found to have hypoxia and a loud murmur. Cardiac catheterization was performed in the general catheterization laboratory, demonstrating a membranous VSD, pulmonary atresia, and MAPCA. We highlight the challenges and limitations that an adult interventional cardiologist may have when encountering these patients.

1. Case Report

A 40-year-old man with scoliosis and developmental delay presented for outpatient evaluation prior to retinal surgery. His physical exam showed a heart rate of 110 bpm, blood pressure of 160/70 mmHg, respiratory rate of 16/minute, oxygen saturation of 84%, clubbing, elevated jugular venous pressure, and a multifocal V/VI systolic murmur radiating to the back. Laboratory tests were remarkable for hemoglobin of 18 g/dL. An echocardiogram demonstrated biventricular hypertrophy, preserved biventricular systolic function, an overriding aorta (Figure 1), and a right-to-left interventricular shunt.

A ventriculogram, right heart catheterization, and oximetry were performed. After initial femoral venous access, there was difficulty passing a J wire and angiography showed an interrupted inferior vena cava (Figure 2). Therefore, access was changed to the internal jugular vein and right heart catheterization demonstrated severely elevated right atrial and ventricular pressures (Figure 3). There was an inability to obtain pulmonary artery waveforms, and a right ventriculogram demonstrated pulmonary atresia. A pigtail catheter was introduced via femoral arterial access, and simultaneous right and left ventricular pressures were obtained. Ventriculography confirmed a membranous VSD. Subsequent root and thoracic aortography showed MAPCA from the lower thoracic aorta connecting to the right upper pulmonary artery branch (Figure 4, Video 1). The main communication to the right lung was cannulated via the MAPCA, and a pulmonary angiogram was performed. There were two areas of stenosis. The pressures in the right upper pulmonary artery branch were measured at 120 mmHg proximal and 18 mmHg distal to the areas of stenosis. Next, the left subclavian artery was engaged, and an angiogram was performed, revealing MAPCA between the left subclavian artery and left and right lower pulmonary artery branches (Figure 5, Video 2).

A discussion was held with the patient and his family including surgical options; however, due to the potentially high operative risks and poor baseline functional capacity, they decided to pursue medical management and focus on quality of life.

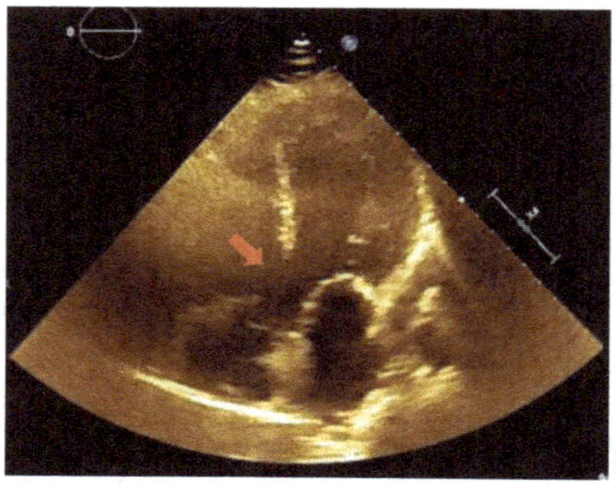

Figure 1: A five-chamber view showing an overriding aorta and ventricular septal defect (red arrow).

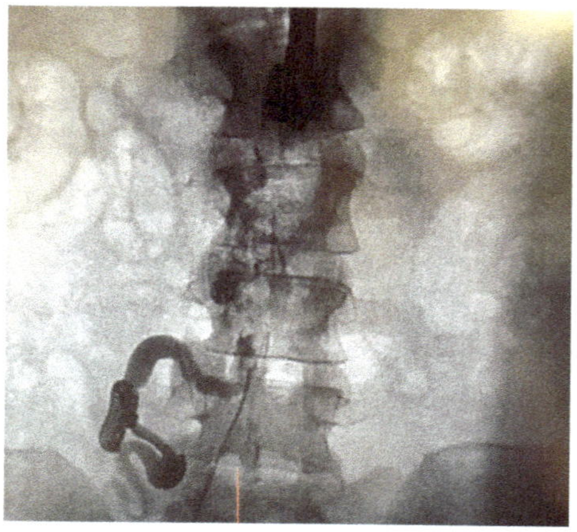

Figure 2: Interrupted inferior vena cava that prompted change from right femoral to right internal jugular access.

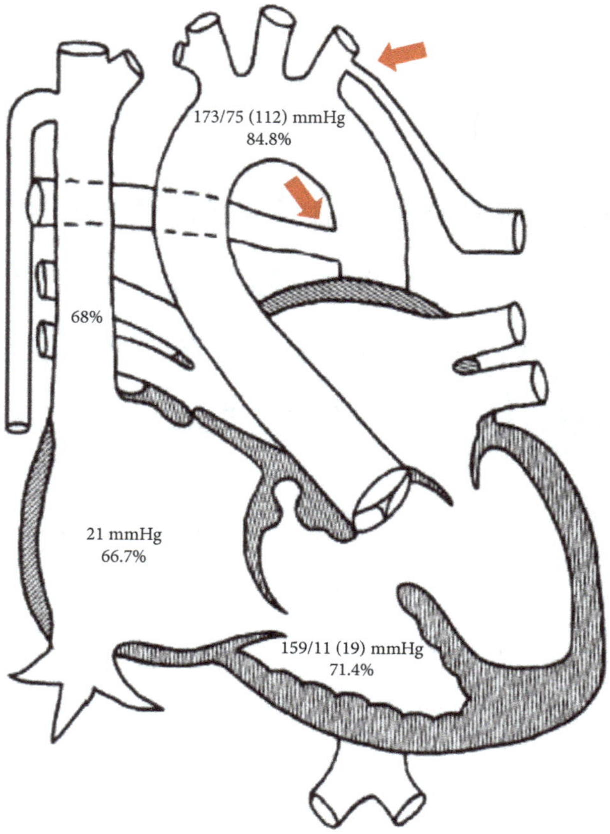

Figure 3: Diagram showing invasive hemodynamics and oximetry. Note that the right MAPCA originates from the descending aorta and the left MAPCA from the left subclavian artery (red arrows).

2. Discussion

Currently, congenital heart disease (CHD) affects more adults than children in the United States [1]. Ideally, patients with complex CHD will be referred to a specialized adult congenital heart disease clinic; however, often this is not possible, and therefore, general and interventional adult cardiologists will inexorably be involved in their care. Thus, awareness about potential challenges and limitations during diagnostic workup of this condition is needed.

The association of pulmonary atresia, VSD, and MAPCA is a complex CHD that occurs in approximately 7 to 10 of 100000 live births [2, 3]. Cyanosis, heart failure, and failure to thrive are the most common initial presentations [3]. If unoperated, it carries a significant mortality of about 40% at 1 year and 80% at 20 years [3]. Thus, encountering adults with this condition is extremely rare, with only a few reports available in the literature and the oldest described patient being 54 years old [4].

Echocardiography is insufficient to fully identify pulmonary atresia, VSD, and MAPCA; however, a dedicated congenital echocardiogram is the preferred first-line imaging in these patients. Cardiac magnetic resonance imaging and computed tomography could supplement anatomic details and even pulmonary blood flow analysis; however, due to the lack of detailed hemodynamic data in these two modalities, cardiac catheterization remains the gold standard for accurately diagnosing this condition [3].

Identification of MAPCA during cardiac catheterization is of exceptional importance, since it will determine treatment strategies. Most MAPCAs have a thoracic origin (descending aorta and subclavian arteries), but they can also arise from cervical vessels [5], the abdominal aorta and even from the coronary arteries in rare cases [6]. In our case, critical attention was paid not only to identify the pulmonary arteries but also to measure hemodynamics.

Surgical management in children could be achieved with native pulmonary artery rehabilitation followed by complete repair, MAPCA unifocalization (anastomosis of ipsilateral MAPCA via patches or conduit, incorporating the ipsilateral native pulmonary artery), or a combined strategy of the two approaches [2]. However, in adults with this condition, pulmonary hypertension may limit the feasibility of the former methods, and medical therapy, combined heart/lung transplant, or palliative care may be the only options.

3. Conclusions

The association of pulmonary atresia, VSD, and MAPCA is a rare complex CHD that is mainly diagnosed with cardiac

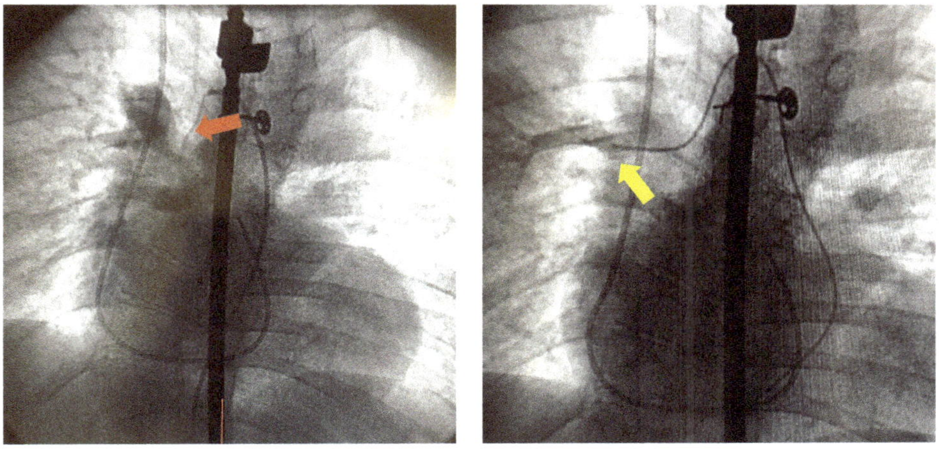

(a) (b)

FIGURE 4: (a) Collaterals (red arrow) from the thoracic aorta. (b) After cannulation of this MAPCA, the right upper pulmonary artery branch was seen (yellow arrow) and had normal systolic pressure.

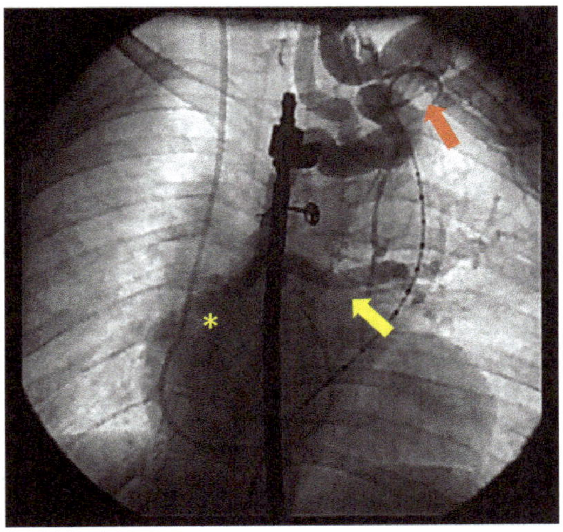

FIGURE 5: Collaterals (red arrow) from the left subclavian artery originating the left (yellow arrow) and right lower (asterisk) pulmonary artery branches.

catheterization. When encountered by an adult interventional cardiologist, obtaining anatomic and hemodynamic details is challenging.

Additional Points

Learning Objective. This case highlights the challenges that an adult interventional cardiologist may have when encountering patients with undiagnosed congenital heart disease.

Supplementary 2. Video 2: subclavian angiogram demonstrating collaterals originating the left pulmonary artery and right lower pulmonary artery branch.

References

[1] S. M. Gilboa, O. J. Devine, J. E. Kucik et al., "Congenital heart defects in the United States: estimating the magnitude of the affected population in 2010," *Circulation*, vol. 134, no. 2, pp. 101–109, 2016.

[2] J. Soquet, D. J. Barron, and Y. d'Udekem, "A review of the management of pulmonary atresia, ventricular septal defect and major aortopulmonary collateral arteries," *The Annals of Thoracic Surgery*, vol. 108, no. 2, pp. 601–612, 2019.

[3] L. B. Presnell, A. Blankenship, S. L. Cheatham, G. E. Owens, and S. L. Staveski, "An overview of pulmonary atresia and major aortopulmonary collateral arteries," *World Journal for Pediatric and Congenital Heart Surgery*, vol. 6, no. 4, pp. 630–639, 2015.

[4] S. Gupta, S. Gupta, A. Miital, and T. Mehta, "Major aorto pulmonary collateral arteries (MAPCA) with tetralogy of Fallot and pulmonary artesia in middle age adult: a rare finding," *Acta Medica Indonesiana*, vol. 47, no. 1, pp. 70-71, 2015.

[5] R. T. Brown and K. E. Fellows, "Cervical collateral arteries in pulmonary atresia with ventricular septal defect," *The American Journal of Cardiology*, vol. 62, no. 17, pp. 1310-1311, 1988.

[6] Z. Amin, D. B. McElhinney, V. M. Reddy, P. Moore, F. L. Hanley, and D. F. Teitel, "Coronary to pulmonary artery collaterals in patients with pulmonary atresia and ventricular septal defect," *The Annals of Thoracic Surgery*, vol. 70, no. 1, pp. 119–123, 2000.

Chyloperirdium due to Subclavian Vein Thrombosis in the Setting of Protein S Deficiency

Ian Jackson,[1] **Yaman Alali**,[1] **Abedel Rahman Anani**,[1] **Ali Nayfeh**,[2] **Arindam Sharma**,[3] **Abhishek Thandra**,[3] **and Amjad Kabach**[3]

[1]*Department of Medicine, Creighton University School of Medicine, Omaha, NE, USA*
[2]*Department of Pulmonary and Critical Care, Creighton University School of Medicine, Omaha, NE, USA*
[3]*Department of Cardiology, Creighton University School of Medicine, Omaha, NE, USA*

Correspondence should be addressed to Ian Jackson; ianjackson@creighton.edu

Academic Editor: Ertugurul Ercan

Background. Chylopericardium is the accumulation of lymphatic fluid in the pericardial cavity. It can be idiopathic or secondary to trauma, cardiothoracic surgery, neoplasm, radiation, tuberculosis, lymphatic duct dysfunction, thrombosis, or other causes. We present a case of chylopericardium due to subclavian vein thrombosis in a patient with protein S deficiency. *Clinical Case.* A 48-year-old man with a history of protein S deficiency presented to the emergency department with shortness of breath and a productive cough. CT of the chest showed pulmonary emboli, moderate pericardial effusion, and a large thrombus of the superior vena cava, brachiocephalic vein, and subclavian veins. He developed echocardiographic evidence of cardiac tamponade so he underwent pericardiocentesis with drainage of milky-appearing fluid. Analysis of the fluid showed elevated triglycerides consistent with chylopericardium. The pericardial effusion reaccumulated, likely secondary to lymphatic duct obstruction due to his subclavian vein thrombus. Catheter-assisted thrombolysis was performed with resolution of the patient's effusion and symptoms. *Conclusion.* Chylopericardium is a rare but important complication of subclavian vein thrombosis. Management is typically with surgical intervention, although our case represents successful treatment with catheter-assisted thrombolysis.

1. Introduction

Chylopericardium is a rare condition characterized by the accumulation of milky fluid rich in triglycerides and chylomicrons in the pericardial cavity. Chylopericardium can be idiopathic or secondary to injury or obstruction of the thoracic duct. The most common causes of secondary chylopericardium are trauma and cardiac or thoracic surgery. Less common causes include neoplasm, radiation therapy, tuberculosis, lymphangiectasis, lymphangioma, cystic hygroma, filariasis, and subclavian vein thrombosis [1, 2].

2. Case Description

A 48-year-old man presented to the emergency department with shortness of breath and a productive cough that had been gradually worsening for the past one week. He had a history of protein S deficiency and numerous associated deep vein thromboses and pulmonary emboli requiring placement of an inferior vena cava filter and long-term anticoagulation. On arrival to the emergency department, he had a heart rate of 101, respiratory rate of 31, blood pressure of 153/110 mmHg, and oxygen saturation of 89% on room air. Physical examination showed lower extremity edema and labored breathing.

Laboratory workup was significant for creatinine of 1.47 mg/dL (normal range 0.60–1.30 mg/dL). A respiratory pathogen screen, severe acute respiratory syndrome coronavirus (COVID-19) PCR testing, and troponin were negative. An electrocardiogram (EKG) showed sinus tachycardia without evidence of ischemia. Computed tomography (CT) of the chest showed pulmonary emboli with involvement of the right middle and lower lobar arteries, a moderate pericardial effusion, and a large, nearly occlusive thrombus in the superior vena cava (SVC) with extension into the right atrium and bilateral brachiocephalic veins. Extensive venous collateralization was also evident and thought to be indicative of obstruction in venous return (Figures 1 and 2). The patient was treated with supplemental oxygen and a heparin infusion.

Vascular surgery determined that the patient's SVC thrombus was likely acute on chronic as it was present but not noted on previous imaging. An initial echocardiogram showed a moderate effusion without evidence of tamponade. However, serial echocardiograms demonstrated increasing size of the effusion with development of right ventricular dilation and collapse. Pericardiocentesis was performed with drainage of 400 mL of chylous-appearing fluid (Figure 3).

Analysis of the pericardial fluid showed 91,000 red blood cells/μL; 26,248 nucleated cells/μL with 62% neutrophils, 36% lymphocytes, and 2% monocytes; protein of 4.8 gm/dL; albumin 2.1 gm/dL; lactate dehydrogenase 373 U/L; glucose 158 mg/dL; amylase 20 U/L; lipase 25 U/L; cholesterol < 200 mg/dL; and triglycerides of 2,726 mg/dL. Gram stain and culture of the fluid were negative for organisms. Cytology was negative for malignancy. Given the results of the pericardial fluid analysis, it was determined that the chylous pericardial effusion was likely due to lymphatic obstruction secondary to subclavian vein thrombus.

The patient was treated with therapeutic doses of enoxaparin for anticoagulation during hospital admission. After pericardiocentesis, he was monitored with serial echocardiograms which showed gradual reaccumulation of his pericardial effusion without evidence of tamponade. A repeat CT of the chest showed worsened venous obstruction with complete occlusion of the left subclavian vein. Vascular and cardiothoracic surgery teams decided that the best treatment option was definitive management of the patient's thrombus as a pericardial window would result in continuous effusion. Despite a high risk of causing pulmonary embolism, the patient underwent catheter-assisted thrombolysis directed at the left subclavian thrombosis.

Following the procedure, a repeat CT angiogram of the chest showed a decrease in clot burden. The patient clinically improved and was discharged without further operative intervention. He was found to have only trace pericardial effusion on echocardiography with no residual symptoms at one-year follow-up.

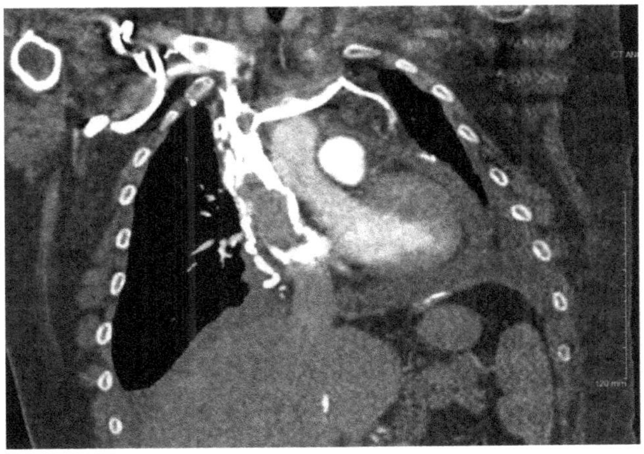

FIGURE 1: CT of the chest with SVC and subclavian thrombus.

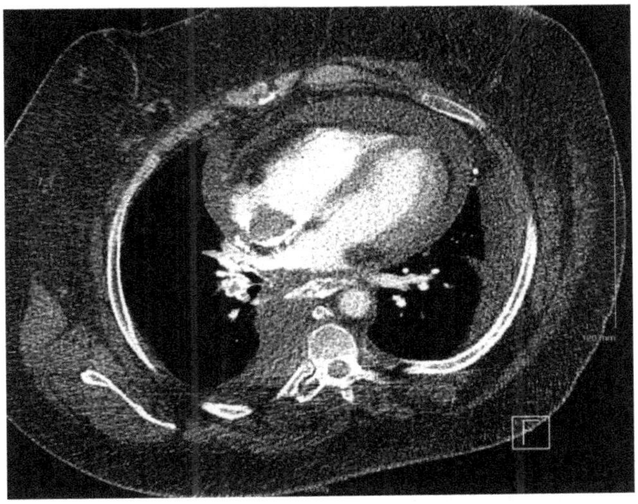

FIGURE 2: CT of the chest with right atrial thrombus and pericardial effusion.

3. Discussion

Secondary chylopericardium is usually due to malignancy or trauma to the thoracic duct during surgery [3]. Rarely, it has been reported to occur secondary to thrombosis of the superior vena cava and subclavian veins, typically due to catheter-related thrombosis [1–3]. One case reported chylopericardium secondary to superior vena cava and brachiocephalic vein thrombosis following community-acquired pneumonia [4]. However, no previous case reports describe secondary chylopericardium due to a hereditary thrombophilia. We report a very rare case of chylopericardium secondary to SVC and left subclavian vein thrombosis in a patient with protein S deficiency.

The cardiac lymphatic vessels normally join as a common trunk and drain into the thoracic duct. In the presented case, venous thrombosis of the SVC, bilateral brachiocephalic veins, and the left subclavian vein likely led to occlusion of ostium of the thoracic duct and consequent increase in thoracic duct pressure [5]. This may have caused reflux of chylous lymph through the lymphatics draining the heart and pericardium, resulting in chylopericardium. This mechanism has been described previously in the literature. Normally, the lymphatic vessels have valves that preclude retrograde flow of chyle unless the pressure increases to the range of 35 to 50 cm water [6, 7]. Additionally, experiments have shown that blocking the thoracic duct alone does not cause chylopericardium due to the presence of several collateral pathways within the venous system, such as the azygous vein and superior vena cava. This indicates the importance of mechanical venous obstruction in the pathophysiology of chyloperdicardium [6, 7]. This also may explain why the presence of collateral venous circulation evident on our patient's chest CT may have prevented the reaccumulation of chyle in the pericardium.

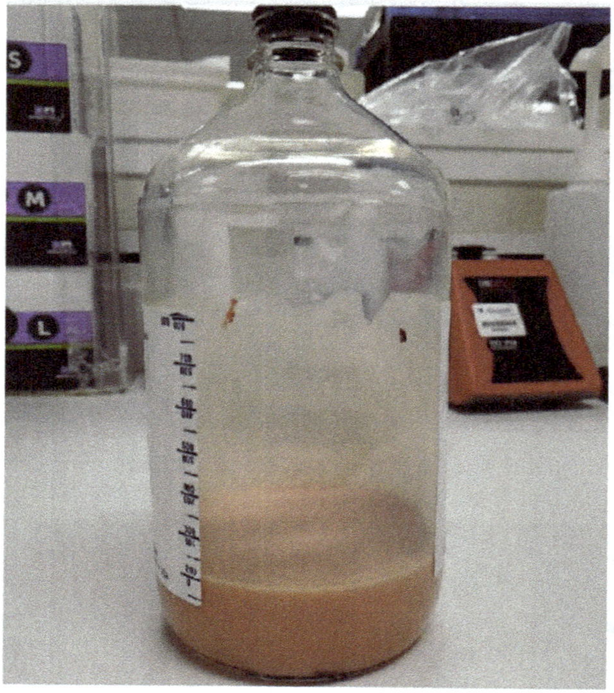

FIGURE 3: Chylous pericardial fluid.

Chylopericardium presents similarly to other causes of pericardial effusion. It varies considerably, ranging from asymptomatic to cardiac tamponade. Fatigue, dyspnea, and cough are the most common symptoms [1–3]. Initial workup includes a chest X-ray which may show an enlarged cardiac silhouette and echocardiography which can confirm the presence of pericardial effusion and evaluate for cardiac tamponade. Pericardiocentesis can be used for both diagnostic and therapeutic purposes. Analysis of the pericardial fluid in chylopericardium typically shows high levels of triglycerides and protein with an elevated lymphocyte count.

Further investigations to determine the underlying cause of chylopericardium should also be pursued. A thorough history can evaluate for recent trauma, thoracic surgery, potential exposure to tuberculosis, or signs of malignancy [1, 2]. Testing for tuberculosis was not done in the presented case as there was no clinical or radiographical evidence to suggest tuberculosis and the patient had no history of travel outside the United States. A lymphangiogram may also be useful in the diagnosis of mediastinal lymphangiomatosis; however, this was not done in this case as the underlying cause for his chylopericardium was established.

A scoring system has been suggested by Dib et al. to assist in the diagnosis of chyloperdicardium [3]. The score is calculated by assigning a point to each of the following features: milky yellowish appearance of fluid, triglyceride level of >500 mg/dL, total cholesterol to triglyceride ratio of <1, and negative fluid bacterial culture with lymphocytic predominance on fluid cell count. A score of two is required for a diagnosis of chylopericardium. The patient in the presented case had a score of four, which is highly indicative of chylopericardium.

Initial management of chylopericardium includes a low-fat diet and initiation of medium-chain triglycerides, which are absorbed via the portal vein rather than via the lymphatic vessels [1–3]. Pericardiocentesis is both diagnostic and therapeutic. Surgical intervention, including pericardial window or thoracic duct ligation, is generally recommended when the daily pericardial drainage is more than 1,500 mL daily, drainage is more than 500 mL daily for five days, or in the setting of malnutrition or recurrent chylopericardium [1, 7].

In the presented case, the cause of chylopericardium was attributed to the extensive venous thrombosis of the patient's SVC and left subclavian vein. Despite anticoagulation with therapeutic enoxaparin, serial imaging showed increasing size of pericardial effusion with evidence of tamponade and progressive thrombosis. Similar cases in the literature were primarily treated with venous stenting or surgical intervention [4, 8]. Although surgical intervention was considered in this case, it was felt that this would only prevent reaccumulation of chyle without addressing the underlying cause. Treatment with catheter-directed thrombolysis was instead pursued. The patient's symptoms resolved, and his chylopericardium did not recur, indicating successful treatment.

4. Conclusion

Chylopericardium is a rare complication of SVC or subclavian vein thrombosis. Our patient with protein S deficiency represents a very rare case of chylopericardium caused by thrombosis secondary to hereditary thrombophilia. Our case also demonstrates that systemic anticoagulation and catheter-directed thrombolysis may be sufficient for treatment without the need for surgical intervention.

References

[1] R. Svedjeholm, K. Jansson, and C. Olin, "Primary idiopathic chylopericardium-a case report and review of the literature," *European Journal of Cardio-Thoracic Surgery*, vol. 11, no. 2, pp. 387–390, 1997.

[2] Z. Han, S. Li, H. Jing, and H. Liu, "Primary idiopathic chylopericardium: a retrospective case series," *BMC Surgery*, vol. 15, no. 1, pp. 1–5, 2015.

[3] C. Dib, A. J. Tajik, S. Park, M. E. Kheir, B. Khandieria, and F. Mookadam, "Chylopericardium in adults: a literature review over the past decade (1996-2006)," *The Journal of Thoracic and Cardiovascular Surgery*, vol. 136, no. 3, pp. 650–656, 2008.

[4] M. Nardini, E. Katsogridakis, M. Migliore, and J. Dunning, "Chylopericardium with symptoms of tamponade on the grounds of extensive neck vein thrombosis," *Journal of surgical case reports*, vol. 2017, no. 1, 2017.

[5] C. S. Thomas Jr. and D. C. McGoon, "Isolated massive chylopericardium following cardiopulmonary bypass," *The Journal of Thoracic and Cardiovascular Surgery*, vol. 61, no. 6, pp. 945–948, 1971.

[6] J. Andrade Santiago, L. Robles, C. Casimiro et al., "Chylopericardium of neoplastic aetiology," *Annals of Oncology*, vol. 9, no. 12, pp. 1339–1342, 1998.

[7] X. Yu, N. Jia, S. Ye, M. Zhou, and D. Liu, "Primary chylopericardium: a case report and literature review," *Experimental and Therapeutic Medicine*, vol. 15, no. 1, pp. 419–425, 2018.

[8] C.-M. Chen, P. M. Ku, Y. Y. Lu, Y. Fong, and T. Y. Huang, "Secondary chylopericardium complicated with cardiac tamponade in a drug addict: a case report," *Journal of Internal Medicine of Taiwan*, vol. 15, pp. 214–218, 2004.

32

A Rare Case of a Right Atrial Paraganglioma in an Individual with the SHDB Mutation

Ian Lancaster, Carlos Nunez, Andrew Willinger, Christiano Caldeira, and Jeffrey Aufman

HCA Healthcare/USF Morsani College of Medicine GME/Largo Medical Center, 201 14th St. SW, Largo, FL 33770, USA

Correspondence should be addressed to Ian Lancaster; ian.lancaster.2@und.edu

Academic Editor: Yi Yan

Paragangliomas are extra-adrenal chromaffin cell tumors. A small percentage of these tumors can be found in the thoracic cavity and, when in the heart, are typically in the left atrium. In this case report, we discuss the case of an individual with a history of several paragangliomas with the *SHDB* mutation who was found to have two cardiac paragangliomas in the right atrium.

1. Introduction

Paragangliomas are extra-adrenal chromaffin cell tumors [1]. The approximate incidence of paragangliomas and pheochromocytomas is approximately 6-7 cases per million individuals per year [2]. The incidence of pheochromocytoma and paragangliomas increases through adulthood until age 60–79 years old, where in the incidence is 8.85 and 14.68 cases per 100,000 people annually for males and females, respectively [2]. In addition, approximately 1.2% of paragangliomas occur in the thoracic cavity [2]. Also, approximately 1% of all paragangliomas are cardiac paragangliomas [2].

There are two general classes of cardiac paragangliomas, sympathetic and parasympathetic. Sympathetic paragangliomas produce catecholamines (particularly norepinephrine or epinephrine) while parasympathetic paragangliomas are usually nonfunctional and mainly located in the head and neck [3]. Cardiac paragangliomas arise from the visceral or branchiomeric autonomic paraganglia resulting in the left atrial and aortic body tumors, respectively [3]. Although cardiac paragangliomas are commonly described in all cardiac chambers, left atrial paragangliomas are the most common, followed by aortic body tumors [3]. Mutations in the succinate dehydrogenase complex unit B (*SDHB*) or succinate dehydrogenase complex subunit D (*SDHD*) genes are common in individuals with thoracic paragangliomas [4].

Frequently, cardiac paragangliomas are close to the great vessels and can involve any of the cardiac cavities [3, 5]. Moreover, these tumors infiltrate cardiac tissues or the pericardial space, which can result in features of cardiac tamponade and make resection challenging [5–7]. In instances when the atrioventricular groove or extracardiac structures are involved, resection may become impossible [5]. Medical management prior to resection of these tumors is aimed at preventing the perioperative complications including hypertensive crisis, cardiac arrhythmias, or even myocardial infarction with the use of alpha- (α-) adrenoceptor and beta- (β-) adrenoceptor blockers at least 2 weeks prior to the surgery [8]. In this case report, we discuss the case of a 26-year-old male whom presented for surgical management of his right atrial paraganglioma.

2. Case Presentation

A 26-year-old male with a past medical history of pheochromocytoma and multiple head and neck paragangliomas presented for worsening shortness of breath for the last "couple of weeks." His dyspnea was present both on exertion and at rest. He had no associated chest pain, palpitations, sweating, nausea, or vomiting. Additionally, he states that he had no similar events to this shortness of breath. He had no reported "significant" change in weight over the last 3 months and states that his hypertension had been "well managed" with his reported systolic blood pressures ranging from 110 to 130 on his current antihypertensive regimen. At an outside facility, an echocardiogram and cardiac magnetic resonance imaging were performed and a right atrial mass was appreciated prompting transfer to a specialized cardiac care center. He did not require supplemental oxygen; his lungs were clear to auscultation bilaterally, and no murmurs were appreciated on physical exam. He was admitted for a planned resection of his cardiac tumor with review of preoperative imaging to be completed for assistance in guiding the operative approach.

As previously stated, his past medical history was significant for multiple paragangliomas in his head and neck, pheochromocytoma requiring adrenalectomy, and an *SDHB* gene mutation. His first case of an identified paraganglioma occurred when he was 14 years of age and was found to have the *SDHB* mutation. Per report, he had undergone at least 6 surgical excisions for a variety of paragangliomas though the dates of these procedures were unknown. His most recent surgical excision was 7 years prior to presentation per patient and family report. In addition, his past medical history also includes adrenal insufficiency following adrenalectomy, hypertension, asthma, and tobacco use. His family history was significant for pheochromocytoma in his sister, father, uncle, and paternal grandfather with each requiring surgical excision and no further recurrences of catecholamine secreting tumors in those family members. Additionally, his mother had a history of hypertension.

His medication regimen as an outpatient included hydrocortisone for adrenal insufficiency as well as carvedilol, amlodipine, and doxazosin for management of his hypertension associated with his paragangliomas.

Lab work following transfer was performed and demonstrated a hemoglobin of 13.9 g/dL, white blood cell count of 7.0×10^9/L, platelet count of 325×10^9/L, sodium of 142 mEq/L, potassium of 3.5 mEq/L, creatinine of 0.91 mg/dL, and blood urea nitrogen (BUN) of 9 mg/dL. His coagulation studies were unremarkable, and liver function studies did not identify any abnormalities. His serum troponin was assessed preoperatively and was less than 0.04 ng/mL. His plasma norepinephrine level was 1186 pg/mL, and plasma normetanephrine level was 283.3 pg/mL. Additionally, his epinephrine level was less than 15 pg/mL and plasma metanephrine was 12.4 pg/mL. His baseline catecholamine levels as an outpatient were not available for review. Radiograph of the chest did not identify an acute cardiopulmonary disease.

For surgical evaluation, review of prior imaging was performed. A transesophageal echocardiogram (TEE) identified two tumors within the right atrium (Figures 1 and 2). The presence of the cardiac tumors was then confirmed with cardiac magnetic resonance imaging.

As an outpatient, the patient had been compliant with his regime of carvedilol, amlodipine, and doxazosin. For preoperative management, he was continued on his outpatient medication regimen.

Following review of the echocardiogram and cardiac magnetic resonance imaging, surgical excision of the two masses were performed. The first tumor was small, measuring 1.0 cm in greatest dimension on the right atrium and close to the atrial appendage on the atrioventricular groove. The second tumor was larger and measured to be 2.5 cm in greatest dimension and attached to the atrioventricular

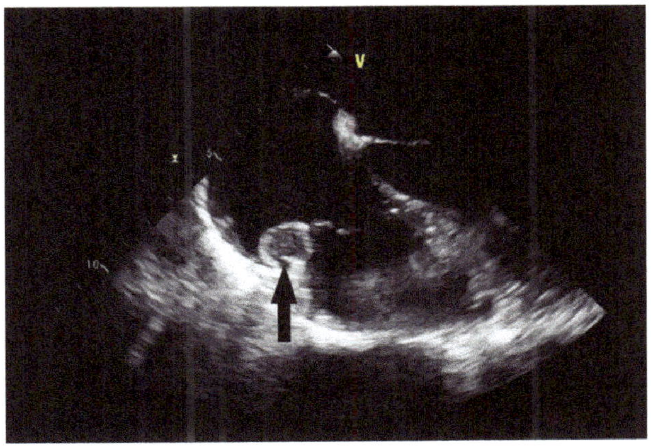

FIGURE 1: TEE horizontal view: right atrial mass (black arrow) in the area adjacent to the tricuspid valve. No visual obstruction of flow was identified on Doppler.

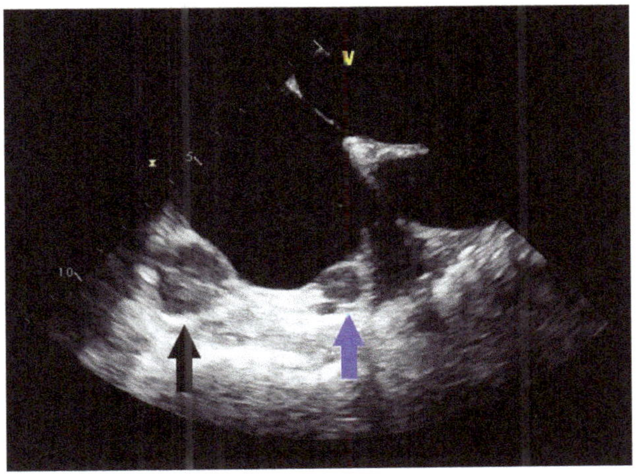

FIGURE 2: TEE horizontal view: right atrial masses in the area of the tricuspid valve and atrioventricular groove (blue arrow) and in the area of the atrioventricular groove (black arrow).

groove, close to the right coronary artery (RCA) on the acute angle of the heart. For excision of the tumors, the patient was placed on full cardiopulmonary bypass. The tumors were then successfully excised and hemostasis was achieved using electrocautery, followed by the placement of several sutures. He had 500 cc of reported fluid loss and did not require transfusion of blood products.

After resection of the tumors, each excised mass was then sent to the pathologist for review. Histologic review confirmed paraganglioma for each of the resected tumors. Immunohistochemistry confirmed neoplastic cells which stained positive for chromogranin and GATA binding protein 3 (GATA-3) and a solid nest-like arrangement partially demarcated by S100-positive sustentacular cells in a "Zellballen" pattern (Figures 3(a), 3(b) and 4).

3. Discussion

Pheochromocytomas are chromaffin cell tumors located within the adrenal medulla while paragangliomas are

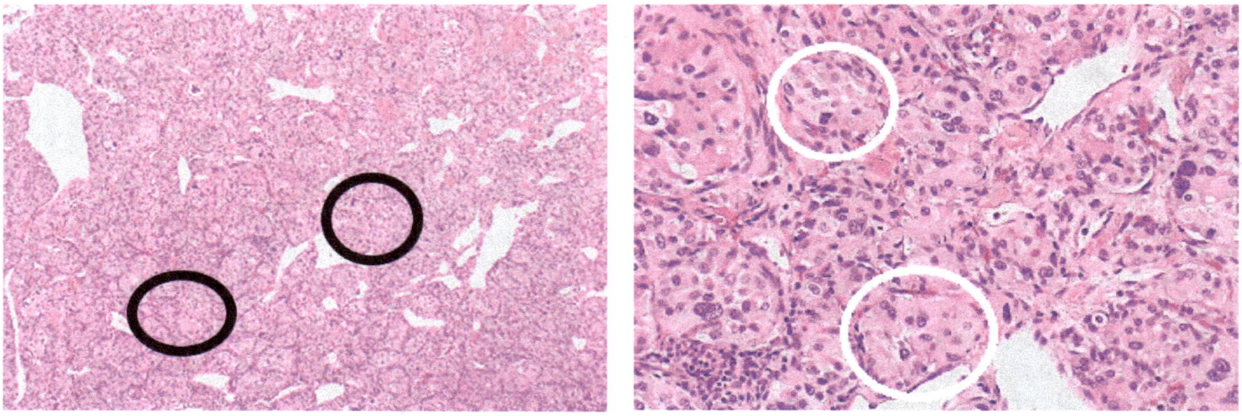

(a) (b)

Figure 3: (a) Cardiac paraganglioma histology. Multiple large groups of characteristic Zellballen morphology (in black circles) with nests of uniform, polygonal chromaffin/chief cells surrounded by sustentacular support cells and well-formed vascular cuffing. (b) Cardiac paraganglioma histology. Characteristic Zellballen morphology (white circles) with nests of uniform, polygonal chromaffin/chief cells surrounded by sustentacular support cells and well-formed vascular cuffing.

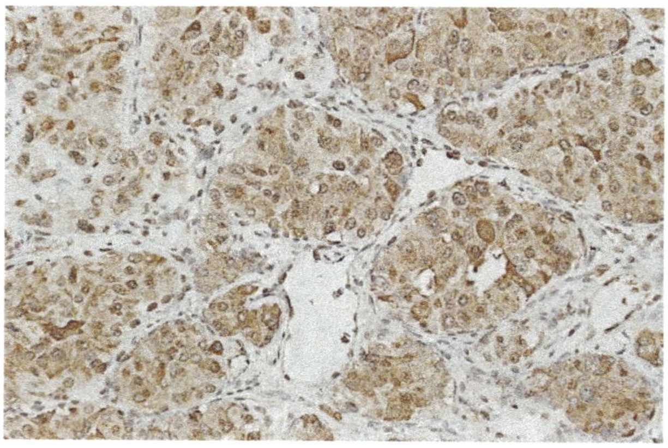

Figure 4: Cardiac paraganglioma histology. Chromaffin cells positive with chromogranin-positive immunohistochemistry stain.

extra-adrenal. Approximately 1.2% of paragangliomas are located within the thoracic cavity, most in the posterior mediastinum [1] and a minority of these tumors are located within the heart [3, 9]. In a prior review of cardiac paragangliomas, it was identified that 85% arise from the epicardium (including interatrial groove and atrioventricular groove) as well as the root of the great vessels (including aorta, pulmonary artery, pulmonary vein, and vena cava) [5]. Typically, these tumors are found in the left atrium, 41.9%, but have been found in all four chambers of the heart and rise to the branchiomeric and visceral autonomic paraganglia [3, 5, 9]. This patient's paragangliomas were found within the right atrium and, to our knowledge, only 6 cases have been reported within the right atrium [5]. Cardiac paragangliomas are highly vascular and derive their blood supply from the coronary circulation [5]. These tumors usually do to not invade to surrounding structures, but their adherence to the surrounding tissues is thought to be due to compression [5]. Upon histologic evaluation, paragangliomas are composed of "chief cells" grouped together in cell clusters referred to as a "Zellballen" surrounded by a capillary network [10].

Evaluation for paragangliomas begins with the patient history and physical exam. Usually, patients complain of episodic headache, diaphoresis, tachycardia, or hypertension; and less commonly can present with palpitations, panic attacks, dyspnea, or orthostatic hypotension [11]. Then biochemical evaluation is performed with 24-hour urine catecholamines and metanephrines or serum metanephrines, with no test being preferred over the other [8]. The elevation in catecholamines is required for the diagnosis [12], but the degree elevation does not predict the invasiveness of the paraganglioma or pheochromocytoma [12, 13]. This is because multiple medications such as antipsychotics, serotonin reuptake inhibitors, and tricyclic antidepressants may alter the serum levels of catecholamines. In this patient's case, he did not complain of new symptomatology other than his shortness of breath. As he was already undergoing treatment for paragangliomas, he did not require biochemical confirmation. Next, imaging for identification of new paragangliomas is performed with either computed tomography (CT) or magnetic resonance imaging (MRI) (Figure 5) [14, 15]. In the case of cardiac paragangliomas both transthoracic and transesophageal echocardiograms can be used for evaluation of the tumor [1, 14]. Additionally, coronary angiography can be considered to outline the vasculature of the tumor prior to surgery as well as the opportunity to embolize potential vascular supplies to the tumor. After the tumor has been identified, further imaging may be required to evaluate for metastatic disease. Previously the 123-I meta-iodobenzyl-guanidine (MIBG) imaging was used to look for metastatic disease [1]. Now, current evaluation methods for detecting metastatic disease include positron emission tomography (PET) with or with computed tomography (CT), somatostatin receptor imaging using indium^{111}- or Tc^{99m}-labeled octreotide or magnetic resonance imaging [5, 16]. This patient had his tumors identified on echocardiogram for evaluation of his dyspnea.

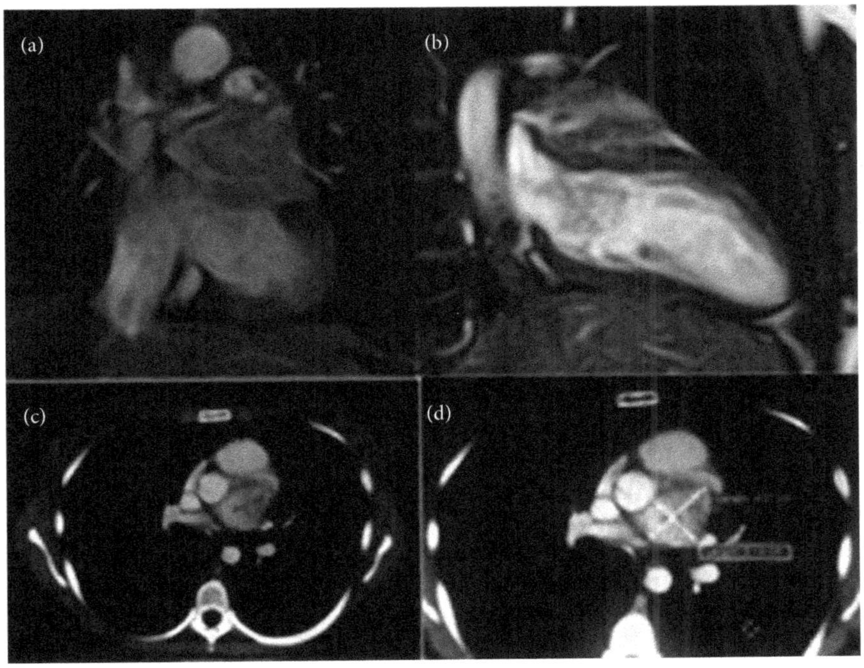

FIGURE 5: An example of Cardiac MRI with a cardiac paraganglioma [10]. (a) Coronal image with mass (isointense) in the area of the left atrium. (b) Two camber longitudinal view with the mass (isointense) in the left atrioventricular groove. (c, d) Axial view demonstrating the mass in relation to the aortic root (c) and pulmonary artery (d), respectively.

These tumors were then confirmed on cardiac magnetic resonance imaging. His outpatient PET scans were not available for review during the hospitalization but were reportedly negative.

The hemodynamic effects and management of cardiac paragangliomas and are dependent on their size, location, and presence of obstruction associated with the tumor. Additionally, paragangliomas are associated most commonly with a catecholamine surge leading to labile elevations in blood pressure which precipitate cardiovascular collapse, pulmonary edema, and occasionally acute respiratory failure [17]. This may be induced by a variety of stimuli of mechanical stressors or by psychological stressors such as anxiety or severe pain [18]. Additionally, hypotension from circulatory collapse is most commonly due to left ventricular dysfunction leading to left ventricular outlet obstruction [19]. In rare instances, the circulatory collapse may due to beta-2 adrenoreceptor stimulation by epinephrine which results in peripheral vasodilation thus precipitating the hypotension [18].

The definitive treatment for cardiac paragangliomas is surgical excision [20]. The major consideration for the majority of patients is the timing of the procedure as well as the surgical approach. The preoperative and intraoperative management of patients with paragangliomas is focused on prevention of hypertensive crises and hypotensive episodes [13]. This is achieved with alpha-blockade followed by beta-blockade and occasional use of dihydropyridine calcium channel blockers for blood pressure control [10]. As an outpatient, the patient was already on metoprolol, doxazosin, and amlodipine. Following admission, intraoperative management with intravenous phenylephrine, esmolol, and nicardipine was undertaken [13]. Due to the heterogeneity of paraganglioma locations in the heart, a wide variety of surgical maneuvers can be employed to achieve surgical excision. Included are transection the inferior vena cava, superior vena cava, pulmonary artery, or aortic root replacement [11, 20]. In the analysis of 100 cardiac paragangliomas requiring surgical excision, approximately 10% had died due to extensive blood loss following surgical excision [4, 20]. In this patient's case, he was placed "off pump" prior to surgical excision and bypass was terminated only after electrocautery and suture placement had finished.

When individuals are considered poor candidates for surgical excision treatment options include chemotherapy and radionuclide therapy. Instances which may exclude patients from surgical excision include the location of the tumor, most typically head and neck paragangliomas; the extent of tumor invasion; and the size of the tumor, especially when greater than 5 cm in diameter [13, 16]. Multiple chemotherapeutic regimens have been developed for paragangliomas and include the CVD regimen of cyclophosphamide, vincristine, and darcarbazine; temozolomide monotherapy; radionuclide pharmacotherapy such as conventional or high-specific activity ^{131}I-MIBG; and peptide receptor radionuclide therapy either alone or in combination with octreotide or low-dose capecitabine [21]. In those with rapidly progressive and metastatic disease, especially in individuals with *SDHB* mutations, combination chemotherapy with CVD followed by temozolomide monotherapy is a first-line option [22]. In the patients who have failed standard temozolomide monotherapy, long-term low-dose temozolomide (metronomic regimen) in combination with lanreotide may be attempted [23]. Alternatively, in patients with slowly progressive metastatic disease, systemic radiotherapy with ^{131}I-MIBG or ^{177}Lu/^{90}Y-DOTA peptides should be considered [16]. With regard to metastatic paragangliomas, treatment will include both surgical excision as well as consideration for treatment with chemotherapy, radionuclide therapy, thermal ablation, or external radiation therapy [13].

Next, identification of primary versus metastatic paragangliomas and pheochromocytomas is challenge. Primary tumors may develop in any location where sympathetic or parasympathetic ganglia are located [24]. Due to the wide dispersion and anatomic locations of both parasympathetic and sympathetic ganglia, the identification of primary versus metastatic tumors is challenging [24]. Thus, World Health Organization (WHO) in 2017 had updated the classification system to define metastatic disease as only sites where normal chromaffin tissue is not present [24]. This was done with the intention of avoiding misclassification of multicentric primary tumors as metastases. In this patient's case, though it had not been confirmed at the time, his tumor most likely represented a primary tumor due to the parasympathetic and sympathetic tissues located within the heart. Lastly, histology is required for a more complete evaluation for presence of metastatic paragangliomas [25]. This has led to the development of scoring systems such as the Grading System for Adrenal Pheochromocytoma and Paraganglioma (GAPP) in an attempt to predict the likelihood of future metastatic disease of a tumor [25]. This scoring system utilizes the histologic pattern, cellularity, presence of necrosis, vascular invasion, Ki67 labeling, and type of catecholamine secreting tumor to predict the likelihood of metastatic behavior [25]. Unfortunately, no single risk stratification has been endorsed for widespread use [26].

The majority of paragangliomas occur sporadically, but up to 30-40% are familial and associated with a variety of genes [27]. For individuals with newly identified paragangliomas, screening for germline mutations is recommended. Currently, the Von Hippel Lindau tumor suppressor gene (VHL); *RET* protooncgene, neurofibromin 1 (NF1); succinate dehydrogenase genes *SDHD*, *SDHAF2*, *SDHC*, *SDHB*, *SDHA*; transmembrane protein 127 (*TMEM127*); and MYC-associated factor X (*MAX*) [13]. The thoracic paragangliomas, including cardiac paragangliomas, are associated mostly with mutations in *SDHB*, *SDHD*, or *VHL* [13]. In our patient, he was previously evaluated to have the *SDHB* mutation. This gene as well as the other succinate dehydrogenase subunits (A, B, C, and D) are proteins within the mitochondria and are involved in both the Krebs cycle and electron transport chain [28]. Patient with the *SDHB*, *SDHC*, and *SDHD* genes are associated with cardiac paragangliomas and the *SDHB* mutation being the having the strongest association with cardiac paragangliomas [28]. Further, the *SDHB* mutation has been associated with extra-adrenal paragangliomas and metastases and is transmitted in an autosomal dominant inheritance pattern [4].

Depending on the patient's genetic mutation that and clinical scenario identified will determine the patient's surveillance and recommended follow-up. For individuals with the *SDHA*, *SDHB*, or *SDHD* mutations, MRI imaging including the skull base and neck, thorax, retroperitoneum and pelvis are recommended [13]. Additionally, it recommended that patients obtain a baseline measurement of metanephrines which is to then be followed by annual metanephrine levels [13]. Following surgical removal of pheochromocytomas or paragangliomas, it recommended to repeat imaging annually for 3 years following excision. In body areas that have had no tumor removal, it is recommended to repeat imaging every 3 years [13]. It is recommended that this follow-up be done with additionally follow-up with an endocrinologist. In our patient, it is recommended that he undergo MRI imaging of his thorax annually given his surgical removal of 2 right atrial paragangliomas in additional to other regularly recommended outpatient monitoring imaging.

For all individuals with first-degree relatives of an individual whom has been diagnosed with a paraganglioma and who also had an identified mutation should be offered predictive (or cascade) testing in the context of genetic counseling [13], the testing of first degree relatives has a 50% likelihood of identifying carriers of a mutation, most of which are typically asymptomatic [13]. These asymptomatic mutation carriers should be offered similar clinical surveillance and management as individuals whom have the mutation and a history of paraganglioma [13, 29].

4. Conclusions

Cardiac paragangliomas are extra-adrenal chromaffin cell tumors which are typically located in the left atrium but can present within all four chambers of the heart as well as the aortic and pulmonic valves. These tumors typically present with episodic tachycardia, hypertension, diaphoresis, and headache. Evaluation of paragangliomas will initially start with biochemical evaluation with 24-hour urine metanephrines or plasma metanephrines followed by magnetic resonance imaging or computed tomography. Treatment of these tumors is complete resection, and preoperative management consists of alpha-blockade followed by beta-blockade with consideration for use of calcium channel blockers for hypertension. When available, genetic analysis is recommended for individuals with paragangliomas and the *SHDB* mutation is associated cardiac paragangliomas.

Disclosure

The views expressed in this publication represent those of the authors and do not necessarily represent the official views of HCA Healthcare or any of its affiliated entities.

Acknowledgments

This research was supported (in whole or in part) by the HCA Healthcare and/or an HCA Healthcare-affiliated entity.

References

[1] R. K. Whalen, A. F. Althausen, and G. H. Daniels, "Extra-adrenal pheochromocytoma," *The Journal of Urology*, vol. 147, no. 1, pp. 1–10, 1992.

[2] A. A. Leung, J. L. Pasieka, M. D. Hyrcza et al., "Epidemiology of pheochromocytoma and paraganglioma: population-based cohort study," *European Journal of Endocrinology*, vol. 184, no. 1, pp. 19–28, 2021.

[3] A. K. Lam, "Update on adrenal tumours in 2017 World Health Organization (WHO) of endocrine tumours," *Endocrine Pathology*, vol. 28, no. 3, pp. 213–227, 2017.

[4] L. Amar, J. Bertherat, E. Baudin et al., "Genetic testing in pheochromocytoma or functional paraganglioma," *Journal of Clinical Oncology*, vol. 23, no. 34, pp. 8812–8818, 2005.

[5] J. G. Wang, J. Han, T. Jiang, and Y. J. Li, "Cardiac paragangliomas," *Journal of Cardiac Surgery*, vol. 30, no. 1, pp. 55–60, 2015.

[6] Y. Y. Chen, W. C. Huang, M. H. Huang, T. M. Lu, and C. P. Hsu, "The intra-pericardial paraganglioma presenting as ascites and hemopericardium with impending tamponade," *International Heart Journal*, vol. 59, no. 3, pp. 664–667, 2018.

[7] H. R. Khan, M. I. Ansari, A. P. Thain, S. Abdullah, R. Parasa, and R. W. Varcoe, "Mediastinal monophasic synovial sarcoma with pericardial extension causing hemodynamic instability," *Oxford Medical Case Reports*, vol. 2018, no. 5, article omy017, 2018.

[8] J. W. Lenders, K. Pacak, M. M. Walther et al., "Biochemical diagnosis of pheochromocytoma: which test is best?," *Journal of the American Medical Association*, vol. 287, no. 11, pp. 1427–1434, 2002.

[9] V. Jeevanandam, M. C. Oz, B. Shapiro, M. L. Barr, C. Marboe, and E. A. Rose, "Surgical management of cardiac pheochromocytoma resection versus transplantation," *Annals of surgery*, vol. 221, no. 4, pp. 415–419, 1995.

[10] I. Mikolaenko, C. A. Galliani, and G. G. Davis, "Pigmented cardiac paraganglioma," *Archives of Pathology & Laboratory Medicine*, vol. 125, no. 5, pp. 680–682, 2001.

[11] W. M. Manger, "The vagaries of pheochromocytomas," *American Journal of Hypertension*, vol. 18, no. 10, pp. 1266–1270, 2005.

[12] A. M. Sawka, R. Jaeschke, R. J. Singh, and W. F. Young Jr., "A comparison of biochemical tests for pheochromocytoma: measurement of fractionated plasma metanephrines compared with the combination of 24-hour urinary metanephrines and catecholamines," *The Journal of Clinical Endocrinology and Metabolism*, vol. 88, no. 2, pp. 553–558, 2003.

[13] H. P. H. Neumann, W. F. Young Jr., and C. Eng, "Pheochromocytoma and paraganglioma," *The New England Journal of Medicine*, vol. 381, no. 6, pp. 552–565, 2019.

[14] M. S. Eigelberger and Q. Y. Duh, "Pheochromocytoma," *Current Treatment Options in Oncology*, vol. 2, no. 4, pp. 321–329, 2001.

[15] L. Arcos, J. Bustos, J. Acuña, A. Cely, J. Forero, and C. Jaimes, "Cardiac paraganglioma: advantages of cardiovascular multimodality imaging," *CASE: Cardiovascular Imaging Case Reports*, vol. 2, no. 6, pp. 266–272, 2018.

[16] S. H. Tella, A. Jha, D. Taïeb, K. A. Horvath, and K. Pacak, "Comprehensive review of evaluation and management of cardiac paragangliomas," *Heart*, vol. 106, no. 16, pp. 1202–1210, 2020.

[17] C. E. Greenleaf, L. A. Griffin, J. G. Shake, and W. S. Orr, "Hypertensive crisis secondary to pheochromocytoma," *Baylor University Medical Center Proceedings*, vol. 30, no. 3, pp. 314-315, 2017.

[18] J. M. Pappachan, N. N. Tun, G. Arunagirinathan, R. Sodi, and F. W. F. Hanna, "Pheochromocytomas and hypertension," *Current hypertension reports*, vol. 20, no. 1, pp. 1–13, 2018.

[19] H. Falhammar, "Pheochromocytoma-and paraganglioma-triggered Takotsubo syndrome," *Endocrine*, vol. 65, no. 3, pp. 483–493, 2019.

[20] S. Yendamuri, M. Elfar, J. C. Walkes, and M. J. Reardon, "Aortic paraganglioma requiring resection and replacement of the aortic root," *Interactive Cardiovascular and Thoracic Surgery*, vol. 6, no. 6, pp. 830-831, 2007.

[21] G. Kong, S. Grozinsky-Glasberg, M. S. Hofman et al., "Efficacy of peptide receptor radionuclide therapy for functional metastatic paraganglioma and pheochromocytoma," *The Journal of Clinical Endocrinology and Metabolism*, vol. 102, no. 9, pp. 3278–3287, 2017.

[22] S. Nölting, A. Grossman, and K. Pacak, "Metastatic phaeochromocytoma: spinning towards more promising treatment options," *Experimental and Clinical Endocrinology & Diabetes*, vol. 127, no. 2-03, pp. 117–128, 2019.

[23] I. Tena, G. Gupta, M. Tajahuerce et al., "Successful second-line metronomic temozolomide in metastatic paraganglioma: case reports and review of the literature," *Clinical Medicine Insights: Oncology*, vol. 12, 2018.

[24] A. S. Tischler, R. R. De Krijger, A. Gill et al., "Phaeochromocytoma," in *WHO Classification of Tumors of Endocrine Organs*, R. V. Lloyd, R. Y. Osamura, and G. Kloppel, Eds., pp. 183–189, International Agency for Research on Cancer, Lyon, France, 4th edition, 2017.

[25] N. Kimura, R. Takayanagi, N. Takizawa et al., "Pathological grading for predicting metastasis in phaeochromocytoma and paraganglioma," *Endocrine-Related Cancer*, vol. 21, no. 3, pp. 405–414, 2014.

[26] J. Turchini, V. K. Y. Cheung, A. S. Tischler, R. R. De Krijger, and A. J. Gill, "Pathology and genetics of phaeochromocytoma and paraganglioma," *Histopathology*, vol. 72, no. 1, pp. 97–105, 2018.

[27] C. C. Boedeker, "Paragangliomas and paraganglioma syndromes," *GMS Current Topics in Otorhinolaryngology - Head and Neck Surgery*, vol. 10, p. Doc03, 2011.

[28] A. P. Gimenez-Roqueplo, P. L. Dahia, and M. Robledo, "An update on the genetics of paraganglioma, pheochromocytoma, and associated hereditary syndromes," *Hormone and Metabolic Research*, vol. 44, no. 5, pp. 328–333, 2012.

[29] J. W. Lenders, Q. Y. Duh, G. Eisenhofer et al., "Pheochromocytoma and paraganglioma: an Endocrine Society clinical practice guideline," *The Journal of Clinical Endocrinology and Metabolism*, vol. 99, no. 6, pp. 1915–1942, 2014.

33

The Slower, the Better: Wide Complex Tachycardia Triggered by Flecainide in an Elderly Female

Ebubechukwu Ezeh,[1] **Maddie Perdoncin**,[1] **Morgan K. Moroi**,[2] **Mohammad Amro**,[3] **Mohammed Ruzieh**,[4] **and Paul I. Okhumale**[5]

[1]*Department of Internal Medicine, Marshall University, Huntington, WV, USA*
[2]*Pennsylvania State University, State College, PA, USA*
[3]*The Palestinian Ministry of Health and Higher Education, State of Palestine*
[4]*University of Florida, Gainesville, FL, USA*
[5]*Cedar Valley Cardiovascular Center, Waterloo, IA, USA*

Correspondence should be addressed to Maddie Perdoncin; perdoncin@marshall.edu

Academic Editor: Gopal Chandra Ghosh

Class IC antiarrhythmics are generally considered a safe means of treating many common arrhythmias such as atrial fibrillation (a-fib), atrial flutter (a-flutter), and paroxysmal supraventricular tachycardia (PSVT). Essentially, flecainide works by binding and blocking sodium channels more effectively at higher heart rates. However, this class of drugs is known to exhibit use dependence which could predispose patients to the development of malignant arrhythmias during episodes of tachycardia. In this case, we present a patient who was being treated with flecainide for a-fib who ultimately developed a wide complex tachycardia after her metoprolol was held.

1. Introduction

Antiarrhythmic medications have been around for over 100 years and are commonly prescribed for conditions such as atrial fibrillation. As the burden of cardiac arrhythmias increases in the United States, these medications have quickly become one of the mainstays of therapy. The primary goal of treatment with these agents in a-fib is to achieve pharmacological cardioversion and limit the number of arrhythmic episodes as well as decrease the number of hospitalizations and mortality associated with atrial fibrillation [1].

The antiarrhythmic medications have historically been classified according to the Vaughan-Williams system, which groups them based on their mechanism of action [2]. Class I antiarrhythmic drugs are known to work by inhibiting cardiac sodium channels. While this group has had a significant impact on patient treatment, it does have significant proarrhythmic side effects. This is particularly pronounced with the class IC antiarrhythmics such as flecainide. Flecainide works in a use-dependent manner, essentially blocking sodium channels more potently at faster heart rates. When this property is not taken into consideration during treatment, malignant arrhythmias can occur [3]. We present the case of a 70-year-old woman treated with flecainide who developed a wide complex tachycardia after her beta blocker therapy was discontinued. This case was presented as an abstract at the 2022 American College of Cardiology conference in Washington, D.C. [4].

2. Clinical Presentation

A 70-year-old woman with paroxysmal a-fib status post direct current cardioversion (DCCV) a few weeks prior presented to the emergency department (ED) with generalized weakness and altered mental status. She had a history of hypertension. A day prior to arriving at the ED, the patient's husband noted that she appeared pale and weak. She was

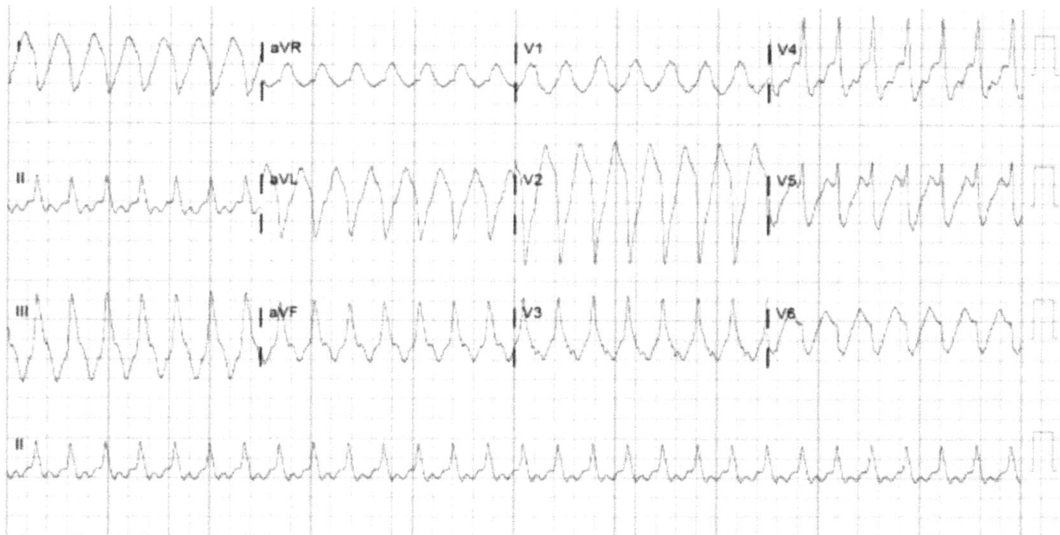

FIGURE 1: Presenting 12-lead electrocardiogram.

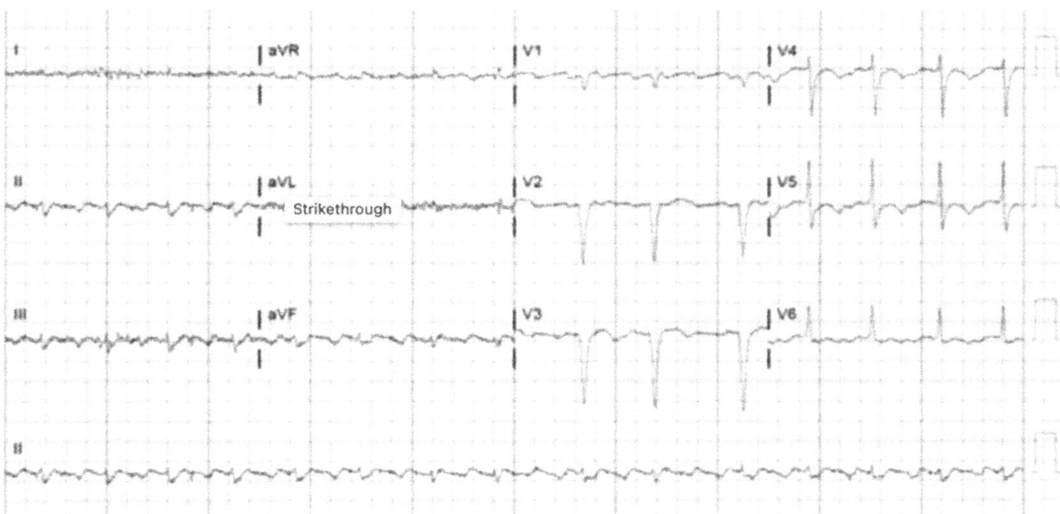

FIGURE 2: ECG showing atrial flutter after administration of metoprolol and amiodarone.

taken to her local pharmacy where her heart rate was found to be 40-45 beats per minute (bpm) and her blood pressure was normal. Her medications included metoprolol 12.5 milligram (mg) twice a day, flecainide 75 mg twice a day, and apixaban 5 mg twice a day. Then, her primary care physician was notified and recommended holding metoprolol and close observation. Her symptoms, however, persisted, and she eventually presented to the emergency department.

Upon initial evaluation, the patient was lethargic but responsive. She denied current feelings of weakness or altered mentation. Electrocardiogram (ECG) revealed wide complex tachycardia with a heart rate of 174 bpm and prolonged QRS of 270 ms (Figure 1), and cardiology was consulted. Serial ECGs continued to show wide complex tachycardia with heart rates between 180 and 190 bpm; the patient remained normotensive. Since the patient was stable, DCCV was deferred. Instead, 150 mg of amiodarone and 5 mg of metoprolol tartrate were given. Within a few minutes, the patient converted to normal sinus rhythm. She was then admitted to the hospital for observation. A transthoracic echocardiogram demonstrated newly depressed left ventricular systolic function.

The ECG revealed a regular wide complex tachycardia at a heart rate of 170 bpm and a prolonged QRS with duration of 270 ms (Figure 1). The following differential diagnosis was entertained including atrial flutter with 1 : 1 atrioventricular (AV) conduction, SVT with aberrancy, QRS widening attributable to flecainide, and ventricular tachycardia. Given the patient's exposure to flecainide and the absence of A-V dissociation (best appreciated in leads II, V3, and V4), atrial tachycardia or atrial flutter with 1 : 1 conduction was the topmost on the differential.

The administration of amiodarone and metoprolol slowed the ventricular rate revealing the flutter waves as shown

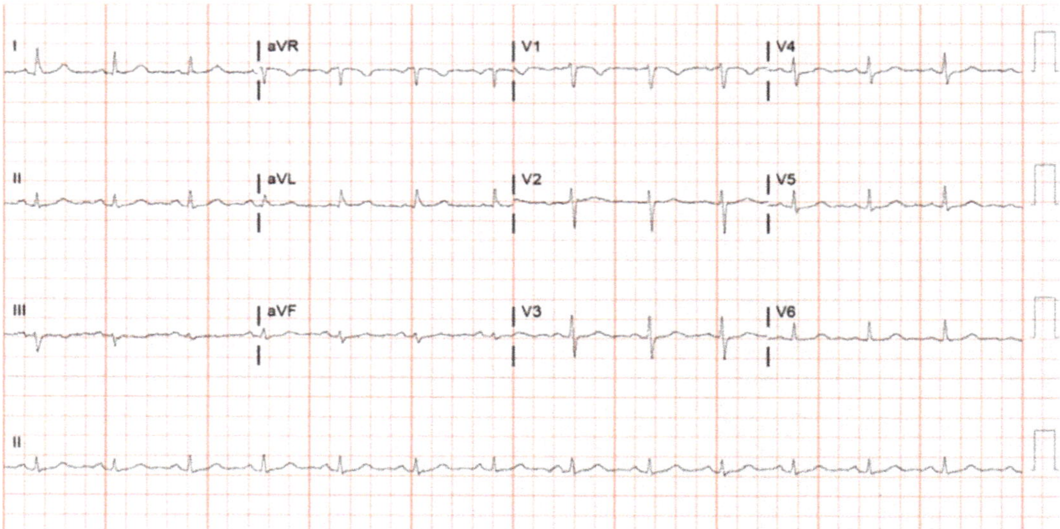

Figure 3: ECG demonstrating sinus rhythm.

in Figure 2. Shortly after, the patient converted to sinus rhythm (Figure 3), and flecainide was stopped. The patient was maintained on continuous IV amiodarone (0.5 mg/min). She was subsequently switched to amiodarone 200 mg twice a day for 10 days followed by 200 mg daily afterwards. Metoprolol tartrate was increased to 50 mg daily. She also underwent an electrophysiology study, which confirmed typical atrial flutter, and had successful cavo-tricuspid-isthmus (CTI) ablation. Given her newly depressed left ventricular function, flecainide was not restarted. She was discharged home on amiodarone and metoprolol without recurrence of arrhythmias on follow-up. The metoprolol dose was halved to 25 mg upon discharge. The patient was also treated for urinary tract infection which was believed to have contributed to her initial weakness.

3. Discussion

Flecainide is a class IC drug that binds open-state sodium channels to increase the effective refractory period and slow conductance in atrial and ventricular tissues. It demonstrates the slowest unbinding kinetics of the class I antiarrhythmic drugs and exhibits use dependence, which captures how the degree of sodium channel blockade increases with increases in heart rate. Essentially, this class of antiarrhythmics is more potent at faster heart rates [5]. Flecainide also blocks the rapid components of the delayed rectifier current and reduces spontaneous calcium release by the sarcoplasmic reticulum through ryanodine receptor inhibition [6].

In terms of noticeable ECG changes, the effect of flecainide is greatly enhanced with higher heart rates and can result in significant intraventricular conduction delays, causing a widened QRS complex [4, 7]. Flecainide can also organize atrial fibrillation into slow atrial tachycardia or atrial flutter due to decreased atrial tissue conductance. While typical atrial flutter usually occurs at rates up to 300 bpm, the atrial rate can be much slower in the presence of flecainide, as seen in our patient. Furthermore, without adequate use of a concomitant AV nodal blocking agent, this slow flutter can be conducted in a 1 : 1 ratio, resulting in a rapid ventricular response [8–10]. Our patient's newly depressed left ventricular function was most likely a result of atrial flutter [11]. Additionally, our patient had a history of hypertension, which could also be a potential etiology of her ventricular dysfunction.

When treating a patient with flecainide, it is important to monitor QRS duration. An increase in QRS duration greater than 15-20% puts the patient at risk for development of arrhythmias and indicates that the dose may need to be lowered [5]. It may also be beneficial to do an exercise stress test prior to starting a patient on flecainide to ensure that elevated heart rates during everyday activities will not significantly prolong the QRS and predispose them to the development of arrhythmias. Additionally, in patients with pacemakers, flecainide increases the pacing threshold [5]. If the pacing is not appropriately adjusted, it may lead to dangerous arrhythmias. Despite these concerns, in general, flecainide assumes a low risk of causing malignant arrhythmias in a structurally normal heart.

4. Conclusion

This case demonstrates the use-dependent properties of the class IC antiarrhythmic medication flecainide. It is important to note that at higher heart rates, flecainide can induce a dangerous arrhythmia by interacting with its target sodium channel more potently. In this case, an elevated heart rate induced by cessation of beta blocker therapy resulted in the development of a wide complex tachycardia.

References

[1] P. Zimetbaum, "Antiarrhythmic drug therapy for atrial fibrillation," *Circulation*, vol. 125, no. 2, pp. 381–389, 2012.

[2] G. S. King, A. Goyal, Y. Grigorova, and M. F. Hashmi, *Antiarrhythmic medications*, StatPearls Publishing, 2022.

[3] G. Kidwell, A. Greenspon, R. Greenberg, and K. Volosin, *Use-Dependent Prolongation of Ventricular Tachycardia Cycle Length by Type I Antiarrhythmic Drugs in Humans*, American Heart Association, 1992.

[4] E. Ezeh, M. Moroi, M. Amro, M. Ruzieh, O. Salem, and P. I. Okhumale, "Wide QRS complex tachycardia in a patient with atrial fibrillation: the use dependence effect of flecainide unmasked in a symptomatic female," *Journal of the American College of Cardiology*, vol. 79, no. 9, p. 2447, 2022.

[5] M. Razavi, "Safe and effective pharmacologic management of arrhythmias," *Texas Heart Institute Journal*, vol. 32, no. 2, pp. 209–211, 2005.

[6] D. O. Kryshtal, D. J. Blackwell, C. L. Egly et al., "RYR2 channel inhibition is the principal mechanism of flecainide action in CPVT," *Circulation Research*, vol. 128, no. 3, pp. 321–331, 2021.

[7] B. Bhardwaj, R. Lazzara, and S. Stavrakis, "Wide complex tachycardia in the presence of class I antiarrhythmic agents: a diagnostic challenge," *Annals of Noninvasive Electrocardiology*, vol. 19, no. 3, pp. 289–292, 2014.

[8] R. Taylor, M. M. Gandhi, and G. Lloyd, "Tachycardia due to atrial flutter with rapid 1:1 conduction following treatment of atrial fibrillation with flecainide," *BMJ*, vol. 340, no. mar10 3, article b4684, 2010.

[9] S. Hegde and V. Kumar, "Wide complex tachycardia in a patient with a history of atrial fibrillation," *JAMA Internal Medicine*, vol. 176, no. 3, pp. 386–388, 2016.

[10] B. Banavalikar, J. Shenthar, and D. Padmanabhan, "Unusual wide complex tachycardia during rhythm control for atrial fibrillation," *Circulation*, vol. 138, no. 5, pp. 537–539, 2018.

[11] B. Brembilla-Perrot, M. Amor, F. Auque et al., "Effect of flecainide on left ventricular ejection fraction," *European Heart Journal*, vol. 8, no. 7, pp. 754–761, 1987.

34

Surgical Treatment of Chronic Giant Left Ventricular Pseudoaneurysm

Roberto Ramos Barbosa,[1,2] Assad Miguel Sassine,[1,2] Vitor Martinelli Batista Rolim,[1] Pietro Dall'Orto Lima,[1] Eduardo Moreno Judice de Mattos Farina,[2] Ramon Chiabai Moura,[2] and Luiz Fernando Machado Barbosa[1,2]

[1]*Department of Cardiology, Santa Casa de Misericórdia de Vitória Hospital, Rua Dr. João dos Santos Neves, 143, Vila Rubim, 29025-023 Vitória, ES, Brazil*
[2]*School of Medicine of Santa Casa de Misericórdia, Av. Nossa Sra. da Penha, 2190, Bela Vista, 29027-502 Vitória, ES, Brazil*

Correspondence should be addressed to Roberto Ramos Barbosa; roberto.cardio@gmail.com

Academic Editor: Kathleen Ngu

Left ventricle pseudoaneurysm is usually a severe complication of acute myocardial infarction, caused by rupture of the myocardial wall with pericardium bleeding. Mortality can reach 50 to 80% within a week if not properly treated. Hemodynamic instability, cardiac tamponade, and cardiac arrest are life-threatening presentations that require surgical treatment. We report a case of a man with a left ventricle chronic giant pseudoaneurysm and unspecific symptoms. After critical judgement on a heart team basis, surgical treatment was successfully performed, with a good long-term clinical outcome.

1. Introduction

Left ventricular pseudoaneurysm (LVPA) is caused by rupture of the left ventricle wall leading to communication between the chamber and the pericardium. It is usually a life-threatening condition presenting after a complicated acute myocardial infarction (AMI). Mortality varies from 50 to 80% within the first week if not treated [1]. The incidence of LVPA is not well known, although it is lower than left ventricle free wall rupture, a critical mechanical AMI complication with a similar mechanism that occurs in 2 to 4% of all AMI cases [2, 3].

Hemodynamic instability with signs of cardiac tamponade is the most common clinical presentation of complicated LVPA, requiring a surgical approach in an emergent setting. In this scenario, the risk of cardiac arrest and death is imminent [4]. Other initial symptoms include pleuritic chest pain, agitation, and vomiting [5], with variable sensibility and specificity. LVPA in a non-AMI clinical context is a rare condition. However, different etiologies such as congenital, traumatic, postoperative, and inflammatory have been described for LVPA and left ventricular true aneurysm [6–8]. We report a challenging case of an elder patient with a giant LVPA accidentally diagnosed, undergoing successful surgical treatment.

2. Case Report

A 77-year-old man with progressive dyspnoea and fatigue at moderate exertion for the last two years was admitted to the Emergency Department on February 5, 2019, with nausea and abdominal pain. He felt the symptoms for three days and reported one episode of syncope after vomiting. He had been a smoker for 58 years and had no history of past AMI or chest pain. Electrocardiogram (ECG) showed a right bundle branch block, cardiac troponins were normal, and serum creatinine was 1.75 mg/dL. When interrogated, he affirmed that he had similar symptoms 45 days before, with nausea, vomiting, and abdominal discomfort followed by syncope. At that time, he was discharged from the Emergency Department after ECG and cardiac troponin dosages.

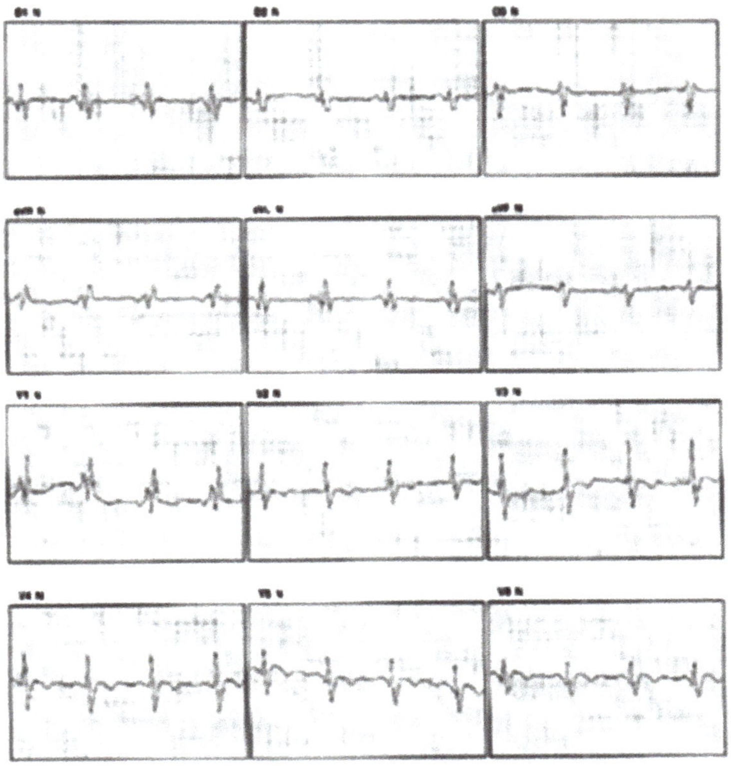

(a)

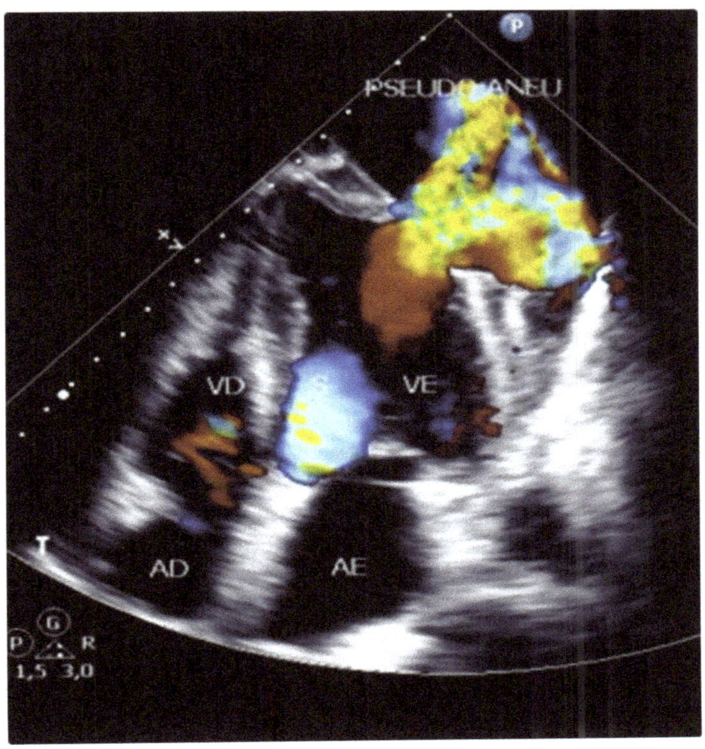

(b)

FIGURE 1: Resting electrocardiogram and transthoracic echocardiogram. (a) Resting electrocardiogram showing right bundle branch block, negative anterior wall T-wave, and lateral wall Q-wave. (b) Transthoracic echocardiogram showing left ventricular pseudoaneurysm and rupture of the apical segment of lateral myocardial wall of the left ventricle. pseudoaneu = pseudoaneurysm; VE = left ventricle; VD = right ventricle; AE = left atrium; AD = right atrium.

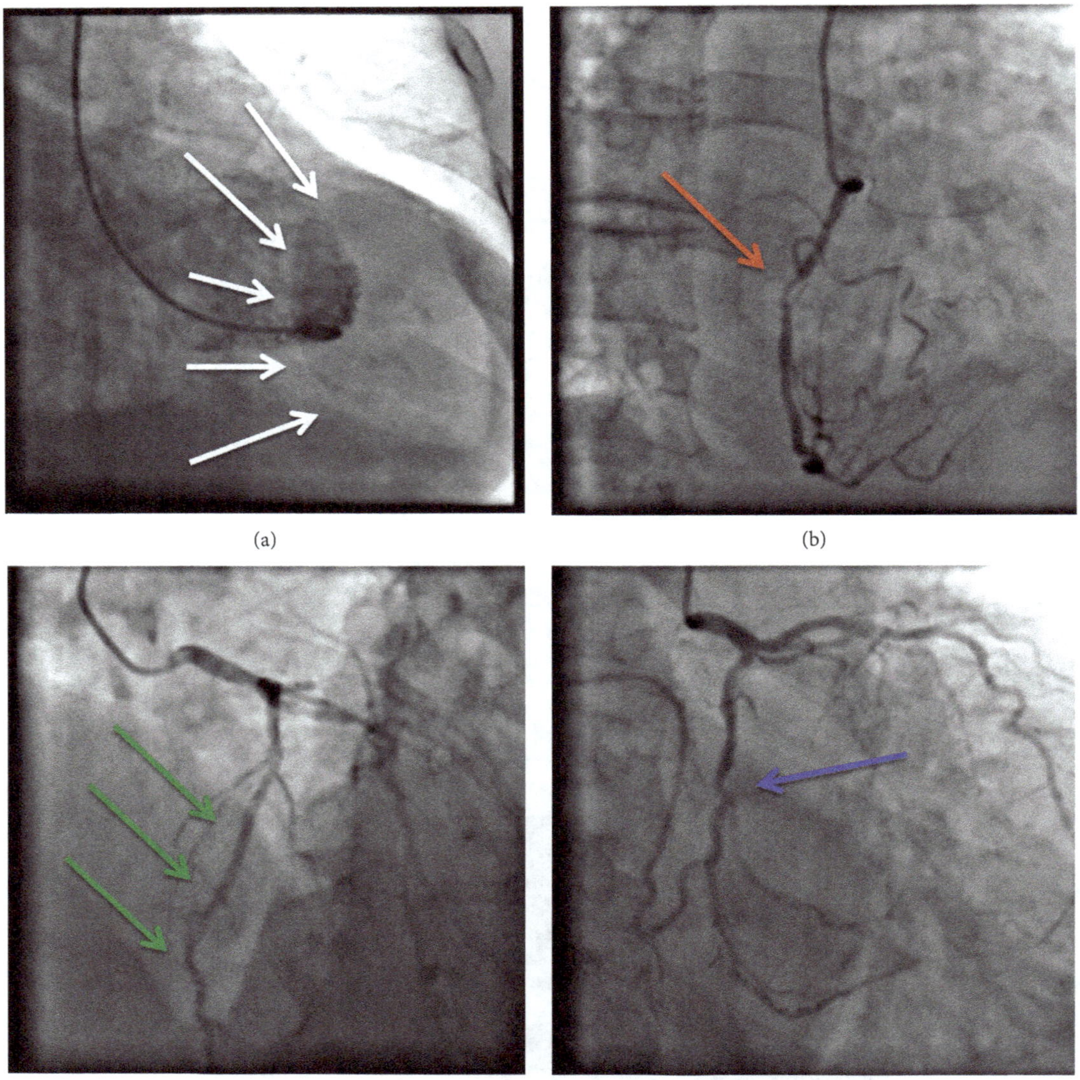

(a) (b) (c) (d)

FIGURE 2: Left ventriculogram and coronary angiogram. (a) Left ventriculogram in right oblique view showing important contrast extravasation from the left ventricle to the pericardium forming a giant pseudoaneurysm (white arrows). (b) Coronary angiogram in right oblique view showing severe stenosis (80% lumen stenosis) in middle segment of the right coronary artery (red arrow). (c) Coronary angiogram in left cranial view showing normal left anterior descending artery (green arrows). (d) Coronary angiogram in right caudal view showing intermediate stenosis (40% lumen stenosis) in the left circumflex artery (blue arrow).

An abdominal ultrasound showed proximal left ureterolithiasis with moderate hydronephrosis. While planning urologic intervention, an abdominal computer tomography (CT) scan was performed and a cardiac enlargement was accidentally found, with mild left pleural effusion. A double-J ureteric catheter was placed, and a cardiac diagnostic workup was electively initiated.

A treadmill exercise test showed a resting ECG with sinus rhythm, right bundle branch block, negative anterior wall T-wave, and lateral wall Q-wave (Figure 1(a)), and no ECG changes were found during exercise. Transthoracic echocardiogram showed rupture of the apical segment of the lateral myocardial wall of the left ventricle, with drainage from the cardiac chamber to an external cavity located on the lateral-inferior-apical region, with bidirectional flow suggesting an LVPA (Figure 1(b)). The ejection fraction via the Teichholz formula was 69%, and it was calculated with exclusion of the pseudoaneurysm.

The patient was referred for cardiac catheterization. Coronary angiogram revealed a normal left anterior descending artery (LAD), intermediate stenosis in the left circumflex artery (LCX) (40% lumen stenosis), and severe stenosis in the right coronary artery (RCA) (80% lumen stenosis). The left ventriculogram showed important contrast extravasation from the left ventricle to the pericardium, with a giant pseudoaneurysm (Figure 2). A contrasted chest CT scan revealed cardiac enlargement with moderate to severe pericardial effusion and a discontinuity area in the left ventricle

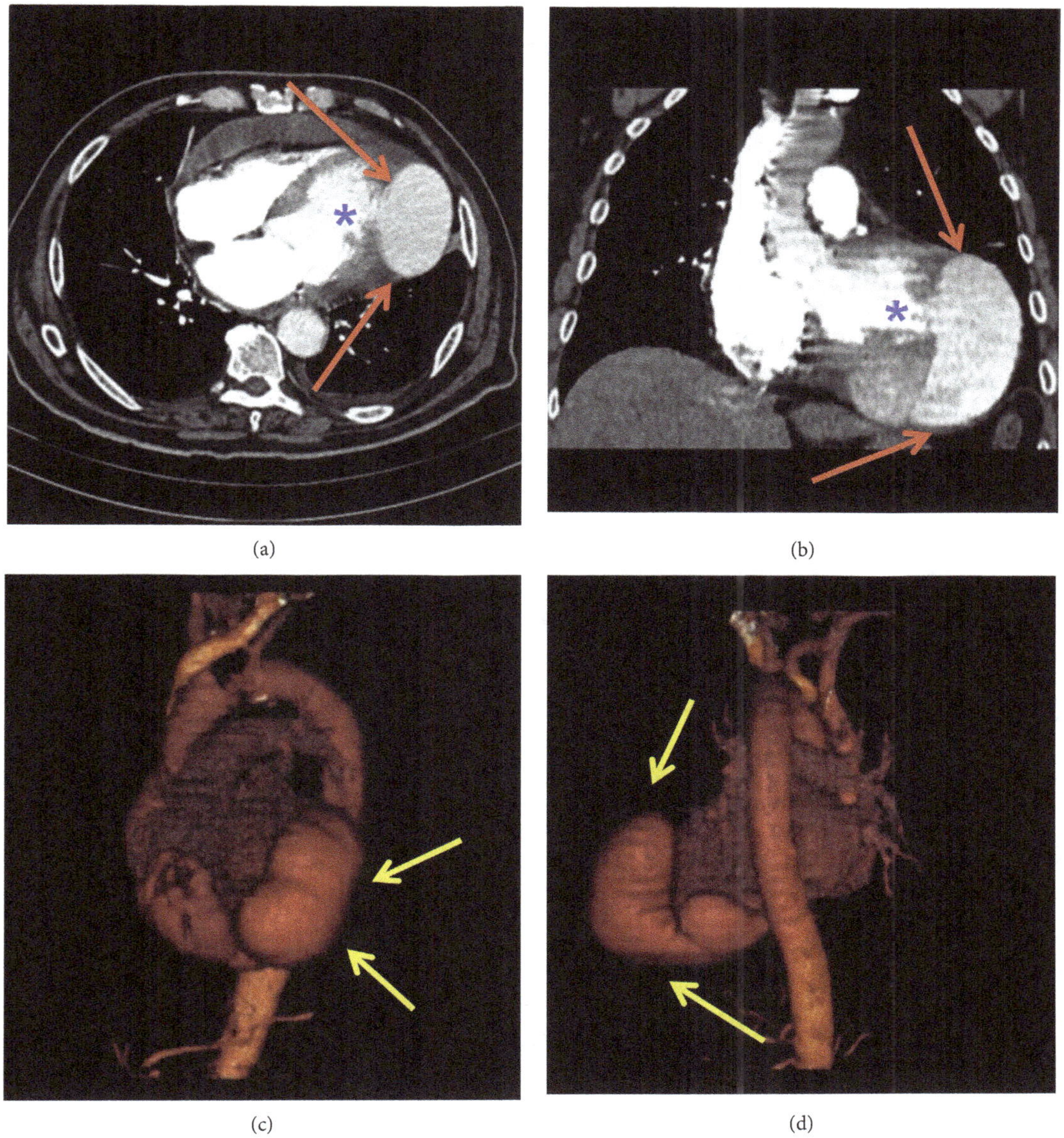

FIGURE 3: Chest computed angiotomography. (a, b) Large pericardial effusion (red arrows) and area of discontinuity in the posterolateral myocardial wall of the left ventricle communicating with the pericardial sac (blue asterisk). (c, d) Three-dimensional reconstruction by computed angiotomography revealing left ventricle giant pseudoaneurysm (yellow arrows).

posterior-lateral wall communicating with the pericardial sac measuring 6.2 cm in its largest transverse diameter (Figure 3).

Surgical treatment was then performed through transsternal thoracotomy. Inspection of the mediastinum revealed severe thickening of the pericardium with adherence of its layers, suggesting constrictive pericarditis (Figure 4(a)). An attempt of dissection was unsuccessful. Transpleural cardiopulmonary bypass was initiated from the aorta to the right atrium, and transpleural access to the LVPA was obtained. Aortic clamping and cardioplegia were performed. Rupture of the left ventricle was noted (Figures 4(b)–4(d)), with fibrous tissue forming three distinct cavities inside the LVPA. Suture of the myocardial lesion and pseudoaneurysm using linear teflon tissue was performed (Figure 5), and anterior pericardiectomy was necessary because of severe pericardial thickening. At last, a bypass saphenous vein graft to the RCA was attempted, but it was impaired due to hostile pericardium anatomy caused by the LVPA.

The patient recovered well after the operation and was discharged from the hospital eight days later. At one-year follow-up, he was asymptomatic, with no signs of heart failure or complications. An echocardiogram showed mild diastolic dysfunction of the left ventricle, with anchoring patch in the lateral-apical wall and no signs of cavitary shunt to the pericardium. Ejection fraction was 72% by the Teichholz formula, and systolic and diastolic left ventricle measurements were, respectively, 32 and 56 mm. A control chest angio-CT scan was considered; however, with a good clinical outcome and serum creatinine persistently between 1.6 and 1.9 mg/dL, the exam was withdrawn. Percutaneous coronary intervention to RCA was deferred for the same reasons added to the lack of symptoms.

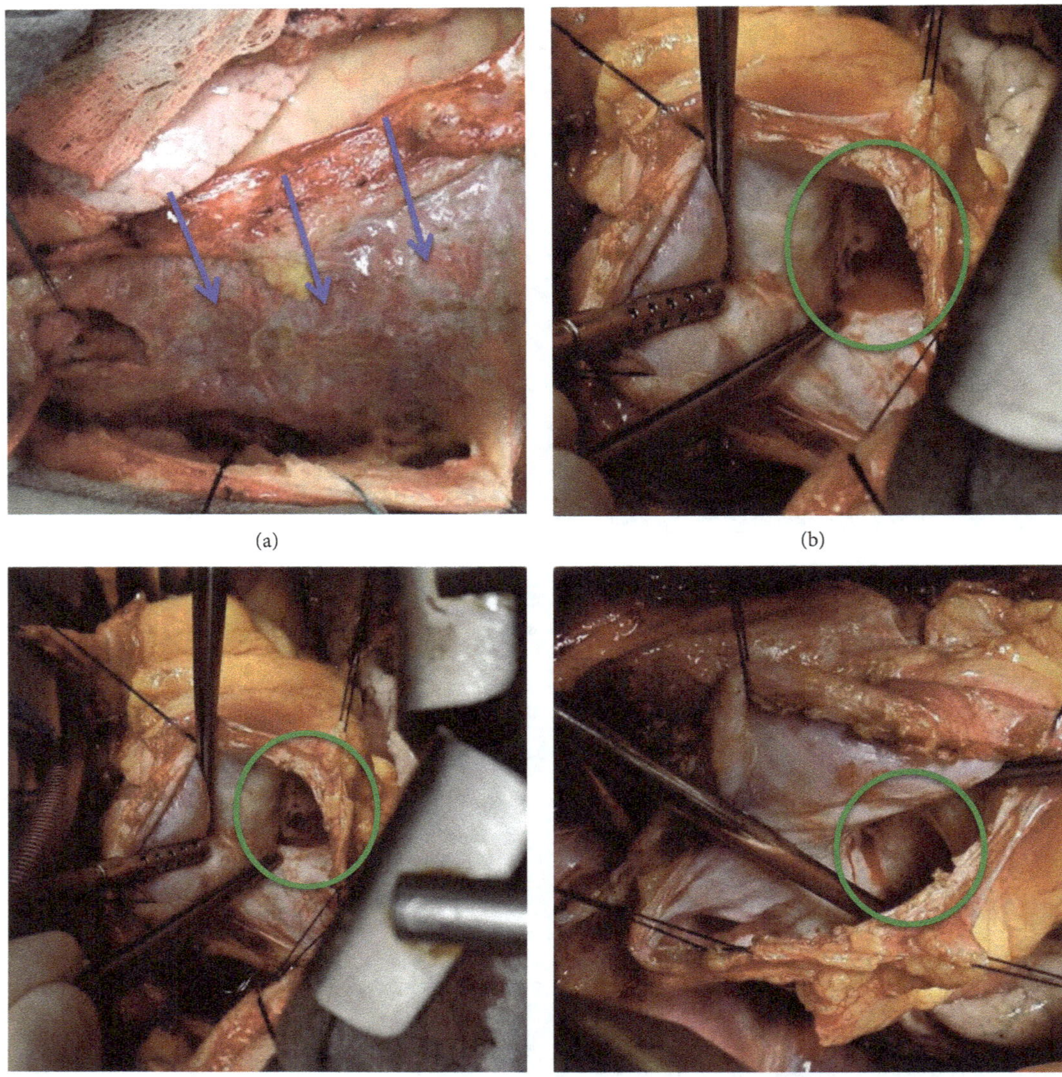

(a) (b) (c) (d)

Figure 4: Intraoperative view. (a) Severe thickening of the pericardium with adherence of its layers (blue arrows), as commonly seen in constrictive pericarditis. (b–d) Rupture of the left ventricle (green circles) communicating the chamber and the pericardial sac.

3. Discussion

In our case, the patient presented a giant chronic LVPA with no clear history of AMI. His symptoms were unspecific, and the diagnosis occurred accidentally after cardiac enlargement was seen in an abdominal CT scan. The rupture of the left ventricular myocardial wall favors ischemic myocardial lesion as etiology. The severe stenosis found in RCA may corroborate this hypothesis. However, diagnosis of the etiology of the LVPA was not clearly determined. Other possible causes previously described are surgical manipulation, penetrating or blunt trauma, and endocarditis with abscess. Due to the imminent risk of complete rupture, cardiac tamponade, and death, we decided for surgical treatment after a thorough heart team discussion.

The diagnosis of LVPA may have no specific symptoms or clinical signs. Chest pain, dyspnoea, or hypotension are common [9]. Pericardial friction and new cardiac murmurs are also possible [10], and sinus bradycardia or junctional rhythm has been reported in LVPA [11]. Most patients with LVPA present recurrent chest pain and signs of heart failure and as much as 10% present cardiac rhythm disturbances and syncope. However, 10% of the patients may be asymptomatic [11]. In the present case, the patient had mostly abdominal symptoms and also syncopes in two episodes.

Initial evaluation is usually done with an echocardiogram. After the suspicion, other imaging modalities offer better diagnostic accuracy, such as cardiac magnetic resonance, angio-CT, or cardiac catheterization [2]. In a case series, Yeo et al. showed that 48% of LVPA cases were incidentally diagnosed, mostly after imaging complementary exams [12]. In our case, the diagnosis of AMI was excluded, and imaging modalities incidentally showed cardiac abnormalities. Cardiac enlargement was found in abdominal CT scan, and then, as initial investigation targeted to heart failure, an echocardiogram revealed LVPA. After cardiac catheterization, the patient

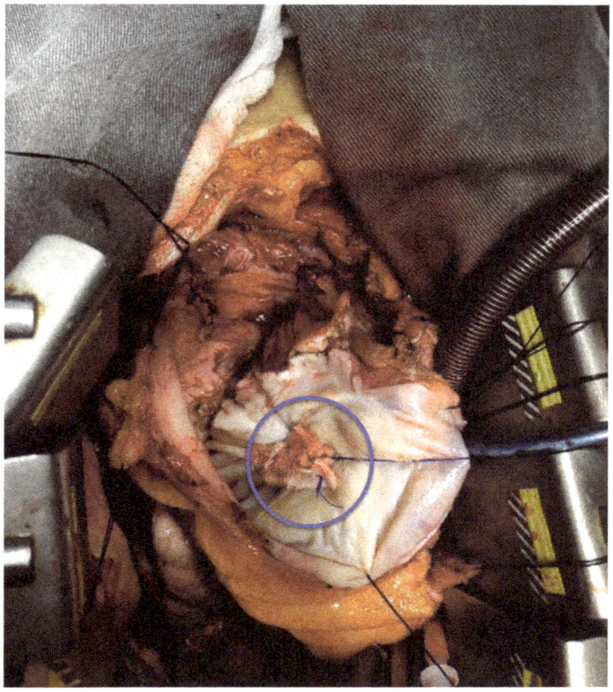

FIGURE 5: Intraoperative view. Suture of the myocardial rupture and pseudoaneurysm using linear teflon tissue (blue circle).

underwent a chest CT scan that provided detailed anatomic features of the LVPA.

The normal ejection fraction was calculated on an echocardiogram via the Teichholz formula, although with exclusion of the pseudoaneurysm. Quantification of systolic function including the area of the pseudoaneurysm could add a surgical value, aiding the prediction of improvement of the ejection fraction. Nevertheless, cardiac magnetic resonance (CMR) might be an important complementary imaging modality, with higher accuracy due to its higher spatial resolution [13]. CMR can distinguish a true left ventricle aneurysm from an LVPA by the finding of late enhancement predominantly in the myocardium or in the pericardium. Besides, CMR imaging is the ideal modality to perform LV function and adds important information on anatomic features of the LVPA [14, 15].

In the 1980s, the first surgical cases of LVPA correction used teflon patches for tamponade of ruptured areas [16]. In 1993, Padró et al. had 100% survival in 13 patients with LVPA after using biological tissue adhesive, with a median follow-up of 26 months [17]. In 2000, Pretre et al. showed better outcomes of surgical treatment over medical expectancy in patients with expanding LVPA, in both acute and chronic cases [18]. However, successful medical conservative treatment has been reported in isolated cases of LVPA [19, 20]. It is still unknown whether a small LVPA is less likely to rupture or which features represent greater risk of rupture and severe complications. Regarding its high surgical mortality, medical treatment may be considered for LVPAs less than 3 mm in size, aimed at decreasing pseudoaneurysm enlargement [14, 21]. Besides, postinfarction LVPAs located on the posteroinferior wall have the anatomical support of the diaphragm, facilitating the restraint of the ventricular cavity by the adjacent pericardium and making it more rupture-resistant [22]. Those favorable features implying stability are common in LVPAs that infrequently are not diagnosed and remain with conservative approaches.

Rupture of an LVPA may occur in 30 to 45% of all cases and is usually dramatic. Thus, the main objective of the surgical approach is to avoid progressive expansion and rupture of an LVPA [23]. Since it is a rare condition, there is a paucity of evidence on guiding therapeutic decisions for LVPA, and most available studies are case reports and case series. Comprehension of the etiology of LVPA is useful to define the best surgical strategy. Moreover, we propose an individual approach and shared understanding for decision-making. Heart team discussion is strongly recommended, including careful investigation on the etiology of LVPA in this process.

References

[1] T. Kjeld, C. Hassager, and V. E. Hjortdal, "Rupture of free left ventricle wall, septum and papillary muscle in acute myocardial infarction," *Ugeskrift for Laeger*, vol. 171, no. 23, pp. 1925–1929, 2009.

[2] S. Bisoyi, A. K. Dash, D. Nayak, S. Sahoo, and R. Mohapatra, "Left ventricular pseudoaneurysm versus aneurysm a diagnosis dilemma," *Annals of Cardiac Anaesthesia*, vol. 19, no. 1, pp. 169–172, 2016.

[3] H. Pollak, H. Nobis, and J. Miczoc, "Frequency of left ventricular free wall rupture complicating acute myocardial infarction since the advent of thrombolysis," *The American Journal of Cardiology*, vol. 74, no. 2, pp. 184–186, 1994.

[4] G. Zoffoli, D. Mangino, A. Venturini et al., "Diagnosing left ventricular aneurysm from pseudo-aneurysm: a case report and a review in literature," *Journal of Cardiothoracic Surgery*, vol. 4, no. 1, 2009.

[5] P. B. Oliva, S. C. Hammil, and W. D. Edwards, "Cardiac rupture, a clinically predictable complication of acute myocardial infarction: report of 70 cases with clinicopathologic correlations," *Journal of the American College of Cardiology*, vol. 22, no. 3, pp. 720–726, 1993.

[6] E. A. Hulten and R. Blankstein, "Pseudoaneurysms of the heart," *Circulation*, vol. 125, no 15, pp. 1920–1925, 2012.

[7] M. A. Ohlow, "Congenital left ventricular aneurysms and diverticula: an entity in search of an identity," *Journal of Geriatric Cardiology*, vol. 14, no. 2, pp. 750–762, 2017.

[8] S. Fox, C. Templeton, and C. Hancock-Friesen, "Commotio cordis and ventricular pseudoaneurysm," *The Canadian Journal of Cardiology*, vol. 25, no. 4, pp. 237-238, 2009.

[9] J. W. Mackenzie and G. M. Lemole, "Pseudoaneurysm of the left ventricle," *Texas Heart Institute Journal*, vol. 21, no. 4, pp. 296-301, 1994.

[10] N. Rasouly, R. Stanekzai, H. Hamidi, and R. Ahamdzai, "Computed tomography features of left ventricular pseudoaneurysm: a case report," *Iranian Journal of Radiology*, vol. 14, no. 2, 2017.

[11] K. Balakumaran, C. J. Verbaan, C. E. Essed et al., "Ventricular free wall rupture: sudden, subacute, slow, sealed and stabilized varieties," *European Heart Journal*, vol. 5, no. 4, pp. 282–288, 1984.

[12] T. C. Yeo, J. F. Malouf, J. K. Oh, and J. B. Seward, "Clinical profile and outcome in 52 patients with cardiac pseudoaneurysm," *Annals of Internal Medicine*, vol. 128, no. 4, pp. 299–305, 1998.

[13] N. Mousavi, R. Buksak, J. R. Walker et al., "Left ventricular pseudoaneurysm: the role of multimodality cardiac imaging," *The Canadian Journal of Cardiology*, vol. 25, no. 11, article e389, 2009.

[14] F. Inayat, A. R. Ghani, I. Riaz et al., "Left ventricular pseudoaneurysm: an overview of diagnosis and management," *Journal of Investigative Medicine High Impact Case Reports*, vol. 6, 2018.

[15] S. G. Coelho, C. F. Jorge, P. B. Carlos, A. Delgado, and L. Vicente, "Evolved inferior wall myocardial infarction with left ventricular pseudoaneurysm: a diagnostic dilemma," *Arquivos Brasileiros de Cardiologia*, vol. 114, no. 4, pp. 730-731, 2020.

[16] R. C. A. Bonini, V. Q. Verazain, R. M. Mustafa et al., "Rupture of the right ventricular free wall after myocardial infarction," *Revista Brasileira de Cirurgia Cardiovascular*, vol. 27, no. 1, pp. 155–159, 2012.

[17] J. M. Padró, J. M. Mesa, J. Silvestre et al., "Subacute cardiac rupture: repair with a sutureless technique," *The Annals of Thoracic Surgery*, vol. 55, no. 1, pp. 20–24, 1993.

[18] R. Pretre, A. Linka, R. Senni, and M. I. Turina, "Surgical treatment of acquired left ventricular pseudoaneurysms," *The Annals of Thoracic Surgery*, vol. 70, no. 2, pp. 553–557, 2000.

[19] D. Ousaka, N. Obara, M. Fujiwara, A. Teraoka, S. Kasahara, and S. Oozawa, "A case of conservative management for left ventricular giant pseudoaneurysm without ST segment changes," *Journal of Cardiology Cases*, vol. 17, no. 5, pp. 167–170, 2018.

[20] R. Moreno, "Long term outcome of patients with postinfarction left ventricular pseudoaneurysm," *Heart*, vol. 89, no. 10, pp. 1144–1146, 2003.

[21] E. Mujanovic, J. Bergsland, S. Avdic, S. Stanimirovic-Mujanovic, T. Kovacevic-Preradovic, and E. Kabil, "Surgical treatment of left ventricular pseudoaneurysm," *Medical Archives*, vol. 68, no. 3, pp. 215–217, 2014.

[22] T. C. Yeo, J. F. Malouf, G. S. Reeder, and J. K. Oh, "Clinical characteristics and outcome in postinfarction pseudoaneurysm," *The American Journal of Cardiology*, vol. 84, no. 5, pp. 592–595, 1999.

[23] C. Frances, A. Romero, and D. Grady, "Left ventricular pseudoaneurysm," *Journal of the American College of Cardiology*, vol. 32, no. 3, pp. 557–561, 1998.

35

Left Atrial Myxoma Presenting as Lateral Medullary (Wallenberg's) Syndrome

Simran Gupta, Ricky Ayala, Aakash Desai, Viraj I. Modi, and Robert J. Nardino

Department of Internal Medicine, University of Connecticut School of Medicine, UCONN Health, Farmington, CT, USA

Correspondence should be addressed to Simran Gupta; sigupta@uchc.edu

Academic Editor: Manabu Shirotani

Myxomas are benign, primary tumors of the heart. Atrial myxomas can present with a variety of clinical features including dyspnea, orthopnea, pulmonary edema, and pulmonary or systemic emboli. Constitutional symptoms such as fever and weight loss may also be present. We report the case of a young female presenting with headache, facial numbness, and vertigo, who was found to have a posterolateral medullary stroke secondary to a large left atrial cardiac myxoma.

1. Learning Objective

Cardioembolic origin is a known cause of ischemic stroke. Differential diagnoses most often include atrial fibrillation and patent foramen ovale. Atrial myxoma is a rare and potentially dangerous cause of ischemic stroke and should be considered on a differential for cardiac etiology.

2. Introduction

The most prevalent primary cardiac tumors, myxomas, most often grow in the atria. About 75% are located in the left atrium and 18% in the right atrium (1, 2). Classically they grow at the fossa ovalis border of the interatrial septum (3). Myxomas most commonly occur in middle age, though rare occurrences in the pediatric population have been reported (1, 3). They are more predominant in women than men (1, 4). Previous studies have shown that patients with myxomas can have a variety of initial presentations, including obstructive symptoms (67%) and embolic symptoms (29%) (5). Other studies have focused on symptoms based on location of the tumor, with septal tumor location strongly associated with congestive heart failure and extraseptal tumors associated with neurological events (6). Most commonly though, most studies conclude that myxoma symptoms can mimic many cardiovascular diseases, and thus a high index of suspicion is important (7). We report the case of young female who presented with a headache, facial numbness, and vertigo who was found to have a posterolateral medullary stroke which was secondary to a large left atrial cardiac myxoma.

3. Case Presentation

A 48-year-old female with a history of hypertension, migraines, anxiety, and depression presented to the Emergency Department with a left-sided occipital headache for one hour (thought to be consistent with her usual migraine presentation) with accompanied numbness of the left face and lips, vertigo, and lightheadedness. Her initial blood pressure was 172/85, and cranial nerves II through XII were intact except for some mildly decreased sensation to light touch on the left side of her face. The patient did note that she felt less vibration from the tuning fork on the left forehead as compared to the right forehead. Cognitive status and language were grossly intact and muscle strength was 5/5 in all extremities. Initial NIH stroke scale was 1. On cardiac examination, the patient had an extra diastolic heart sound, interpreted as a splitting of S2, without murmurs, gallops, or rubs. Given concern for a stroke, an initial computed tomography (CT) scan of the head was performed and was found to be negative for an acute, evolving cerebrovascular accident. It was thought that the symptoms were most likely related to a migraine, but the patient was admitted to the floors for further workup. Over the next 24 hours, the patient's clinical condition continued to deteriorate with a worsened neurological exam now including diplopia, left-sided dysmetria, more pronounced vertigo, and difficulty swallowing. A stroke alert was called and magnetic resonance imaging (MRI) of the brain was performed, which showed focal restricted diffusion within the left posterolateral aspect of the medulla with associated focal heterogeneous hyperintense signal, indicative of an evolving focal subacute cerebrovascular accident (Figure 1). The patient was transported to the step-down unit with an NIH stroke scale score of 2 for neurological checks every two hours. It was noted that the patient was not a candidate for tPA at this time due to presence of symptoms ongoing for over 24 hours.

Given her presentation and imaging findings, she underwent further workup including a transthoracic echocardiogram (TTE). TTE demonstrated a large, 5.7 cm × 1.9 cm, mobile mass on the left side of the interatrial septum consistent with a myxoma (echocardiographic contrast reveals vascularity of the mass). The mass traveled along the anterior mitral leaflet and plopped in and out of the left ventricle (Figure 2). The patient's left ventricular ejection fraction was preserved, and there was no wall motion abnormality. Based on location and size of the mass, there was serious concern for complete obstruction of blood flow through the heart. Further history elicited from the patient at this time revealed that she had a long-standing history of dizziness and lightheadedness.

Cardiothoracic surgery was consulted and they took the patient to the operating room within 12 hours of echocardiography. The surgeons used a median sternotomy technique to enter the chest cavity, the aorta was cross clamped, and the heart was arrested with 1 liter of antegrade first warm then cold hyperkalemic blood cardioplegia. The right atrium was entered and the incision was carried cephalad toward the interatrial septum. The roof of the left atrium was then incised and the incision was carried toward the fossa ovalis, at which point the tumor was carefully excised off the septum. The incisions were closed carefully and the heart was deaired and the aortic cross clamp was removed. The heart did not require defibrillation and spontaneously returned to normal sinus rhythm. Upon reaching normothermia, the patient was easily weaned from cardiopulmonary bypass on no pressors or ionotropes. The patient tolerated the procedure well and was monitored in the intensive care unit for 24 hours and then transferred to a monitored step-down unit. Her stroke symptoms continued to persist through the postoperative stay, with some resolution of diplopia. She was discharged after two days in step-down to a long-term acute care facility for extensive rehabilitation of her stroke symptoms. A repeat transthoracic echocardiogram obtained one month after surgery showed no evidence of myxoma recurrence, with a normal left ventricular ejection fraction.

4. Discussion

Stroke, or central nervous system infarction, is broadly defined as brain, spinal cord, or retinal cell death (8). Ischemic stroke in particular is defined as "an episode of neurologic dysfunction caused by focal cerebral, spinal, or retinal dysfunction." Cardioembolic origin accounts for approximately 14-30% of ischemic strokes, with atrial fibrillation being the most common (45%) underlying condition (9). Other common etiologies include infective endocarditis, valvular heart disease, and much more rarely, cardiac myxoma. Previous research has shown that cardiac myxomas account for only approximately 0.5% of strokes (9, 10). The classic triad of symptoms of cardiac myxomas includes obstructive, embolic, and constitutional manifestations (2). Obstructive symptoms, which are the most common initial symptoms, include dyspnea, cough, and heart failure (4). Embolic symptoms usually present as peripheral, pulmonic, or cerebral. Constitutional symptoms are thought to be driven by tumor cell release of IL-6 and include arthralgias, fatigue, weight loss, fever, and Raynaud's phenomenon (5). Patients often have some or all of these symptoms on initial presentation, and severity depends on the tumor size, location, and mobility. Our patient, with a large obstructing left atrial myxoma accompanied by lightheadedness and stroke, displayed obstructive and embolic symptoms.

Lateral medullary, or Wallenberg's, syndrome is defined as a neurological condition due to a stroke in the vertebral or posterior inferior cerebellar artery of the brain stem (11). Symptoms may include difficulty of swallowing, dizziness, nausea and vomiting, decreased pain and temperature sensation on one side of the face and opposite side of the body, and problems with coordination. During her hospital course, our patient noted almost all of the above symptoms. Treatment is predominantly symptomatic, and prognosis is dependent on size and location of the affected brain stem area. To our knowledge, this is only the second reported case of Wallenberg's syndrome as the initial presentation in a patient with a left atrial myxoma. Cerebral vascular accidents in general are a known complication, however, of atrial myxomas, particularly those of the left atrium. Regardless of presenting symptoms, research has shown that it is important to consider myxoma on the differential diagnosis of stroke origin. The American Heart Association guidelines propose that initial evaluation of an embolic event should include echocardiography to investigate intracardiac causes (12). A study of 24 patients with cardiac myxomas in Taiwan also suggests that echocardiography is the most useful diagnostic tool for cardiac myxomas and serial echocardiograms (every six to twelve months) may be needed after resection to monitor recurrence. (7).

Siminelakis et al. showed that urgent surgical resection via median sternotomy with the patient on cardiopulmonary bypass under mild hypothermia is the treatment of choice (2). Using a technique described by Siminelakis et al. (2), they suggest the ideal approach to a left atrial myxoma occupying the majority of the left atrium is an incision starting from the pulmonary vein continuing vertically to the interatrial septum and the free wall of the right atrium. This would allow complete visualization and opening of the left atrium. As described above, this was the surgical technique employed by the cardiothoracic surgeons for our patient. Other studies have shown that the ideal surgical technique is right atriotomy with excision of the fossa ovalis and surrounding tissues and closure with a pericardial patch (2). Regardless of

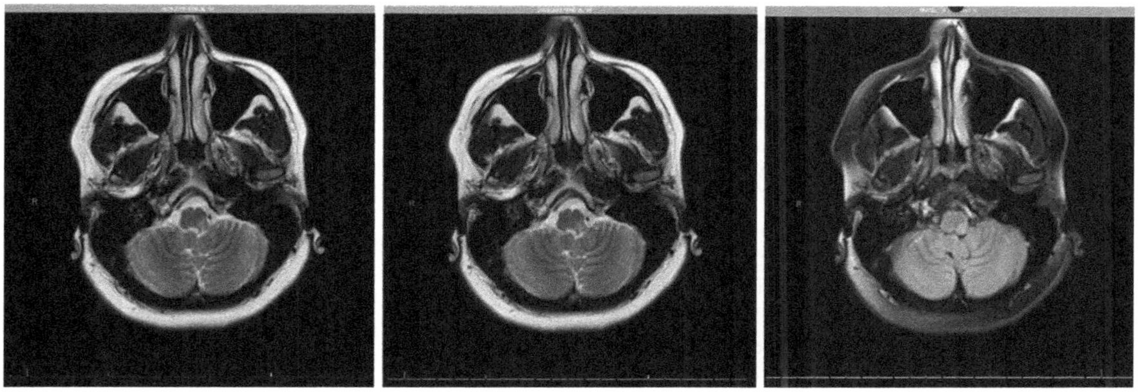

FIGURE 1: MRI of the brain with and without contrast showing focal restricted diffusion within the left posterolateral aspect of the medulla with associated focal heterogeneous T2 hyperintense signal, indicative of an evolving focal subacute cerebrovascular accident. Alternatively, this finding may represent an acute-subacute focus of demyelination in the proper clinical setting.

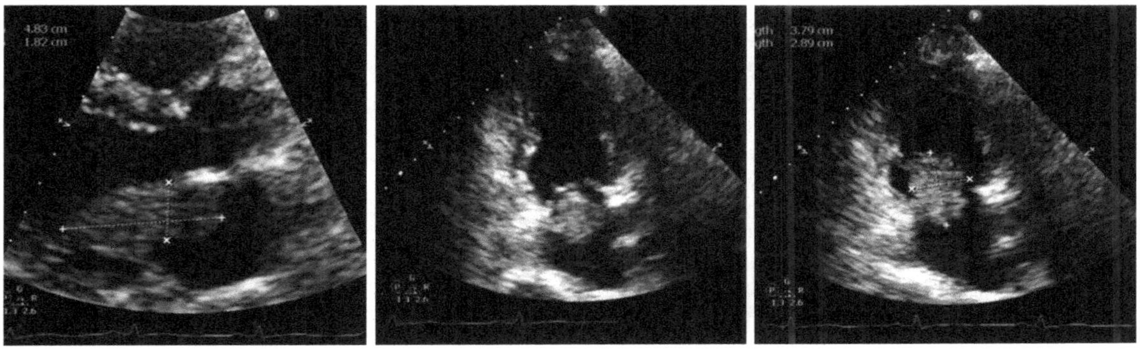

FIGURE 2: Transthoracic echocardiogram. There is a large, 5.7 $cm\ (L) \times 1.9\ cm\ (W)$, mobile mass on the left side of the interatrial septum; the appearance is consistent with myxoma (echocardiographic contrast reveals vascularity of the mass). The mass travels along with the anterior mitral leaflet and plops in and out of the left ventricle. Transvalvular velocity of the mitral valve is within the normal range, and there is no evidence of stenosis. Left ventricular ejection fraction was in the range of 55% to 60%.

technique, it is important to achieve complete resection of the tumor with a margin of safety to minimize chance of recurrence (13). With complete resection of the tumor, the risk of recurrence is approximately 3% (14, 15). Regular and long-term follow-up with clinical examinations and serial echocardiography is highly recommended (16), though a consensus on total duration of follow-up time has not been established.

5. Conclusion

This case highlights the variety of presentations that can be associated with cardiac myxomas and emphasizes the need for obtaining an echocardiogram as well as considering cardiac myxoma as a possible differential diagnosis for stroke. Our patient was a young, relatively healthy female with few risk factors for stroke. However, she did have a long-standing history of dizziness, a symptom that could be explained by the tumor. Given the size of her myxoma, a delay in diagnosis could have been fatal. In a patient without major risk factors, who has an unusual or unclear presentation, it is imperative to consider myxoma as a part of cardiac etiologies and intervene early.

References

[1] A. Hoffmeier, J. R. Sindermann, H. H. Scheld, and S. Martens, "Cardiac Tumors," *Deutsches Ärzteblatt International*, vol. 111, no. 12, pp. 205–211, 2014.

[2] S. Siminelakis, A. Kakourou, A. Batistatou et al., "Thirteen years follow-up of heart myxoma operated patients: what is the appropriate surgical technique?," *Journal of Thoracic Disease*, vol. 6 Suppl 1, Supplement 1, pp. S32–S38, 2014.

[3] B. Thyagarajan, M. P. Kumar, S. Patel, and A. Agrawal, "Extracardiac manifestations of atrial myxomas," *Journal of the Saudi Heart Association*, vol. 29, no. 1, pp. 37–43, 2017.

[4] D. Hi, A. Yoon, and W. C. Roberts, "Sex distribution in cardiac myxomas," *The American Journal of Cardiology*, vol. 90, no. 5, pp. 563–565, 2002.

[5] L. Pinede, P. Duhaut, and R. Loire, "Clinical presentation of left atrial cardiac myxoma. A series of 112 consecutive cases," *Medicine (Baltimore)*, vol. 80, no. 3, pp. 159–172, 2001.

[6] M. F. Swartz, C. J. Lutz, V. S. Chandan, S. Landas, and G. W. Fink, "Atrial myxomas: pathologic types, tumor location, and presenting symptoms," *Journal of Cardiac Surgery*, vol. 21, no. 4, pp. 435–440, 2006.

[7] B. R. Fang, C. W. Chiang, J. S. Hung, Y. S. Lee, and C. S. Chang,

"Cardiac myxoma - clinical experience in 24 patients," *International Journal of Cardiology*, vol. 29, no. 3, pp. 335–341, 1990.

[8] R. L. Sacco, S. E. Kasner, J. P. Broderick et al., "An updated definition of stroke for the 21st century: a statement for healthcare professionals from the American Heart Association/American Stroke Association," *Stroke*, vol. 44, no. 7, pp. 2064–2089, 2013.

[9] S. M. Yuan and G. Humuruola, "Stroke of a cardiac myxoma origin," *Revista Brasileira de Cirurgia Cardiovascular*, vol. 30, no. 2, pp. 225–234, 2015.

[10] W. T. Browne, E. F. Wijdicks, J. E. Parisi, and R. W. Viggiano, "Fulminant brain necrosis from atrial myxoma showers," *Stroke*, vol. 24, no. 7, pp. 1090–1092, 1993.

[11] *Wallenberg's Syndrome Information Page*, National Institute of Neurological Disorder and Stroke, 2019, May 2019, https://www.ninds.nih.gov/Disorders/All-Disorders/Wallenbergs-Syndrome-Information-Page.

[12] M. D. Cheitlin, J. S. Alpert, W. F. Armstrong et al., "ACC/AHA Guidelines for the Clinical Application of Echocardiography: a report of the American College of Cardiology/American Heart Association Task Force on Practice Guidelines (Committee on Clinical Application of Echocardiography) Developed in Collaboration With the American Society of Echocardiography," *Circulation*, vol. 95, no. 6, pp. 1686–1744, 1997.

[13] G. Samanidis, K. Perreas, P. Kalogris et al., "Surgical treatment of primary intracardiac myxoma: 19 years of experience," *Interactive Cardiovascular and Thoracic Surgery*, vol. 13, no. 6, pp. 597–600, 2011.

[14] A. W. Elbardissi, J. A. Dearani, R. C. Daly et al., "Survival after resection of primary cardiac tumors: a 48-year experience," *Circulation*, vol. 118, 14 Suppl, pp. S7–15, 2008.

[15] M. D. P. Oliveira, A. O. Tamazato, F. R. de Fazzio, L. J. Kajita, E. E. Ribeiro, and P. A. Lemos, "Left atrial myxoma hypervascularized from the right coronary artery: an interesting cath lab finding," *Case Reports in Cardiology*, vol. 2016, Article ID 4865439, 3 pages, 2016.

[16] A. Karabinis, G. Samanidis, M. Khoury, G. Stavridis, and K. Perreas, "Clinical presentation and treatment of cardiac myxoma in 153 patients," *Medicine*, vol. 97, no. 37, article e12397, 2018.

36

Multisystem Myotilinopathy, including Myopathy and Left Ventricular Noncompaction, due to the *MYOT* Variant c.179C>T

Josef Finsterer,[1] Claudia Stöllberger,[2] Matthias Hasun,[2] Korbinian Riedhammer,[3,4] and Mathias Wagner[3]

[1]*Krankenanstalt Rudolfstiftung, Messerli Institute, Vienna, Austria*
[2]*2nd Medical Department with Cardiology and Intensive Care Medicine, Krankenanstalt Rudolfstiftung, Vienna, Austria*
[3]*Institute of Human Genetics, Germany*
[4]*Department of Nephrology, Klinikum Rechts der Isar, School of Medicine, Technical University of Munich, Munich, Germany*

Correspondence should be addressed to Josef Finsterer; fipaps@yahoo.de

Academic Editor: Kuan-Rau Chiou

Left ventricular hypertrabeculation/noncompaction is a myocardial abnormality of unknown etiology/pathogenesis, which is frequently associated with neuromuscular disorders or chromosomal defects. LVHT in association with a *MYOT* mutation has not been reported. The patient is a 72-year-old male with a history of strabismus in childhood, asymptomatic creatine-kinase elevation since age 42 years, slowly progressive lower limb weakness since age 60 years, slowly progressive dysarthria and dysphagia since age 62 years, and recurrent episodes of arthralgias and myalgias since age 71 years. He also had arterial hypertension, diverticulosis, hyperlipidemia, coronary heart disease, and a hiatal hernia with reflux esophagitis. Clinical exam revealed mild quadruparesis and proximal wasting of the legs. Whole exome sequencing revealed a known variant in the *MYOT* gene. Muscle biopsy, previously assessed as inclusion body myopathy, was compatible with the genotype after revision. Cardiologic work-up revealed a left anterior hemiblock, mild myocardial thickening, and noncompaction. This case shows that myotilinopathy may manifest as a multisystem disease, including noncompaction.

1. Introduction

Left ventricular hypertrabeculation (LVHT), also known as left ventricular noncompaction (LVNC), is a myocardial anomaly characterised by hypertrabeculation of the left ventricular apex [1]. It is frequently associated with monogenic disease or chromosomal defects, but a causal relation has not been established [1]. If neuromuscular disorders (NMDs) are systematically screened for LVHT, up to 80% of the NMD patients show LVHT on echocardiography or cardiac MRI [1, 2]. Though LVHT has been associated with a number of NMDs, myotilinopathy (myopathy due to a variant in the *MYOT* gene most frequently manifesting as limb girdle muscular dystrophy type 1A (LGMD1A)) has not been reported in association with LVHT. Additionally, long-term, slowly progressive creatine-kinase (CK) elevation, which may be the first sign in LGMDs, has been only rarely reported as a manifestation of myotilinopathy. Here, we present a patient in whom a pathogenic variant in the *MYOT* gene was detected by whole exome sequencing (WES), who presented with late-onset, slowly progressive myopathy and LVHT.

2. Case Report

The patient is a 72-year-old Caucasian male, height 186 cm, weight 94 kg, and with a previous history of strabism since childhood resulting in impaired vision of the right eye, asymptomatic CK elevation first detected at age 42 years, arterial hypertension since age 57 years, diverticulosis of the sigma detected at age 57 years, slowly progressive weakness of the lower limbs since the age of 60 years, slowly progressive dysarthria and dysphagia since age 62 years, and hyperlipidemia since the age of 62 years. At age 66 years, a drug-eluting stent (DES) was implanted into the left anterior descending (LAD) coronary artery. Despite stenting, the patient experienced a non-ST elevation myocardial infarction (NSTEMI)

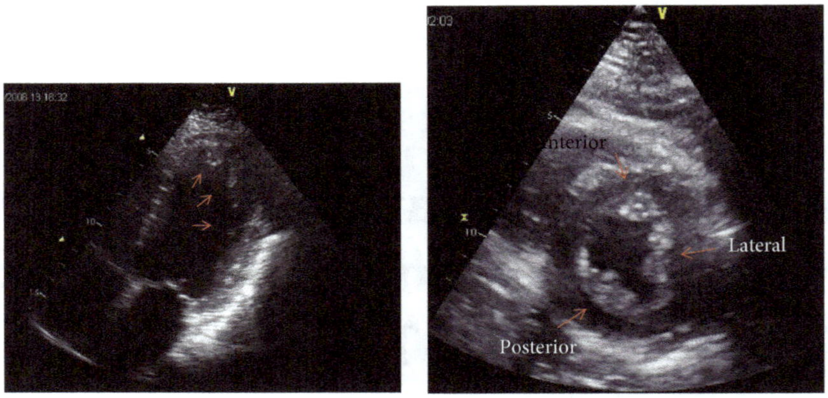

(a) (b)

FIGURE 1: Echocardiographic apical 4-chamber view showing left ventricular hypertrabeculation/noncompaction affecting the apex of the left ventricle (a). Echocardiographic short axis view of the left ventricle with hypertrabeculation/noncompaction affecting the anterior, lateral, and posterior walls (b).

due to coronary two-vessel disease 6 months later. The history was further positive for hiatal hernia with reflux disease since age 68 years and for resection of a left transverse colon polyp at age 66 years. Five months prior to the last presentation, the patient experienced recurrent episodes of arthralgias and myalgias together with chills. Three months prior to the last presentation, he was able to climb stairs upwards only with a rail and used two sticks for walking on an even floor. The patient was regularly taking acetyl-salicylic acid, ticagrelor, esomeprazole, ramipril, nebivolol, and evolocumab since he did not tolerate statins. The family history was positive for CK elevation in his son who refused to undergo diagnostic work-up for myotilinopathy.

A clinical neurologic exam at age 72 years revealed weakness for hip extension (right M5-, left M4), for knee extension (right M5-, left M4+), for knee flexion (M4+ bilaterally), and for foot extension (right M4+, left M5-), diffuse wasting of the lower limb muscles with proximal predominance, hypoesthesia of the lateral left lower limb, absent tendon reflexes on the lower limbs, mild edema of the feet and ankles, bilateral contractures of the Achilles tendons with incipient tiptoe walking, and missing pulses of the dorsalis pedis arteries bilaterally.

CK was elevated to values between 200 and 500 U/L. There was recurrent elevation of CK-MB and troponin, but proBNP was either normal or only mildly elevated. Nerve conduction studies revealed symmetric, axonal polyneuropathy. Muscle MRI revealed marked wasting and replacement of the muscle tissue by fat in the proximal limb muscles, most pronounced in the lateral, intermedius, and medial vastus muscles; the semimembranosus and semitendinosus muscles; and the adductors but largely sparing the gracilis and the sartorius muscles. Muscle biopsy from the left lateral vastus muscle at age 60 years revealed fiber size variation, numerous atrophic fibers, regenerating fibers, fiber necrosis, some ragged-red and COX-negative fibers, and large rimmed vacuoles with APP-, tau-, and ubiquitin-positive depositions. In the vicinity of these vacuoles, tubulofilamentous inclusions were seen on electron microscopy. This is why initially, inclusion body myopathy was suspected [3].

ECG revealed a left anterior hemiblock. Holter ECG and 24 h blood pressure monitoring were normal. Transthoracic echocardiography showed normal systolic function but thickening of the left ventricular myocardium and LVHT (Figure 1). LVHT was confirmed by cardiac MRI at age 71 years (Figure 2). A CT scan of the brain was normal. MRI of the brain at age 61 years revealed spot-like, T2-hyperintense lesions of the white matter and some lacunas in the left crus cerebrum. Carotid ultrasound showed only mild atherosclerosis. Videocinematography only revealed impaired motility of the esophagus. Impedance manometry revealed ineffective motility of the bolus along the esophagus. WES at age 79 years revealed the known missense variant c.179C>T in the *MYOT* gene.

3. Discussion

The presented patient is interesting for several aspects. First, the variant c.179C>T has been only occasionally described in patients with myotilinopathy. Generally, *MYOT* variants manifest phenotypically as myofibrillar myopathy [4, 5], spheroid-body myopathy [6], pseudohypertrophy and muscle stiffness [7], distal myopathy [8, 9], or as LGMD1A [10, 11]. Since there is a broad overlap between these phenotypes, they are summarised under the term myotilinopathies [12]. The variant found in the index patient has been previously reported in a patient with myofibrillar myopathy [11], in a French family with late onset nonspecific myopathy [13], and in a patient with severe proximal muscular dystrophy [10]. Additionally, the variant has been reported in two British patients with late onset myofibrillar myopathy [14]. The first homozygous (recessive) *MYOT* variant was detected in a German patient with progressive myofibrillar myopathy [4]. The variant c.179C>T is listed in ClinVar as pathogenic.

Second, the initial manifestation was long-term CK elevation, which has not been described in myotilinopathy before. However, CK elevation in the absence of any other clinical manifestation is often the first sign in limb girdle muscular dystrophies.

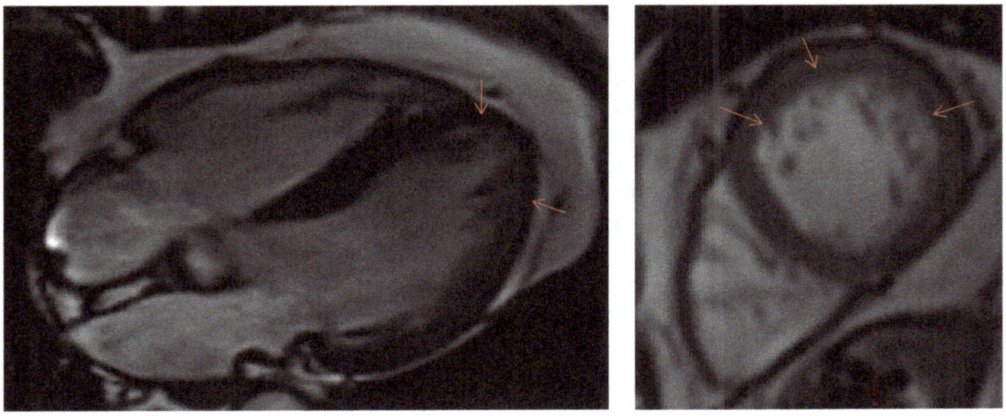

FIGURE 2: Cardiac MRI (3T, true fisp) showing left ventricular hypertrabeculation/noncompaction in the end-diastolic 4-chamber view (a) and in the apical short axis view (b).

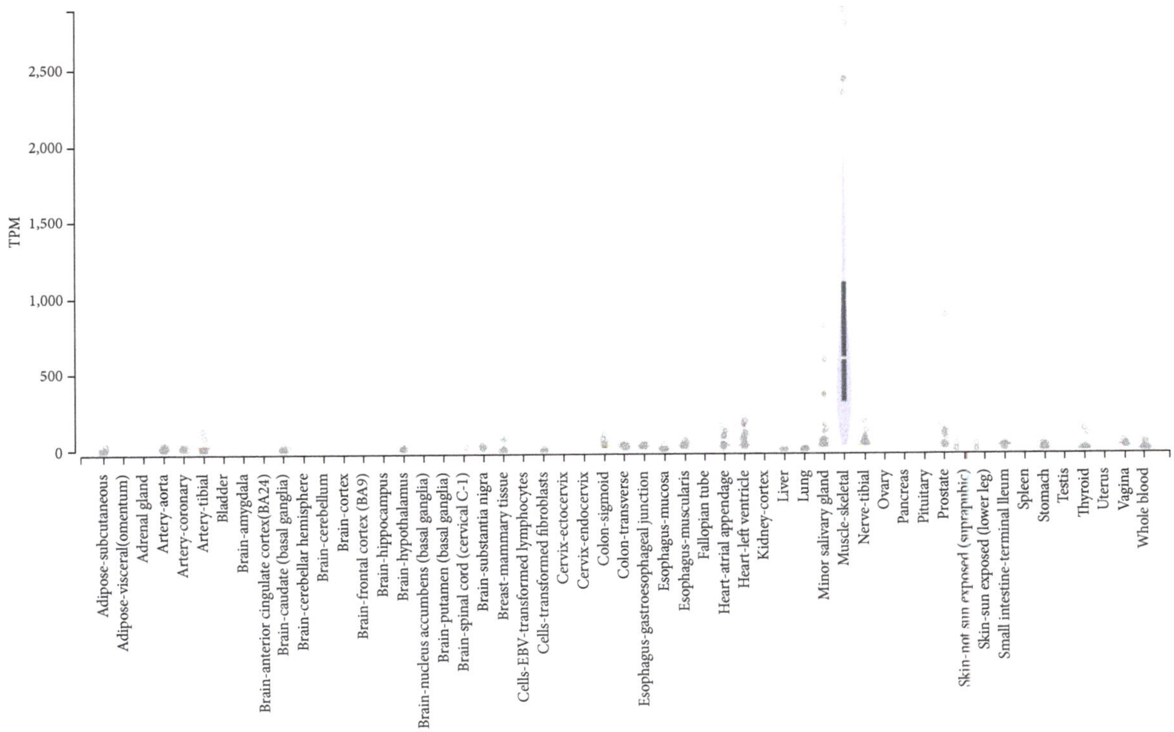

FIGURE 3: Gene expression for MYOT (ENSG00000120729.5).

Third, the patient manifested with a multisystem disease, affecting not only the muscles but also the brain (dysarthria, dysphagia), heart (myocardial thickening, LVHT), and peripheral nerves (axonal polyneuropathy). A multisystem disease due to *MYOT* variants affecting the skeletal muscles as well as other organs (heart, peripheral nerves) has been previously reported although myotilin is predominantly expressed in the skeletal muscle (Figure 3). Phenotypes of previously reported patients with myotilinopathy [11] showed similarities with the index patient. In accordance with the index patient, patients carrying other *MYOT* variants manifested in the peripheral nerves as polyneuropathy [11], as cardiomyopathy [11], or as dysphagia or dysarthria [15]. In a French family with myotilinopathy [13], muscle biopsy showed large rimmed vacuoles similar to those found in the index patient. Whether hiatal hernia and diverticulosis were related to the *MYOT* variant remains speculative, but affection of the autonomous innervation is more likely than affection of the smooth muscle cells as myotilin is not expressed in smooth muscle cells. Tightened heel cords are, on the contrary, frequently seen in patients with myotilinopathy [15]. Not only patients with late onset and slow progression of the phenotype have been reported, but also patients with early onset [15] and rapid progression [16]. Atherosclerosis, manifesting as a coronary heart disease and arterial occlusive disease, was regarded as unrelated to the *MYOT* variant.

Arrhythmias or LVHT have not been reported in association with *MYOT* variants. LVHT in the index patient represents a unique phenotypic feature but nonetheless needs to be recognised since it may strongly influence the outcome of these patients. LVHT is well-known for complications such as cardioembolism, heart failure, or ventricular arrhythmias potentially leading to sudden cardiac death [1]. Cardioembolism can be prevented by oral anticoagulation, systolic dysfunction may respond to heart failure therapy, and arrhythmias may respond to antiarrhythmics or device implantation. LVHT has not been reported in any other limb girdle muscular dystrophy before.

In conclusion, this case shows that myotilinopathy may manifest with LVHT and not only in the skeletal muscle but also in the brain, heart, and peripheral nerves. Patients with myotilinopathy should be investigated by not only the neurologist but also the cardiologist.

Additional Points

Highlight. MYOT mutations may manifest with left ventricular noncompaction. Myotilinopathies may manifest with mild, long-term creatine-kinase elevation. Myotilinopathies may manifest as a multisystem disease.

Authors' Contributions

JF was responsible for patient care, design, literature search, discussion, and the first draft; CS was responsible for patient care, literature search, discussion, and critical comments; and KR and MW were responsible for genetic investigations, discussion, and critical comments. All authors contributed equally to this work.

References

[1] J. Finsterer, "Cardiogenetics, neurogenetics, and pathogenetics of left ventricular hypertrabeculation/noncompaction," *Pediatric Cardiology*, vol. 30, no. 5, pp. 659–681, 2009.

[2] C. Stöllberger, J. Finsterer, and G. Blazek, "Left ventricular hypertrabeculation/noncompaction and association with additional cardiac abnormalities and neuromuscular disorders," *The American Journal of Cardiology*, vol. 90, no. 8, pp. 899–902, 2002.

[3] J. Finsterer, C. Stöllberger, and R. Höftberger, "Left ventricular hypertrabeculation/noncompaction in hereditary inclusion body myopathy," *International Journal of Cardiology*, vol. 150, no. 2, pp. e67–e69, 2011.

[4] J. Schessl, E. Bach, S. Rost et al., "Novel recessive myotilin mutation causes severe myofibrillar myopathy," *Neurogenetics*, vol. 15, no. 3, pp. 151–156, 2014.

[5] R. Ebrahimzadeh-Vesal, A. Teymoori, A. M. Dourandish, and M. Azimi-Nezhad, "Identification of a novel nonsense mutation in kyphoscoliosis peptidase gene in an Iranian patient with myofibrillar myopathy," *Genes Dis*, vol. 5, no. 4, pp. 331–334, 2018.

[6] T. Foroud, N. Pankratz, A. P. Batchman et al., "A mutation in myotilin causes spheroid body myopathy," *Neurology*, vol. 65, no. 12, pp. 1936–1940, 2005.

[7] J. Gamez, J. Armstrong, A. Shatunov et al., "Generalized muscle pseudo-hypertrophy and stiffness associated with the myotilin Ser55Phe mutation: a novel myotilinopathy phenotype?," *Journal of the Neurological Sciences*, vol. 277, no. 1-2, pp. 167–171, 2009.

[8] A. McNeill, D. Birchall, V. Straub et al., "Lower limb radiology of distal myopathy due to the S60F myotilin mutation," *European Neurology*, vol. 62, no. 3, pp. 161–166, 2009.

[9] J. Berciano, E. Gallardo, R. Domínguez-Perles et al., "Autosomal-dominant distal myopathy with a myotilin S55F mutation: sorting out the phenotype," *Journal of Neurology, Neurosurgery, and Psychiatry*, vol. 79, no. 2, pp. 205–208, 2008.

[10] G. Rudolf, T. Suominen, S. Penttilä et al., "Homozygosity of the dominant myotilin c.179C>T (p.Ser60Phe) mutation causes a more severe and proximal muscular dystrophy," *Journal of Neuromuscular Diseases*, vol. 3, no. 2, pp. 275–281, 2016.

[11] D. Selcen and A. G. Engel, "Mutations in myotilin cause myofibrillar myopathy," *Neurology*, vol. 62, no. 8, pp. 1363–1371, 2004.

[12] M. Olivé, L. G. Goldfarb, A. Shatunov, D. Fischer, and I. Ferrer, "Myotilinopathy: refining the clinical and myopathological phenotype," *Brain*, vol. 128, no. 10, pp. 2315–2326, 2005.

[13] I. Pénisson-Besnier, K. Talvinen, C. Dumez et al., "Myotilinopathy in a family with late onset myopathy," *Neuromuscular Disorders*, vol. 16, no. 7, pp. 427–431, 2006.

[14] A. E. Vincent, J. P. Grady, M. C. Rocha et al., "Mitochondrial dysfunction in myofibrillar myopathy," *Neuromuscular Disorders*, vol. 26, no. 10, pp. 691–701, 2016.

[15] M. A. Hauser, C. B. Conde, V. Kowaljow et al., "Myotilin mutation found in second pedigree with LGMD1A," *American Journal of Human Genetics*, vol. 71, no. 6, pp. 1428–1432, 2002.

[16] P. Reilich, S. Krause, N. Schramm et al., "A novel mutation in the myotilin gene (MYOT) causes a severe form of limb girdle muscular dystrophy 1A (LGMD1A)," *Journal of Neurology*, vol. 258, no. 8, pp. 1437–1444, 2011.

Recurrent Coronary Thrombus in a Patient with Chronic Immune Thrombocytopenia with Treatment using Eltrombopag

Terumori Satoh,[1] Masao Saotome,[1] Kenichiro Suwa,[1] Hayato Ohtani,[1] Yasuyuki Nagata,[2] Takaaki Ono,[2] and Yuichiro Maekawa[1]

[1]*Department of Cardiology, Internal Medicine 3, Hamamatsu University School of Medicine, Hamamatsu, Japan*
[2]*Department of Hematology, Internal Medicine 3, Hamamatsu University School of Medicine, Hamamatsu, Japan*

Correspondence should be addressed to Masao Saotome; msaotome@hama-med.ac.jp

Academic Editor: Tayfun Sahin

Background. Eltrombopag, a nonpeptide thrombopoietin receptor agonist (TPO-RA), has been reported to be an effective therapy for chronic immune thrombocytopenia (ITP). However, a higher incidence of arterial and venous thromboembolic events was reported after using eltrombopag. *Case Presentation.* A 67-year-old man, treated with eltrombopag due to chronic ITP, was admitted due to acute coronary syndrome (ACS). Although coronary angiography revealed no occlusion, cardiac magnetic resonance imaging suggested a myocardial infarction in the territory of the left circumflex coronary artery. Three months after the ACS event, the obtuse marginal branches exhibited significant stenosis; hence, a percutaneous coronary intervention (PCI) was performed to implant a zotarolimus-eluting stent under the treatment of a dual antiplatelet therapy. However, stent thrombosis occurred 3 hours after PCI and required three other PCIs during the eltrombopag treatment. *Conclusion.* We present a case of an ITP patient, who experienced repeated coronary and stent thrombosis during the treatment with eltrombopag. We propose that the risk of ACS and consequent coronary stent thrombosis should be considered before the introduction of eltrombopag.

1. Introduction

Chronic immune thrombocytopenia (ITP) is an autoimmune syndrome, which is caused by the development of an autoantibody against structural platelets. Although bleeding is a major symptom of ITP, a thrombophilia condition can be promoted in ITP patients by excess activated platelet function. Since platelets play critical roles in the progression of atherosclerosis, cardiovascular events have often been reported in ITP patients. Thus, the safety and recommended strategy in percutaneous coronary intervention (PCI) and subsequent antiplatelet therapies toward ITP patients have remained a matter of debate.

Currently available treatments of ITP include corticosteroids, splenectomy, immunosuppressants, and thrombopoietin receptor agonist (TPO-RA). Eltrombopag, a nonpeptide TPO-RA, has been reported to be effective as a second-line therapy for ITP. However, previous reports indicated a higher incidence of arterial and venous thromboembolic events, including myocardial infarction, after using eltrombopag [1]. In this report, we showed a case of recurrent coronary thrombosis in a patient with ITP who was treated with eltrombopag. We also reviewed the previous reports of PCI and antiplatelet therapy during and after PCI, in ITP patients.

2. Case Presentation

A 67-year-old man, who was suffering from long-lasting (>2 hours) severe chest pain, was admitted in our hospital. He was an ex-smoker (between the ages of 20 and 25 years) and had been treated for hypertension and hyperlipidemia. He was diagnosed with ITP 6 months before admission and maintained his platelet count between 10.0×10^9/L and 15.0×10^9/L by receiving prednisolone (10 mg daily) and eltrombopag (50 mg daily). He was immediately relieved of chest pain after admission, and there was no significant finding on a 12-lead electrocardiogram except a left axis

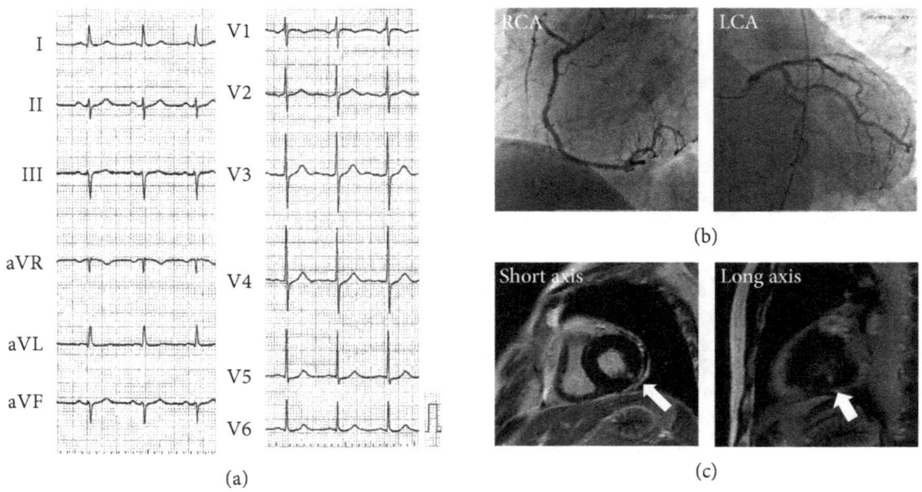

FIGURE 1: Electrocardiography (ECG), coronary angiography (CAG), and cardiac magnetic resonance imaging (C-MRI) on the first admission. (a) ECG on admission revealed no significant change except a left axis deviation. (b) CAG revealed no coronary artery occlusion either in the right coronary artery (RCA: left anterior oblique 50° view) or the left coronary arteries (LCA: caudal 30° view). (c) C-MRI of short and long axis view. The arrows indicate the delayed enhancement of the myocardium.

deviation (Figure 1(a)). However, a cardiac catheterization was performed urgently due to the significant increase of serum myocardial enzymes (troponin-I 1.56 ng/mL, creatine kinase (CK) 233 IU/L, and CK-muscle/brain 20 IU/L). Although coronary angiography (CAG) revealed no artery occlusion (Figure 1(b)), left ventriculography showed mild hypokinesis in the posterior wall, and cardiac magnetic resonance imaging exhibited a delayed gadolinium enhancement in the posterior wall area (Figure 1(c)), suggesting myocardial infarction in the territory of the left circumflex coronary artery (LCX).

Because the patient persistently complained of chest pain even after discharge, the second CAG was performed 3 months after the discharge. CAG revealed de novo stenosis in the obtuse marginal branches (#12: 75% with haziness, Figure 2(a)), and adenosine stress myocardial perfusion scintigraphy (Tc-99m tetrofosmin) showed myocardial ischemia in the posterior wall area (Figure 2(b)), where the tracer uptake was reduced at stress and restored at rest. Thus, the first PCI was planned for #12, and a dual antiplatelet therapy (aspirin 100 mg daily and clopidogrel 75 mg daily) was started more than 1 month before the procedure, where his platelet was kept at 27.4×10^9/L by eltrombopag (50 mg daily). The first PCI toward #12 was successfully performed by implantation of a zotarolimus-eluting stent (3.0 × 12 mm) and CAG revealed no residual stenosis (Figure 3(a)). However, the patient complained of severe chest pain with significant ST depression after returning to his hospital room (3 hours after the PCI). The emergent CAG demonstrated a stent thrombosis at the proximal edge of the stent (Figure 3(b)). Although the intravascular ultrasound imaging exhibited neither the underexpansion of the prior-implanted stent nor the coronary artery dissection around the stent, it showed new lining thrombus (white arrows) at the proximal edge of the stent (Figure 3(c)). An additional drug-eluting stent (3.0 × 12 mm, everolimus-eluting stent) was implanted at the proximal edge of the prior stent lesion of #12 (Figure 4(a), second PCI) under the support of an intra-aortic balloon pumping. To avoid further stent thrombosis, the antiplatelet agent was changed from clopidogrel (75 mg daily) to prasugrel (3.75 mg daily). However, CAG, performed 3 days after the second PCI, revealed a massive thrombus with 75% stenosis in #12 (Figure 4(b)). Urokinase (UK 240.000 U) was selectively injected into the LCX, instead of balloon inflation for the third PCI, because recurrent coronary thrombosis was occurring at the area of the dual stent implantation. CAG after the UK injection revealed the residual stenosis (50%) in #12. The follow-up CAG, which was performed 14 days after the third PCI, again revealed the recurrence of stent thrombosis with 75% stenosis in #12 (Figure 4(c)). Subsequently, a coronary thrombus aspiration was performed as the fourth PCI. The final CAG after coronary thrombus aspiration exhibited 50% residual stenosis. Since his platelet maintained at $>39.3 \times 10^9$/L by eltrombopag during all PCIs, the association between a recurrence of coronary thrombosis and inappropriate platelet increase induced by eltrombopag was suspected. Thus, we transiently ceased eltrombopag, and his platelet promptly decreased to 8.0×10^9/L after 7 days of cessations. CAG, after the cessation of eltrombopag, showed 50% of residual stenosis with thrombus; hence, we did not perform further PCI to #12 (Figure 4(d)). In addition, after he received a splenectomy to cease eltrombopag, he has not complained of any chest pain, and CAG after splenectomy revealed no thrombus in #12.

3. Discussion and Conclusions

We report a rare case of recurrent coronary thrombosis in a patient with ITP who was treated with eltrombopag. Despite the thrombocytopenic condition, acute coronary syndrome (ACS) events have been reported in ITP patients. ITP patients could experience comorbid thromboembolic events (TEEs) because ITP itself affords an inflammatory condition

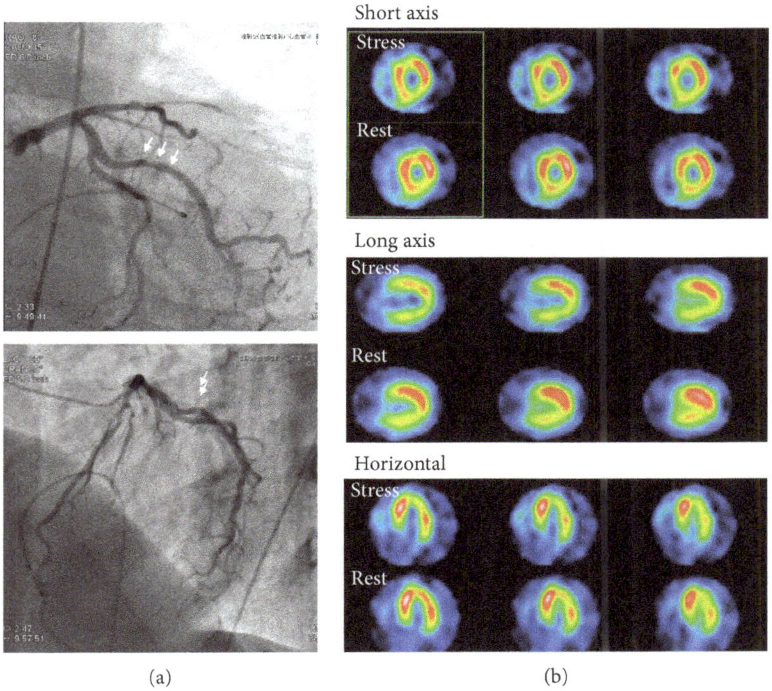

FIGURE 2: Second CAG and adenosine stress myocardial perfusion scintigraphy. (a) The second CAG was performed to investigate the acetylcholine-induced vasospasm. Although the coronary arteries did not exhibit vasospasm induced by acetylcholine, CAG revealed de novo stenosis in #12. (b) The adenosine stress myocardial perfusion scintigraphy (Tc-99m tetrofosmin) showed the myocardial ischemia in the posterior wall area, suggesting myocardial ischemia in #12.

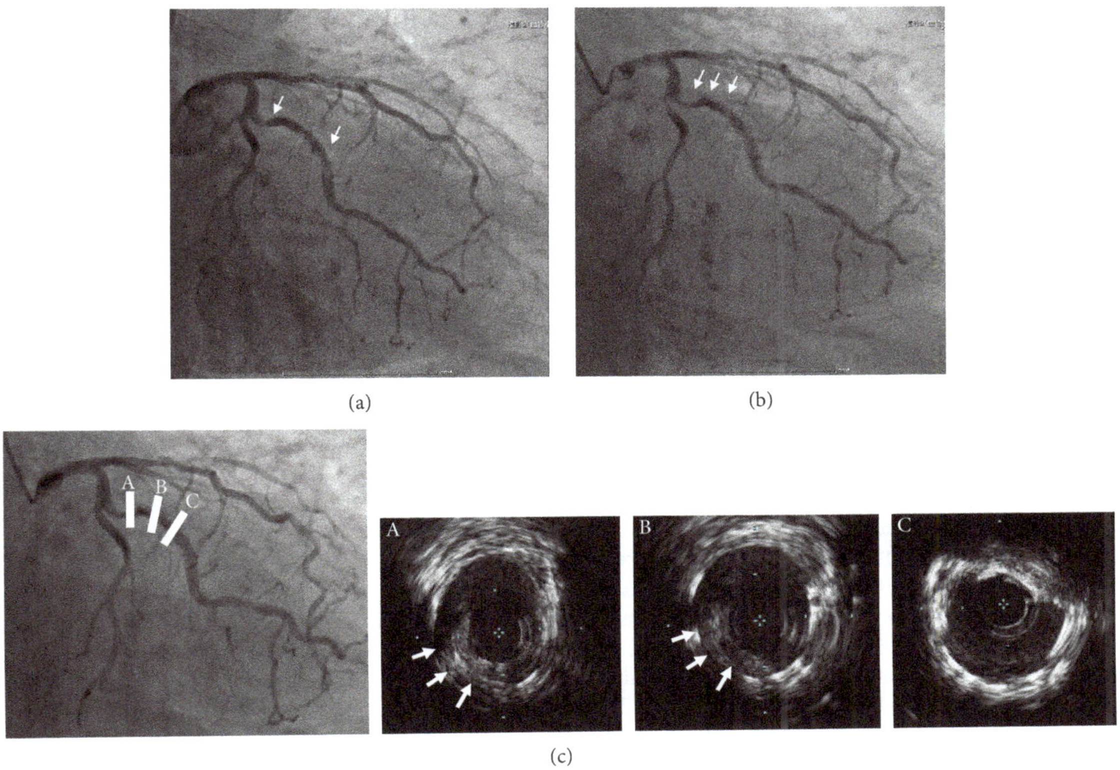

FIGURE 3: CAG and intravascular ultrasound images during PCI. In the first PCI, a zotarolimus-eluting stent (3.0 × 12 mm) was implanted in #12 (a, between white arrows). Emergent CAG, which was performed 3 hours after the first PCI, revealed massive thrombus in the stent lesion (b, white arrows). The intravascular ultrasound study (c) showed the new lining thrombus (white arrows) in the stent proximal (A and B), whereas not in the distal (C).

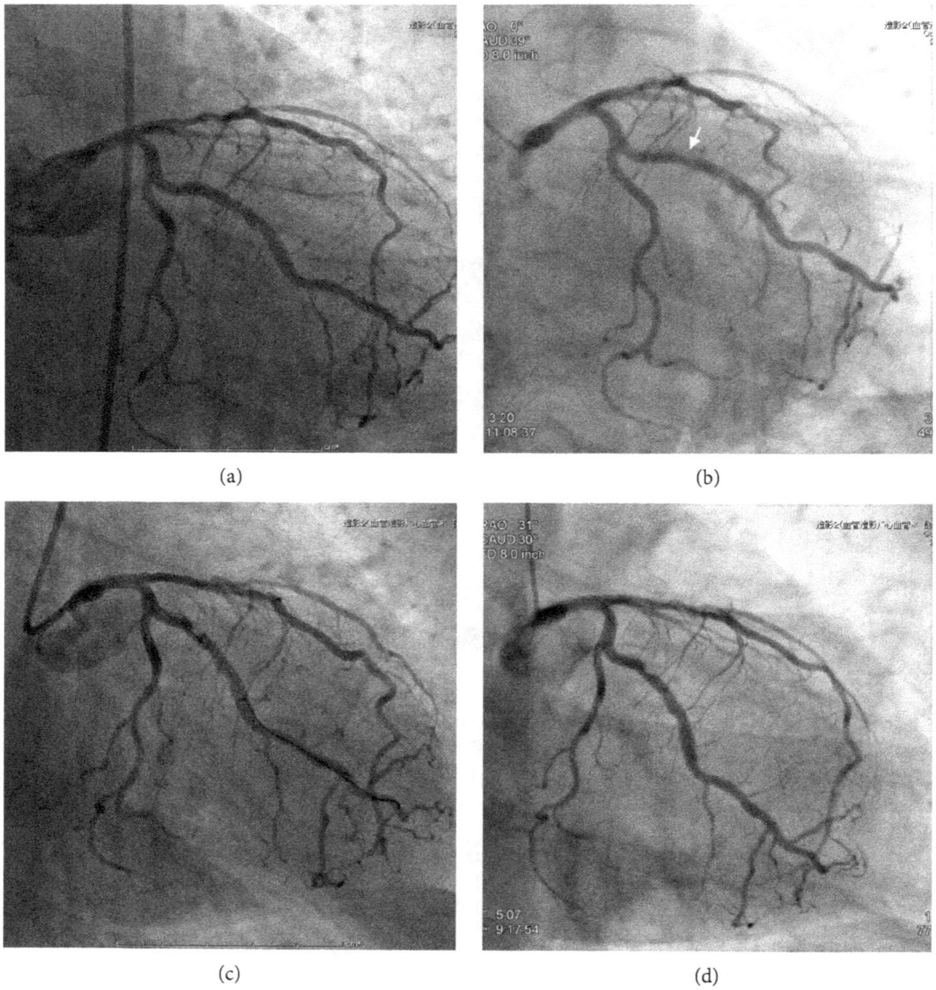

FIGURE 4: CAG findings after second PCI. Although an additional drug-eluting stent sized 3.0×12 mm was implanted in #12 (a), CAG performed 3 days after the second PCI revealed the recurrence of thrombus (white arrow) with 75% haziness stenosis in #12 (b). Another CAG performed 14 days after the third PCI again revealed recurrence of stent thrombosis with 75% stenosis in #12 (c). The final CAG, which was performed after the fourth PCI, showed 50% of residual stenosis with thrombus, and we decided not to perform further PCI to #12 (d).

and promotes an aberrant platelet condition, with larger, younger, and more adherent platelets. In addition, the multifactorial predisposing factors, such as prednisolone treatment and atherosclerotic comorbidities, facilitate the trigger of TEEs.

Although eltrombopag has been commonly used as a second-line therapy of ITP, it may enhance the ITP-specific characteristics of thromboembolism, which may increase the incidence of ACS events in ITP patients. Previous reports described cardiac manifestation, such as tachycardia, cyanosis, QT interval prolongation, pulmonary thromboembolism, and ACS after the use of eltrombopag. A pooled data analysis from five eltrombopag RCTs exhibited that the overall TEE rate was 4.5% (27 cases) in the eltrombopag-treated ITP patients, whereas there was none in the placebo groups, and four patients had ACS event [2]. Previously, three ACS events in patients with ITP were reported, which are suspected to be associated with eltrombopag. No association seems to be seen in the ACS event with the treatment duration (1 to 12 months), the platelet counts (107 to 437×10^9/L), and the atherosclerotic risk factors among them [3–5]. Although the mechanism, by which eltrombopag causes ACS event, remains elusive, a rapid platelet increase induced by eltrombopag (0.8×10^9/L to 10.5×10^9/L per month) may affect the ACS events in the present case.

Since platelets play critical roles in the progression of atherosclerosis, as well as vascular healing, after stent implantation, PCI and the antiplatelet therapies in ITP patient have been a matter of debate for a long time [6]. The present case showed recurrent coronary thrombosis in the LCX even under dual antiplatelet therapy (DAPT—both clopidogrel plus aspirin and prasugrel plus aspirin), suggesting that DAPT may not be effective for activated platelets induced by eltrombopag. Thus, when ITP patients using eltrombopag have a coronary event, it might be safe to avoid any nonurgent PCI. If possible, PCI should be performed with other supporting treatments, such as corticosteroids, splenectomy, and immunosuppressants. Even in an evitable condition, such as ACS, it might be better to avoid any implantation of drug-eluting stent because they might have a poor response to DAPT, which results in repetitive coronary thrombosis. Furthermore, even in ITP patients not receiving eltrombopag treatment, adding eltrombopag before PCI is not recommended. The DAPT treatment for ITP patients has been commonly accepted if ITP patients have a sufficient platelet count ($>50 \times 10^9$/L) [7]. Even in severe thrombocytopenic conditions, major bleeding was rarely reported in the previous cases [6].

Accordingly, when ITP patients present any risk factors for thromboembolism or atherosclerosis, we recommend careful consideration of the risk-benefit balance before the introduction of eltrombopag. Further investigation is required to detect the eltrombopag-specific factors which increase the TEEs.

Abbreviations

ACS: Acute coronary syndrome
CAG: Coronary angiography
CK: Creatine kinase
DAPT: Dual antiplatelet therapy
ITP: Immune thrombocytopenia
LCX: Left circumflex coronary artery
TPO-RA: Thrombopoietin receptor agonist
TEEs: Thromboembolic events.

Acknowledgments

This work was supported by JSPS KAKENHI Grant number JP16K09428 (to M. S).

References

[1] F. Catalá-López, I. Corrales, C. de la Fuente-Honrubia et al., "Risk of thromboembolism with thrombopoietin receptor agonists in adult patients with thrombocytopenia: systematic review and meta-analysis of randomized controlled trials," *Medicina Clínica*, vol. 145, no. 12, pp. 511–519, 2015.

[2] J. B. Bussel, G. Cheng, M. N. Saleh, B. Mayer, S. Y. Vasey, and A. Brainsky, "Incidence of thromboembolic events across eltrombopag clinical trials in chronic immune thrombocytopenia (ITP)," *Blood*, vol. 116, no. 21, p. 70, 2010.

[3] J. Teichman, A. Taher, A. Hashi, A. Bagai, and M. Sholzberg, "A sticky situation: myocardial infarction in a young woman with immune thrombocytopenia on eltrombopag and a history of mediastinal radiation," *Journal of Thrombosis and Thrombolysis*, vol. 45, no. 1, pp. 192–195, 2018.

[4] S. Sert, H. Ozdil, and M. Sunbul, "Acute myocardial infarction due to eltrombopag therapy in a patient with immune thrombocytopenic purpura," *Turkish Journal of Haematology*, vol. 34, no. 1, pp. 107-108, 2017.

[5] H. Gunes and T. Kivrak, "Eltrombopag induced thrombosis: a case with acute myocardial infarction," *Current Drug Safety*, vol. 11, no. 2, pp. 174–176, 2016.

[6] G. Li-Sha, C. Peng, and L. Yue-Chun, "Recurrent acute coronary syndrome and restenosis after percutaneous coronary intervention in a patient with idiopathic thrombocytopenic purpura: a case report and literature review," *BMC Cardiovascular Disorders*, vol. 15, no. 1, p. 101, 2015.

[7] A. Russo, M. Cannizzo, G. Ghetti et al., "Idiopathic thrombocytopenic purpura and coronary artery disease: comparison between coronary artery bypass grafting and percutaneous coronary intervention," *Interactive Cardiovascular and Thoracic Surgery*, vol. 13, no. 2, pp. 153–157, 2011.

38

Inappropriate Defibrillator Shocks due to Mechanical Inference from an Investigational Device

Ying chi Yang,[1] Thein Tun Aung,[1] and Abdul Wase[2]

[1]*University of Iowa Hospitals and Clinics, Iowa City, IA, USA*
[2]*Dayton Heart and Vascular Hospital, Dayton, OH, USA*

Correspondence should be addressed to Ying chi Yang; myomintun3@gmail.com

Academic Editor: Hajime Kataoka

Cardiac contractility modulation (CCM) is an investigational device-based therapy to enhance ventricular contractility in systolic heart failure patients who are not candidates for cardiac resynchronization therapy (CRT) owing to the absence of wide QRS complexes or who have failed to respond on CRT. The principal mechanism is based on the stimulation of cardiac muscles by nonexcitatory electrical signals to augment the influx of calcium ions into the cardiomyocytes. The majority of patients receiving CCM therapy have concurrent implantable cardioverter defibrillators, and the manufacturer declares both devices can be used in parallel without any interactions. Nevertheless, proper lead positioning of both devices are crucial, and it is mandatory to check device-device interactions during each and every cardiac electronic implantable device-related procedure to prevent adverse outcomes.

1. Introduction

Cardiac contractility modulation (CCM) can be attained by an investigational device designed to improve the strength of myocardial contractility by delivering nonexcitatory electrical signals to increase calcium ion influx into the cardiomyocytes during the absolute refractory period of the cardiac cycle. The CCM device, Optimizer, is accepted in the United States as an investigational device to treat systolic heart failure patients with narrow QRS complexes or who are nonresponders of cardiac resynchronization therapy (CRT). A CCM unit includes a pulse generator and three pace-sense leads; a sensing lead in the right atrium and two signal-delivering leads implanted at the right ventricular (RV) septum. The manufacturer declares that CCM devices work in parallel with any kinds of implantable cardioverter defibrillator (ICD) system without affecting the ICD function. We present a case in which CCM leads chatter with the ICD lead in the RV which resulted in inappropriate sensing of the CCM signals by the ICD with subsequent delivery of inappropriate shocks.

2. Case Presentation

A 72-year-old male with past medical history of myocardial infarction status postpercutaneous coronary intervention, chronic systolic heart failure secondary to ischemic cardiomyopathy, received a single chamber Biotronik implantable cardioverter defibrillator (ICD) with a Medtronic single-coil defibrillator lead (model 6949-65) in 2005. A year later, the patient also received an investigational device, Optimizer III (Impulse Dynamics, Orangeburg, NY) (model #CCMX8), assembled with St. Jude Medical active fixation pace-sense leads (Model 1388-T), one lead in the right atrium and two in the upper and lower interventricular septum. Prominent electrical signals were identifiable on the patient's surface EKG when CCM was activated.

In August 2014, the old Medtronic lead (Model 6949-65) was found to have a sudden increase in RV impedance to >2000 Ohms with "RED" alert warning of the Biotronik device. The particular Medtronic lead was also a subject of a Class-I recall by the Food and Drug Administration. Subsequently, he underwent laser lead extraction and replacement for a new ICD lead, Medtronic Sprint Quattro (Model 6947) dual coil defibrillation lead. The procedure was uneventful. The function of the new ICD system was assessed, and all the device parameters were found within normal limits. Patient's CCM was eight years old at that time and was found no longer functional due to battery depletion. Hence, the device-device interaction with the concurrent CCM unit was not evaluated.

In earlier 2015, the patient presented with receipt of six ICD shocks without prior symptoms. Interrogation of the ICD disclosed intermittent, noncyclical, and nonphysiologic noise signals. The intracardiac electrogram recording was shown (Figure 1). All the device parameters were found within normal limits.

Lead failure was unlikely as all sensing and pacing parameters including lead impendence of the new Medtronic Sprint Quattro lead were normal. The signals (Figure 2) were noncyclical and very chaotic, ruling out the T-wave oversensing or crosstalk from far-field P-wave sensing. The noise signals were not suggestive of electromagnetic interference since external interferences are often repetitive high-frequency signals. The signals were not reproducible with isometric arm exercises. The patient was not physically active prior to or during the delivery of inappropriate shocks excluding the possibility of interference from pectoral myopotentials.

The patient underwent fluoroscopic examination (Figure 3) on which right ventricular leads of the CCM unit were found to be chattering with the newly inserted dual-coil ICD lead at the tricuspid annulus. Intracardiac mechanical interference/lead chattering was the cause of inappropriate sensing to result in an inappropriate ICD firing. The intermittent noise signals seen on the device intracardiac electrogram were coincidental with the leads chattering on the fluoroscopy.

The CCM device along with two St. Jude Medical right ventricular pace-sense leads was extracted, but the same ICD unit was left in place. During the follow-ups over two years, no further noise signals had been detected by his ICD and the patient had not received any more inappropriate shocks.

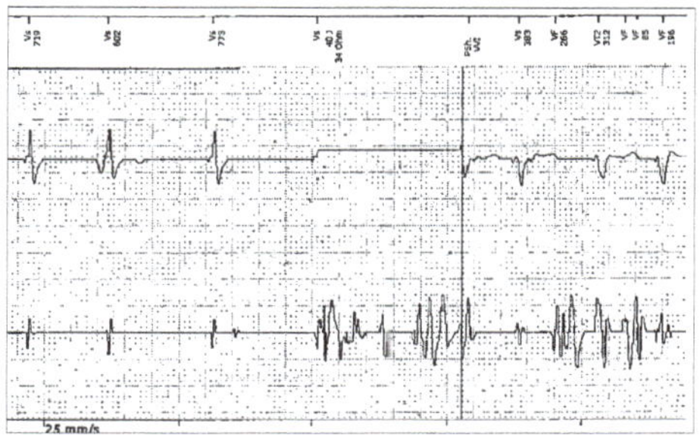

Figure 1: Delivery of 40-joule shock despite resolution of inappropriate VF sensing prior to the committed nature of therapy. Note that due to shock delivery, vigorous ventricular contraction occurs that resumes the lead chattering inappropriate sensing as VF (from top to bottom: marker channel, RV shock electrogram, and RV sense electrogram).

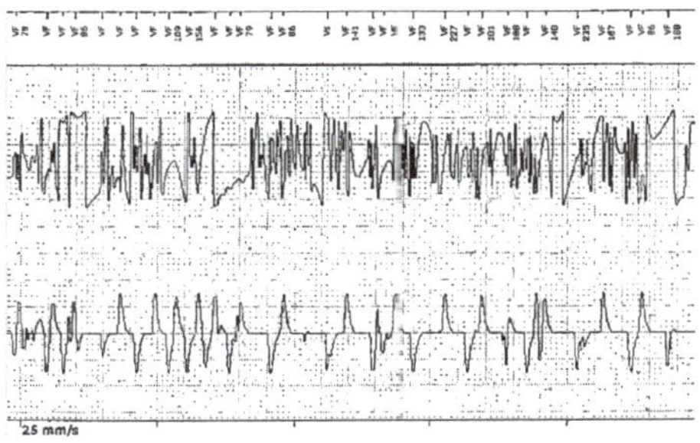

Figure 2: Intermittent nonphysiologic noise signals upon ICD interrogation (from top to bottom: marker channel, RV shock electrogram, and RV sense electrogram).

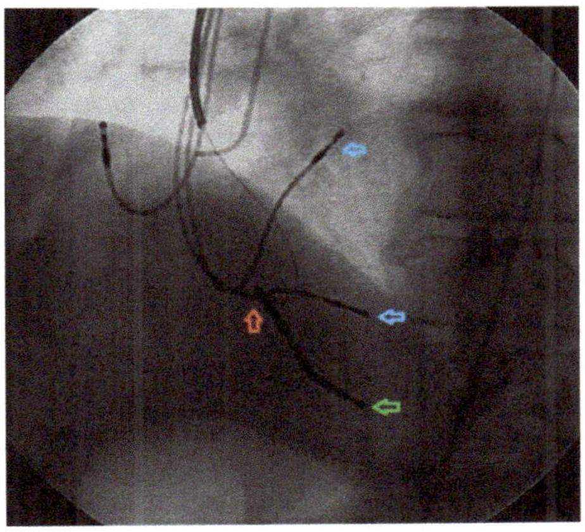

Figure 3: CCM signal-delivering leads in the upper and middle septum (blue arrows) and single chamber ICD lead at RV apex (green arrow) chattering each other at tricuspid annulus (red arrow).

3. Discussion

Cardiac contractility modulation (CCM) device is designed to enhance ventricular contractility in a subgroup of systolic heart failure patients who are not candidates for cardiac resynchronization therapy (CRT) owing to the absence of wide QRS complexes or who have failed to respond on CRT. Although CCM therapy falls under the investigational category in the United States, it is approved as one of the device-based therapy for heart failure in Europe. CCM therapy can provide a better quality of life and NYHA functional class by improving peak venous oxygen (pVO_2), Minnesota Living with Heart Failure Questionnaires (MLWHFQ) in narrow QRS systolic heart failure patients despite its lack in mortality benefits or all-cause hospitalizations [1–3]. Also, improved myocardial contractility induced by CCM was not found in association with an increase in myocardial oxygen consumption [4, 5].

The Optimizer CCM system includes a pulse generator and three leads. Current available CCM devices use three pace-sense leads with one lead in the right atrium and two in the right ventricular septum with a minimum of 1-2 cm apart. The right atrial lead detects atrial signals and transmits to the pulse generator. Based on atrial signals and predetermined measurements, the pulse generator generates the CCM signals to the right ventricle during the absolute refractory period [6–8].

As the primary use of CCM is for systolic heart failure, most of the patients on CCM therapy have a concomitant ICD device. The manufacturer of Optimizer CCM declares that the system is designed to work in parallel with any CEIDs (cardiac electronic implantable devices) including ICDs and generally does not cause any interruption with ICD functions. However, functional testing of both Optimizer CCM and ICD systems is crucial and mandated to conduct during every procedure including the time of CCM implantation, an addition or revision of a lead(s) to ensure there is neither oversensing of CCM signals by the ICD nor any device-device interactions. It is important to allow an optimal spacing between the ICD lead and the CCM signal-delivering leads to prevent chattering each other in the RV.

To our best knowledge, the consequences of CCM-ICD leads chattering as an outcome of inappropriate delivery of ICD shocks which even warranted the extraction of the CCM device have never been reported. In our case, CCM and the old ICD units were working in parallel without any interactions until the ICD lead was replaced. The diagnosis was challenging since signals were similar to those of ICD lead dysfunction but the leads parameters were normal. Under fluoroscopic examination, it was found that all the leads were implanted 1-2 cm apart as recommended by the manufacturer. However, there was the excessive redundancy of some of the leads, and it was believed to be the etiology of leads chattering and oversensing by the ICD. Our case gives us a valuable lesson regarding the crucial role of CCM-ICD leads positioning and mandatory testing of device-device interactions during each and every CEID procedure.

4. Conclusion

Optimizer is an investigational device based on the concept of cardiac contractility modulation. It is designed to improve myocardial contractility without increasing cardiac oxygen consumption by facilitating the calcium handling of cardiomyocytes. The device has a potential to fill up the present therapeutic gap in the treatment of systolic heart failure patients who have narrow QRS complexes or failed to CRT. The majority of patients receiving CCM therapy have concurrent ICD and the manufacturer declared both devices can be used in parallel without any interaction in between. Nevertheless, proper leads positioning of both devices are crucial, and it is mandatory to check device-device interactions during each and every CEID procedure to prevent adverse outcomes.

References

[1] F. Giallauria, C. Vigorito, M. F. Piepoli, and A. J. Stewart Coats, "Effects of cardiac contractility modulation by non-excitatory electrical stimulation on exercise capacity and quality of life: an individual patient's data meta-analysis of randomized controlled trials," *International Journal of Cardiology*, vol. 175, no. 2, pp. 352–357, 2014.

[2] A. Kadish, K. Nademanee, K. Volosin et al., "A randomized controlled trial evaluating the safety and efficacy of cardiac contractility modulation in advanced heart failure," *American Heart Journal*, vol. 161, no. 2, pp. 329–337.e2, 2011.

[3] W. T. Abraham, K. H. Kuck, R. L. Goldsmith et al., "A randomized controlled trial to evaluate the safety and efficacy of cardiac contractility modulation," *JACC: Heart Failure*, vol. 6, no. 10, pp. 874–883, 2018.

[4] G. Goliasch, A. Khorsand, M. Schütz et al., "The effect of device-based cardiac contractility modulation therapy on myocardial efficiency and oxidative metabolism in patients with heart failure," *European Journal of Nuclear Medicine and Molecular Imaging*, vol. 39, no. 3, pp. 408–415, 2012.

[5] C. Butter, E. Wellnhofer, M. Schlegl, G. Winbeck, E. Fleck, and H. N. Sabbah, "Enhanced inotropic state of the failing left ventricle by cardiac contractility modulation electrical signals is not associated with increased myocardial oxygen consumption," *Journal of Cardiac Failure*, vol. 13, no. 2, pp. 137–142, 2007.

[6] S. Mohri, J. Shimizu, Y. Mika et al., "Electric currents applied during refractory period enhance contractility and systolic calcium in the ferret heart," *American Journal of Physiology-Heart and Circulatory Physiology*, vol. 284, no. 4, pp. H1119–H1123, 2003.

[7] T. Kleemann, "Cardiac contractility modulation. A new form of therapy for patients with heart failure and narrow QRS complex?," *Herz*, vol. 40, no. 7, pp. 945–951, 2015.

[8] A. R. Lyon, M. A. Samara, and D. S. Feldman, "Cardiac contractility modulation therapy in advanced systolic heart failure," *Nature Reviews Cardiology*, vol. 10, no. 10, pp. 584–598, 2013.

Description of Ventricular Arrhythmia after Taking Herbal Medicines in Middle-Aged Couples

Mohammad Ali Zakeri[1,2] **Vahid Mohammadi**[3] **Gholamreza Bazmandegan**[4,5] **and Maryam Zakeri**[6]

[1]*Social Determinants of Health Research Center, Rafsanjan University of Medical Sciences, Rafsanjan, Iran*
[2]*Non-Communicable Diseases Research Center, Rafsanjan University of Medical Sciences, Rafsanjan, Iran*
[3]*Department of Cardiology, Ali-Ibn Abi-Talib Hospital, School of Medicine, Rafsanjan University of Medical Sciences, Rafsanjan, Iran*
[4]*Clinical Research Development Unit, Ali-Ibn Abi-Talib Hospital, Rafsanjan University of Medical Sciences, Rafsanjan, Iran*
[5]*Department of Family Medicine, Ali-Ibn Abi-Talib Hospital, School of Medicine, Rafsanjan University of Medical Sciences, Rafsanjan, Iran*
[6]*Physiology-Pharmacology Research Center, Research Institute of Basic Medical Sciences, Rafsanjan University of Medical Sciences, Rafsanjan, Iran*

Correspondence should be addressed to Mohammad Ali Zakeri; mazakeri@rums.ac.ir

Academic Editor: Christopher S. Snyder

Medicinal herbs and some derivatives have been used in the treatment of heart disease which is rarely responsible for ventricular arrhythmias and cardiac arrest. Ventricular tachycardia (VT) increases the risk of sudden cardiac death (SCD). However, only a few reports are available about the cardiac ventricular arrhythmia followed by taking herbal medicines. We present two patients (a couple) without a history of heart disease who referred to the hospital with ventricular arrhythmia.

1. Introduction

VT is caused by the activity of abnormal ventricular foci. It is mostly developed due to either acute myocardial infarction or advanced cardiomyopathy [1]. VT maybe increased the risk of SCD [2]. According to SCD reports, the prevalence of cardiac arrest (CA) is 45-83.7 per 100,000 individuals [3, 4]. A study has shown stable polymorphic VT, ventricular fibrillation, and patient death due to herbal medicines [5]. Medicinal herbs and some derivatives have been used in the treatment of heart disease, including congestive heart failure, hypertension, angina, atherosclerosis, cerebral insufficiency, venous insufficiency, and arrhythmias [6]. However, many plants and some supplements used in cardiovascular therapies have potentially serious side effects and complications that need to be evaluated through clinical experiments [7]. Many herbal medicines have not been scientifically evaluated, and some of them can cause serious toxic effects and major drug interactions [6]. We will present an interesting case of ventricular arrhythmia following the use of herbal medicines to better understand the complications, diagnosis, and treatment in the early acute stages.

2. Case Presentation

Patients were a middle-aged couple with a history of hypertension who referred to a public hospital with acute abdominal pain and periodic palpitation. Acute abdominal pain in both patients was due to the consumption of herbal medicines for reducing emotional stress including (a) Echium amoenum (containing saponins, flavonoids, unsaturated terpenoids, and sterols [8]), (b) Citrus aurantifolia (containing flavonoids including apigenin, hesperetin, kaempferol, nobiletin, quercetin, and rutin [9]), (c) Citrus aurantium (containing limonene, β-myrcene, α-pinene, and β-pinene [10]), and (d) Matricaria chamomilla L. (containing sesquiterpenes, flavonoids, coumarins, and polyacetylenes [11]). These drugs were taken arbitrarily and without a doctor's prescription. The two patients had an acute fever, numbness, sweating, dryness, tingling, and abdominal pain. They used a combination of these herbal medicines only once (for the first time) and had no previous use of it.

Ventricular arrhythmia (an automatic focus, monomorphic, and nonsustained VT) without hemodynamic effects was seen in the male and female case for 24 hours and 1 hour, respectively, after receiving the first dose of amiodarone. Ultrasound, abdominal X-ray, exercise test, and echocardiography were performed in both patients, showing normal results. The patients' electrocardiogram (ECG) was normal on the second day of hospitalization, at the time of discharge, and 3 months later. After the treatment and discharge, the patients were followed up for three months (monthly) with Holter monitoring for 24 hours. No sign of arrhythmia was observed. Follow-up was performed to test the herbal medicines used; however, we did not access them.

2.1. Case 1. A 64-year-old male patient with no medical or coronary heart disease history referred to a public hospital for acute abdominal pain. A specialist in the emergency department clinically examined the patient's abdominal pain, weakness, and numbness. The patient had abdominal pain, weakness, numbness, sweating, dryness, and burning mouth for 1 hour. The abdominal pain was localized to the epigastric region spread to the back and got worse with 7/10 intensity after lying down. The patient reported no change in his bowel habits, no nausea and vomiting, and no history of trauma to his chest or abdomen. He also had no history of substance or alcohol use.

Abdominal pain and its symptoms appeared after drinking medicinal herbs. The abdomen was soft without tenderness and rebound tenderness. Gastrointestinal consultation showed no abnormality. The patient had a blood pressure of 80/50 and a heart rate of 115 beats per minute (bpm). The lung and heart sounds were normal and the pulse of the distal organs was full and symmetrical. The patient was also evaluated for myocardial infarction (MI), and the troponin test was negative. An irregular heartbeat was observed in the patient's ECG and cardiac monitoring (Figure 1). Ventricular arrhythmia (an automatic focus, monomorphic, variable cycle length, and nonsustained VT) with a stable hemodynamic state was diagnosed. Oxygen therapy and antiarrhythmic treatment were prescribed in the emergency department. 150 mg amiodarone was used to control the patient's arrhythmia. The patient was referred to the Coronary Care Unit(CCU) for further evaluation. He was hospitalized in the CCU for 48 hours, evaluated for any arrhythmia, and received cardiac medication. One mg/min amiodarone was used to control the patient's arrhythmia for 6 hours, and then, 0.5 mg/min amiodarone was used for 18 hours. The probabilities of cardiomyopathy as well as toxicity were rejected. Finally, the patient was discharged after 72 hours after taking the necessary examinations.

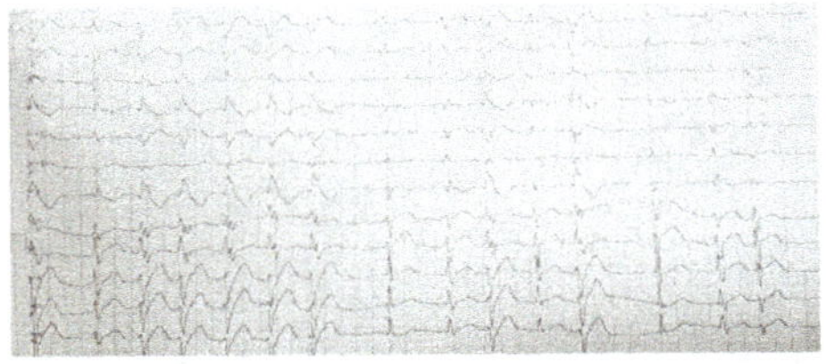

FIGURE 1: Male patient's ECG, ventricular arrhythmia (run of VT).

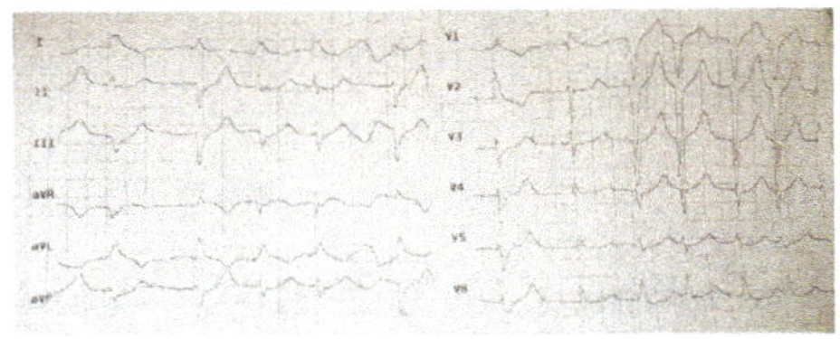

FIGURE 2: Female patient's ECG, ventricular arrhythmia (run of VT).

2.2. Case 2. A 50-year-old woman with no family history of coronary heart disease referred to a public hospital for acute abdominal pain for 1 hour. The specialist in the emergency department examined the patient. She complained of abdominal pain, fatigue, and generalized weakness without dizziness. The patient had tingling and numbness of the lower jaw and hands.

The abdominal pain was localized to the epigastric region with 6/10 intensity, which was constant in nature and did not radiate elsewhere. The patient had no recent travel and no sign of substance or alcohol use.

Abdominal pain and associated symptoms appeared after drinking medicinal herbs. The patient's abdomen was soft with no tenderness. She had a history of hypothyroidism and hysterectomy. Her blood pressure was 95/50 mmHg with a heart rate of 92 bpm. Gastrointestinal counseling showed no abnormality. The patient's ECG showed ventricular arrhythmia (monomorphic with fusion beats, an automatic focus, variable cycle length, and nonsustained VT) at a rate of 92 bpm (Figure 2). Oxygen therapy and antiarrhythmic treatment were provided in the emergency department. The patient was evaluated for MI. Troponin test results were negative for the patient. 150 mg amiodarone was used to control the patient's arrhythmia in the emergency department. She was immediately transferred to the cardiac care unit and received 1 mg/min amiodarone for 6 hours and then 0.5 mg/min for 18 hours. The probability of toxicity was rejected. Finally, the patient was discharged after 72 hours with necessary clinical examinations.

3. Discussion

Herbal medicines have been used for centuries over time. However, the side effects associated with them need to be evaluated and understood [12]. Two important herbal medicines used to treat heart disease are Echium amoenum and Citrus aurantium in the southern regions of Iran [13]. Studies have shown the positive role of Echium amoenum in cardiac remodeling in an animal model with MI and congestion [14]. The effect of Echium amoenum on the blood pressure and heart rate in an animal model was studied. This plant did not cause significant damages to the heart tissue. Significant changes in erythrocytes and related parameters were observed. High doses of Echium amoenum should be used with caution due to its blood toxicity [15]. However, Hamidi and Khaksari showed the effect of Echium amoenum and Citrus aurantiflia on animal blood pressure and heart rate. Echium amoenum has a hypertensive effect, so it is not recommended. Compound consumption of Echium amoenum and Citrus aurantiflia is effective in reducing heart rate [16]. These findings indicate different effects of these plants on the heart. Therefore, the hypothesis that "compound effects of herbal medicines may be different from those of the herbal medicines alone" is strengthened.

Citrus aurantium extract contains p-synephrine. It is generally assumed that p-synephrine will increase heart rate and blood pressure [17, 18]. However, Seifert et al. showed that Citrus aurantium extract did not lead to increased cardiovascular stress (hypertension and heart rate) [19]. Moreover, Stohs showed that the adverse effects of Citrus aurantium extract were unjustified [20]. However, a 22-year-old healthy man was reported to develop myocardial infarction after taking dietary supplements containing Phenorex, the main ingredient of Citrus aurantium. Although the use of these plants separately has been associated with adverse cardiac events, no sufficient information is available about the concomitant use of these plants [21]. Khouri et al. studied the cardiac effects of Citrus aurantium and showed that it inhibited the electrophysiological properties of the ventricular lobe in a concentration-dependent, time-dependent, and rapidly unrelated model. It also had inhibitory and antiarrhythmic effects when used for treating supraventricular tachyarrhythmia in animal models [22].

Jambi studied the cardiac effects of Matricaria chamomilla L. and showed the effectiveness of this extract in reducing doxorubicin-induced cardiac toxicity [23]. Furthermore, Chamomile tea can reduce the severity of short breath and anxiety in patients with chronic heart failure [24]. No further study on the cardiac effects of Matricaria chamomilla L. was found. While herbal products are mainly used for their therapeutic effects, the use of multiple medicines increases the risk of drug interactions and side effects [25]. The present study demonstrated the erythema caused by some herbal medicines. Medications have diverse effects, and several herbal medicines can be used simultaneously. However, these effects cannot be attributed to one or even all herbal medicines. Few studies have investigated and reported side effects of herbal medicines. This being so, further studies are required due to lack of scientific evidence about the safety and side effects of such medicines.

4. Conclusion

Since herbal medicines are widely used for treating various diseases, it is necessary to pay attention to their toxic effects on cardiac function. Health professionals should consider the use of herbal medicines and their effects on the diagnosis and treatment of patients. The evaluation of the patients showing herbal side effects can provide valuable insights to better understand clinical effects of these medicinal plants and identify adverse cardiovascular reactions.

Consent

Written informed consent was obtained from the patients for publication of this case series and accompanying images.

Acknowledgments

The authors would like to thank the Clinical Research Development Unit for its support and collaboration (IR.RUMS.REC.1399.152) in Ali-Ibn Abi-Talib Hospital, Rafsanjan University of Medical Sciences, Rafsanjan, Iran.

References

[1] B. P. Jong-Ming and M. Green, "Epidemiology of ventricular tachyarrhythmia," *Herzschrittmachertherapie & Elektrophysiologie*, vol. 28, no. 2, pp. 143–148, 2017.

[2] F. D'Ascenzi, A. Zorzi, F. Alvino, M. Bonifazi, D. Corrado, and S. Mondillo, "The prevalence and clinical significance of premature ventricular beats in the athlete," *Scandinavian journal of medicine & science in sports*, vol. 27, no. 2, pp. 140–151, 2017.

[3] J. Berdowski, R. A. Berg, J. G. Tijssen, and R. W. Koster, "Global incidences of out-of-hospital cardiac arrest and survival rates: systematic review of 67 prospective studies," *Resuscitation*, vol. 81, no. 11, pp. 1479–1487, 2010.

[4] C. Sasson, M. A. Rogers, J. Dahl, and A. L. Kellermann, "Predictors of survival from out-of-hospital cardiac arrest: a systematic review and meta-analysis," *Circulation: Cardiovascular Quality and Outcomes*, vol. 3, no. 1, pp. 63–81, 2010.

[5] A. Strzelecki, N. Pichon, J. M. Gaulier, J. B. Amiel, P. Champy, and M. Clavel, "Acute toxic herbal intake in a suicide attempt and fatal refractory ventricular arrhythmia," *Basic & clinical pharmacology & toxicology*, vol. 107, no. 2, pp. 698-699, 2010.

[6] N. H. Mashour, G. I. Lin, and W. H. Frishman, "Herbal medicine for the treatment of cardiovascular disease," *Archives of internal Medicine*, vol. 158, no. 20, pp. 2225–2234, 1998.

[7] K. L. Miller, R. S. Liebowitz, and L. K. Newby, "Complementary and alternative medicine in cardiovascular disease: a review of biologically based approaches," *American heart journal*, vol. 147, no. 3, pp. 401–411, 2004.

[8] B. Shafaghi, N. Naderi, L. Tahmasb, and M. Kamalinejad, "Anxiolytic effect of Echium amoenum L. in mice," *Iranian Journal of Pharmaceutical Research*, vol. 1, pp. 37–41, 2010.

[9] N. Narang and W. Jiraungkoorskul, "Anticancer activity of key lime, Citrus aurantifolia," *Pharmacognosy reviews*, vol. 10, no. 20, pp. 118–122, 2016.

[10] F. Azimi and M. Fatemi, "Multivariate curve resolution-assisted GC-MS analysis of the volatile chemical constituents in Iranian Citrus aurantium L. peel," *RSC advances*, vol. 6, no. 112, pp. 111197–111209, 2016.

[11] O. Singh, Z. Khanam, N. Misra, and M. K. Srivastava, "Chamomile (Matricaria chamomilla L.): an overview," *Pharmacognosy reviews*, vol. 5, no. 9, pp. 82–95, 2011.

[12] L.-F. Shyur, *Recent Trends in Medicinal Plants Research*, Academic Press, Elsevier Science, 2012.

[13] F. Behrooznia, "Herbal plant for heart disease," *Plant Biotechnology Persa*, vol. 1, no. 1, pp. 39–41, 2019.

[14] J. dos Santos Maldonado-Menetti, T. Vitor, R. C. L. Edelmuth, F. A. Ferrante, P. R. de Moraes Souza, and M. K. Koike, "Borage oil attenuates progression of cardiac remodeling in rats after myocardial infarction," *Acta cirurgica brasileira*, vol. 31, no. 3, pp. 190–197, 2016.

[15] P. Sadighara, A. Araghi, B. Tajdar-oranj, L. P. Roudsari, A. Mohajer, and R. Behzadi, "The effect of borage (Echium amoenum) on the mouse heart and hematology parameters," *Cardiovascular & Hematological Disorders-Drug Targets*, vol. 19, no. 2, pp. 154–159, 2019.

[16] E. Hamidi and M. Khaksari, *The effects of aqueous extracts of Echium amoenum and citrus aurantiflia on blood pressure and heart rate before and after phynelephrine injection in rat*, 2014.

[17] S. R. Penzak, M. W. Jann, J. A. Cold, Y. Y. Hon, H. D. Desai, and B. J. Gurley, "Seville (sour) orange juice: synephrine content and cardiovascular effects in normotensive adults," *The Journal of Clinical Pharmacology*, vol. 41, no. 10, pp. 1059–1063, 2001.

[18] A. Fugh-Berman and A. Myers, "Citrus aurantium, an ingredient of dietary supplements marketed for weight loss: current status of clinical and basic research," *Experimental biology and medicine*, vol. 229, no. 8, pp. 698–704, 2016.

[19] J. G. Seifert, A. Nelson, J. Devonish, E. R. Burke, and S. J. Stohs, "Effect of acute administration of an herbal preparation on blood pressure and heart rate in humans," *International journal of medical sciences*, vol. 8, no. 3, pp. 192–197, 2011.

[20] S. J. Stohs, "Assessment of the adverse event reports associated with Citrus aurantium (bitter orange) from April 2004 to October 2009," *Journal of Functional Foods*, vol. 2, no. 4, pp. 235–238, 2010.

[21] T. B. Smith, B. A. Staub, G. M. Natarajan, D. M. Lasorda, and I. G. Poornima, "Acute myocardial infarction associated with dietary supplements containing 1, 3-dimethylamylamine and Citrus aurantium," *Texas Heart Institute Journal*, vol. 41, no. 1, pp. 70–72, 2014.

[22] V. Khouri, M. Nayebpour, E. Rakhshan, A. Mirabbasi, and M. Zamani, *The effect of essence of Citrus aurantium on the electrophysiological properties of isolated perfused rabbit AV-node*, 2006.

[23] H. A. Jambi, "Matricaria chamomilla extract ameliorates doxorubicin-induced cardiac dysfunction in male rats," *World Applied Sciences Journal*, vol. 33, no. 8, pp. 1267–1278, 2015.

[24] M. Rahimi, A. Sanagoo, Z. A. S. Fatah, N. Bahnampour, and L. Jouybari, "Effect of Chamomile tea on the severity of dyspnea and anxiety in patients with chronic heart failure: a clinical trial study," *Journal of Gorgan University of Medical Sciences*, vol. 20, no. 1, pp. 9–15, 2018.

[25] A. Tachjian, V. Maria, and A. Jahangir, "Use of herbal products and potential interactions in patients with cardiovascular diseases," *Journal of the American College of Cardiology*, vol. 55, no. 6, pp. 515–525, 2010.

Recurrent Episodes of Fluid Retention in a Patient with Heart Failure and Chronic Kidney Disease: The Additional Value of Implantable Monitoring Systems

Marc Vanderheyden,[1] **Sofie Verstreken**,[1] **and Richard Houben**[2]

[1]*Cardiovascular Center, Onze Lieve Vrouwziekenhuis, Aalst, Belgium*
[2]*2BMedical, Maastricht, Netherlands*

Correspondence should be addressed to Marc Vanderheyden; marc.vanderheyden@olvz-aalst.be

Academic Editor: Takatoshi Kasai

The additional role of continuous monitoring of filling pressures and impedance in heart failure patients with chronic kidney disease remains undetermined. In this case report, the effects of diuretic therapy and renal replacement therapy by hemodialysis upon right ventricular filling pressures and impedance are described in a patient with end-stage heart failure and end-stage chronic kidney disease (grade 5). We demonstrated that unloading of the heart by hemodialysis partly restored the blunted Frank-Starling relationship.

1. Introduction

Chronic heart failure (CHF) has emerged as a major public health problem affecting close to 12 million Europeans and North Americans each year while the health care cost of these patients almost doubled [1, 2]. Despite new and more effective pharmacological and nonpharmacological therapeutic strategies, the prognosis of CHF patients remains poor [3, 4]. Because of its progressive and unstable nature, many patients, although often affected by significant comorbidities, require multiple hospital admissions for CHF decompensation, contributing to increasing health care costs. These episodes of decompensation result from high cardiac filling pressures and concomitant volume overload [5, 6].. Therefore, effective management of heart failure is primarily aimed at reducing the filling pressures and improving ventricular performance [7].

There is growing body of evidence that continuous monitoring of the filling pressures with implantable hemodynamic monitors (IHM) plays an important role in the management of the patient with heart failure. Observational as well as randomized studies revealed that trends in monitored pressures precede hospitalization by as much as 4 days and that strategies based on these data could optimize treatment and reduce hospitalizations [8, 9]. Retrospective analysis of the COMPASS study data revealed a 36% relative risk reduction ($p = 0.03$) in time to first HF hospitalization in the patients in whom the management was guided by pressure data obtained from the Chronicle IHM (Medtronic Inc. Minneapolis MN, USA) [10]. Recently, Adamson et al. found that assessment of daily changes in estimated pulmonary artery diastolic pressure (ePAD) allowed to predict a heart failure hospitalization a median of 21 days prior to the clinical event with a sensitivity of 86% and specificity of 90% [9, 11, 12].

2. Case Report

We report on a 75-year-old male patient who participated in a clinical investigational prospective nonrandomized study comparing OptiVol™ intrathoracic impedance measurements (InSync Sentry™, Medtronic Inc. Minneapolis, MN, USA) to right ventricular (RV) pressure hemodynamics obtained by an implantable hemodynamic monitor (Chronicle™, Medtronic Inc. Minneapolis, MN, USA). During the first 6 months of the trial, investigators were blinded to the

Table 1: Clinical characteristics, lab results, medical therapy, and echocardiographic and device parameters. NYHA: New York Heart Association class; ABPsyst: systolic arterial blood pressure; ABPdiast diastolic arterial blood pressure; Creat: creatinine; MDRD: modified diet renal disease; EF: ejection fraction; MR: mitral regurgitation; TR: tricuspid regurgitation; VCI: inferior caval vein; RV: right ventricular; BiV: biventricular; Na: not available; JVP: jugular venous pressure.

	Implant	1 month postimplant	AE1: bronchitis		AE2: AHF	AE3: dialysis	
			Onset	Resolved		Start dialysis	2-month dialysis
Clinical exam							
NYHA	3	1	4	2	3	4	1
Body weight (kg)	70	67	68	67	71	73	67
Heart rate (beats/min)	60	70	80	70	70	70	70
ABPsyst (mmHg)	110	120	100	130	120	120	110
ABPdiast (mmHg)	70	80	70	70	70	70	60
JVP	Elevated	No	No	No	Elevated	Elevated	No
Leg edema	Present	No	No	No	Present	Present	No
Lung sounds/rales	Present	No	No	No	Present	Present	No
Lab results							
Creat (mg/ml)	4.50	3.80	5.25	3.53	4.50	6.00	Na
MDRD (ml/min/ 1.73 m^2)	13	18	10	20	13	8	Na
Nt-proBNP (pg/ml)	8070	2509	32404	6732	29574	/	Na
Medical therapy							
Carvedilol	6.25 mg twice	6.25 mg twice	Stop	6.25 mg twice	6.25 mg twice	6.25 mg twice	6.25 mg twice
Bumetanide	2 mg	2 mg	2 mg	1.5 mg	2 mg	Dialysis	Dialysis
Echocardiography							
EF (%)	15	15	15	15	15	15	18
MR (grade)	3	2	2	2	3	3	2
TR (grade)	3	2	3	3	3	2	1
VCI	Dilated	Not dilated	Not dilated	Not dilated	Dilated	Dilated	Not dilated
RV systolic pressure (mmHg)	60	38	57	36	65	58	37
E/*e*	18	9	12	12	18	20	10
Device parameters							
% BiV pacing	/	99	93	94	96	97	94
ePAD (mmHg)	25	12	18	14	35	26	15
Impedance (Ohm)	/	60	56	62	53	46	63

implanted device parameters for clinical decision-making. After 6 months, information acquired by the devices was available for clinical management [13].

The patient had a history of ischemic heart disease treated by CABG with recurrent admissions for heart failure which was associated with the development of renal insufficiency grade IV. Because of recurrent episodes of heart failure, the presence of a wide QRS complex with LBBB morphology (QRS duration: 157 msec) and first-degree AV block (PR-interval: 230 msec) on the standard ECG, episodes of nonsustained ventricular tachycardia, and an ejection fraction (EF) of 15%, he fulfilled all criteria for implantation of a cardiac defibrillator with cardiac resynchronization therapy (CRT-D) (Medtronic InSync Sentry™). Along with the CRT-D, an implantable hemodynamic monitor (IHM- Medtronic Chronicle™) was implanted in the contralateral region.

At the time of implant, the patient was in NYHA class III heart failure with a weight of 70 kg, blood pressure of 110/70 mmHg, and a heart rate of 60 bpm. The central venous pressure was elevated (jugular venous height 1/2 to the jaw), and heart auscultation revealed a mitral pansystolic murmur grade 2. Blood chemistry showed an elevated NT-proBNP level of 8070 pg/ml together with a creatinine level of 4.5 mg/dl with modified diet renal disease (MDRD) of 13 ml/min/1.73 m^2. The patient was on optimal medical therapy with a potassium-sparing and a loop diuretic and a beta blocker (Table 1). No ACE inhibitors or angiotensin receptor blockers were prescribed because of the advanced renal dysfunction.

One month following implantation (Jan 3), the patient's hemodynamic situation improved as evidenced by the rise in pulse pressure, the drop in weight and jugular vein

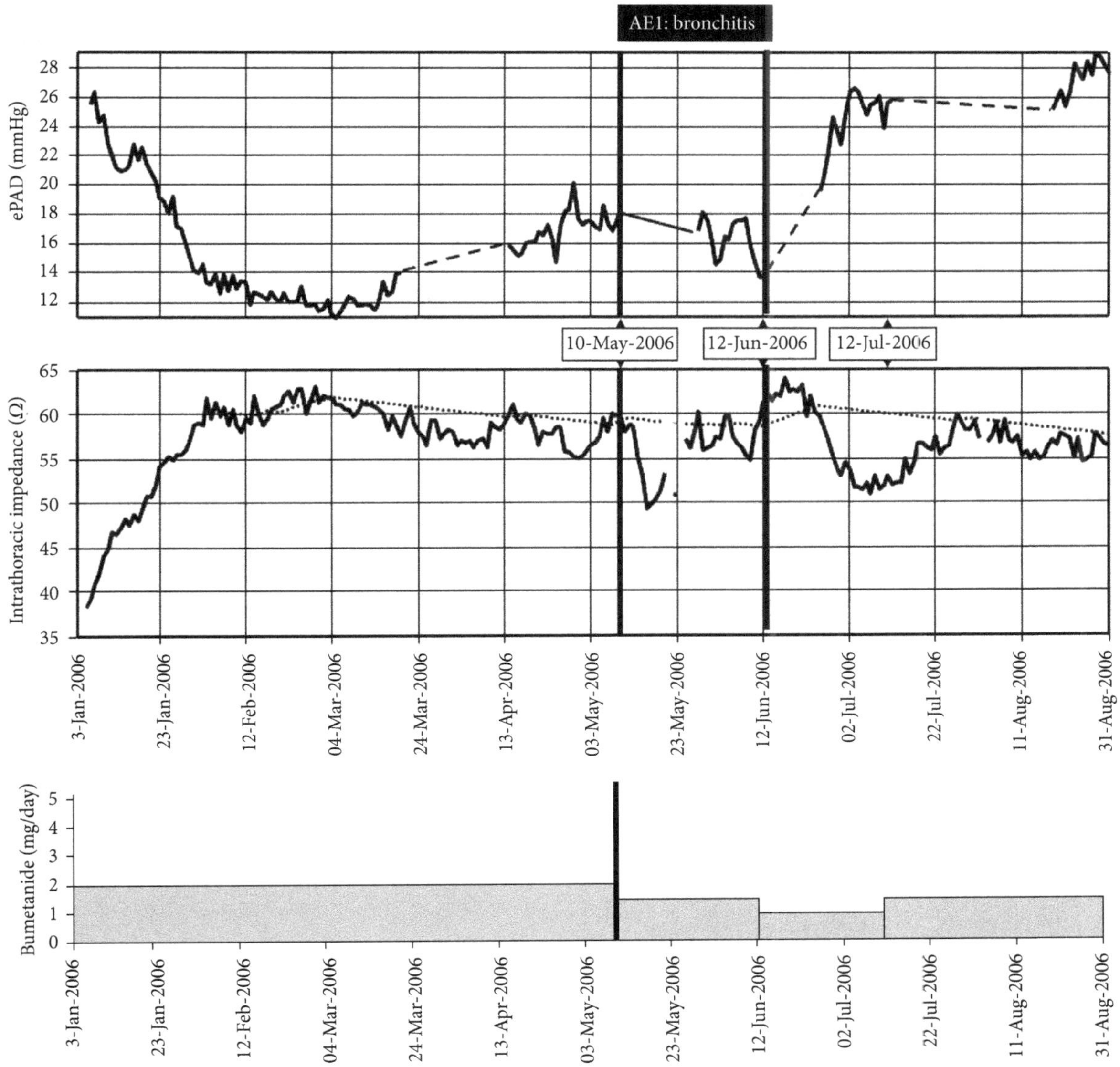

FIGURE 1: (a) Daily averaged estimated pulmonary artery diastolic pressure (ePAD). (b) Intrathoracic impedance (Ω) with reference line (dotted). (c) Diuretic dose (bumetanide, mg/day). AE: adverse event. Dashed lines indicate loss of long-term trend data because of remote patient hospitalization and noncompliance.

distention (JVD), and the disappearance of leg edema and dyspnea. This hemodynamic improvement was associated with a moderate MDRD improvement and a decrease in Nt-proBNP levels to 2509 pg/ml.

Retrospective analyses of the Chronicle and InSync Sentry™ device data confirmed this favorable response: during the first month, ePAD decreased to 12 mmHg while intrathoracic impedance increased (Figure 1, Table 1). However, five months after enrollment, the patient was hospitalized with an acute lower respiratory tract infection necessitating artificial ventilation, inotropic support, and antibiotic treatment (AE1). On admission, an increase in ePAD till 18 mmHg without major changes in impedance was noted (Table 1). Because of low blood pressures and clinical signs of dehydration, the beta blockers were temporary discontinued, and diuretics were reduced from 2 to 1.5 mg/day. As this resulted in a sudden drop of impedance from 59 Ω to 50 Ω (Figure 1, Table 1) without major change in ePAD, we speculated that the increase in lung water content secondary to the bronchitis rather than fluid overload due to heart failure accounted for this observation.

On June 12, the patient was euvolemic as evidenced by the gradual increase in impedance and decrease in ePAD. Therefore, the dose of the diuretic (bumetanide) could be further decreased to 1 mg/day and beta blockade was restarted (carvedilol; 6.25 mg/twice daily) (Figure 1). Interestingly, this resulted in a significant rise in the ePAD by 11 mmHg together with a reduction of the intrathoracic impedance, suggestive for volume overload which prompted us to adjust the diuretic regimen to 1.5 mg/day which resulted in an increase of the intrathoracic impedance to 57 Ω (+5 Ω (Table 1)).

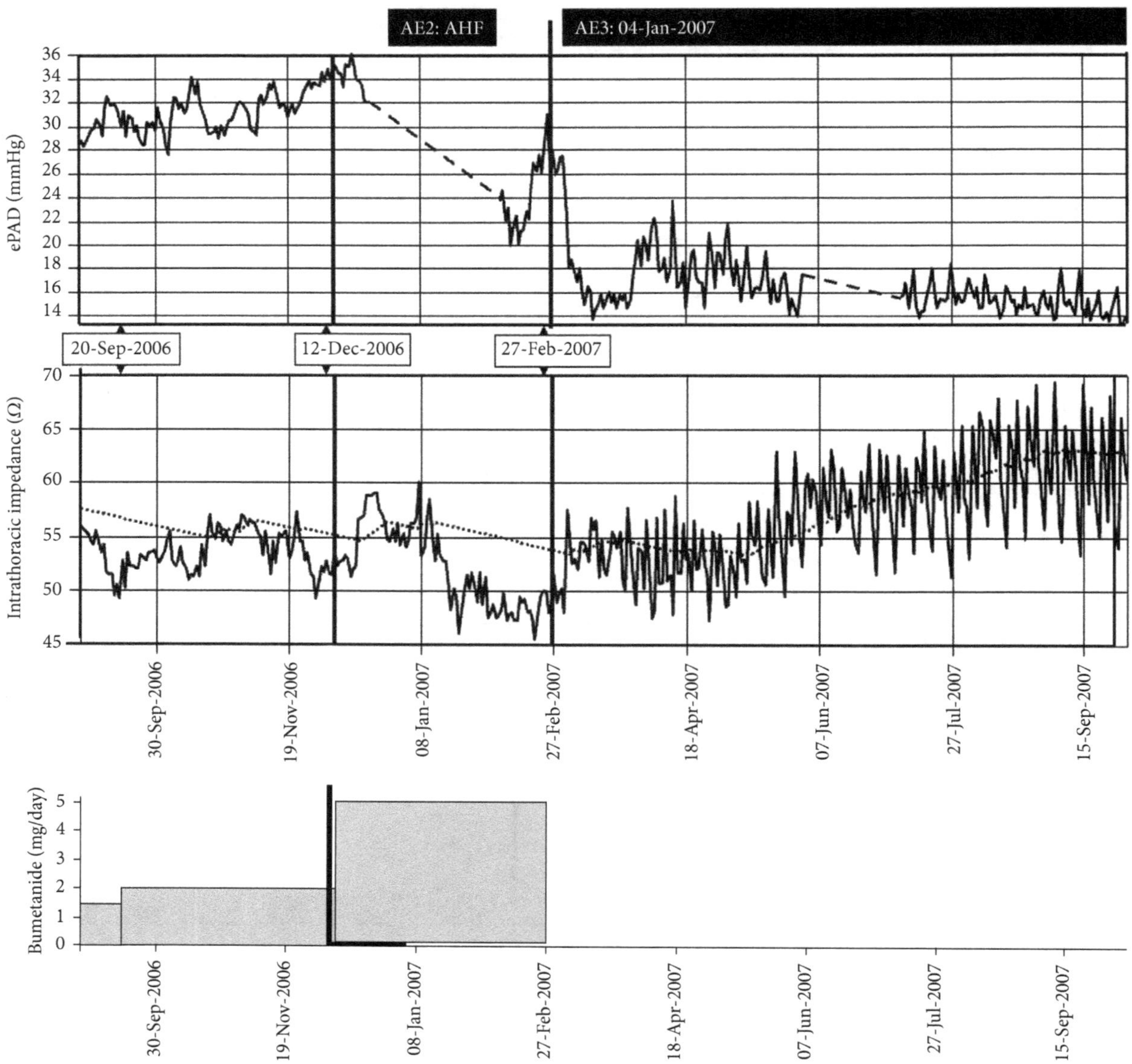

FIGURE 2: (a) ePAD (mmHg). (b) Intrathoracic impedance (Ω) with reference line (dotted). (c) Diuretic dose (bumetanide, mg/day). AE: adverse event. Dashed line indicates loss of ePAD data.

In summary, the clinically guided adjustment of the diuretics resulted in appropriate changes in impedance and pressure with sharp fall in intrathoracic impedance, together with a gradual increase in ePAD after increase of diuretics and vice versa.

However, in December 7th, uptitration of the diuretic regimen to the initial dose (2 mg/day) because of worsening heart failure did not increase impedance and even resulted in a paradoxical increase in ePAD from 28 to 35 mmHg, together with worsening renal function and the development of acute heart failure (AE2) (Figure 2). The patient was hospitalized, the bumetanide dosage was increased till 5 mg/day, and inotropic support with dobutamine was started resulting in a transient hemodynamic improvement as evidenced by the rise in intrathoracic impedance.

Because of drug-resistant heart failure and the development of grade 5 renal insufficiency (February 27, 2007; AE3) unresponsive to diuretic therapy, the decision was taken to initiate hemodialysis three times a week. Over the following months, a typical sawtooth pattern of intrathoracic impedance and ePAD (Figure 2) was noted with higher ePAD and lower impedance the days before dialysis. Over time, there were a transient decrease in ePAD towards 15 mmHg and a corresponding increase in intrathoracic impedance from 46 to 63 Ω (Table 1).

3. Discussion

The correlation between right ventricular filling pressures, measured by the IHM and the intrathoracic fluid content, assessed by the intrathoracic impedance provides interesting insights in the complex interplay between both the heart and kidney in a patient with concomitant end-stage heart failure and kidney disease.

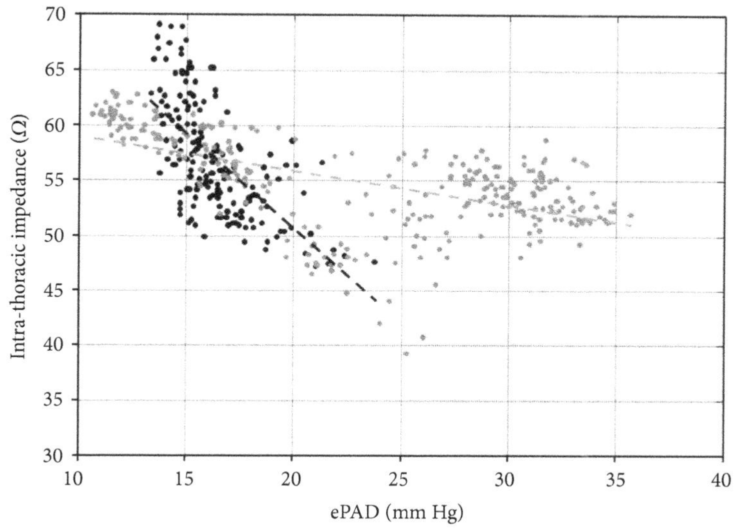

FIGURE 3: Daily averaged ePAD (mmHg) vs. intrathoracic impedance (Z; Ω). Two subpopulations of points relating ePAD to Z coupled to episodes before (grey) and during dialysis (black) can be identified. A significant relation ($r = -0.56$) but with only a moderate negative slope (-0.31) was found between ePAD and Z before dialysis ($n = 282$ days). During dialysis, a stronger negative relation was observed ($r = -0.68$; slope = −1.71, $n = 179$ days).

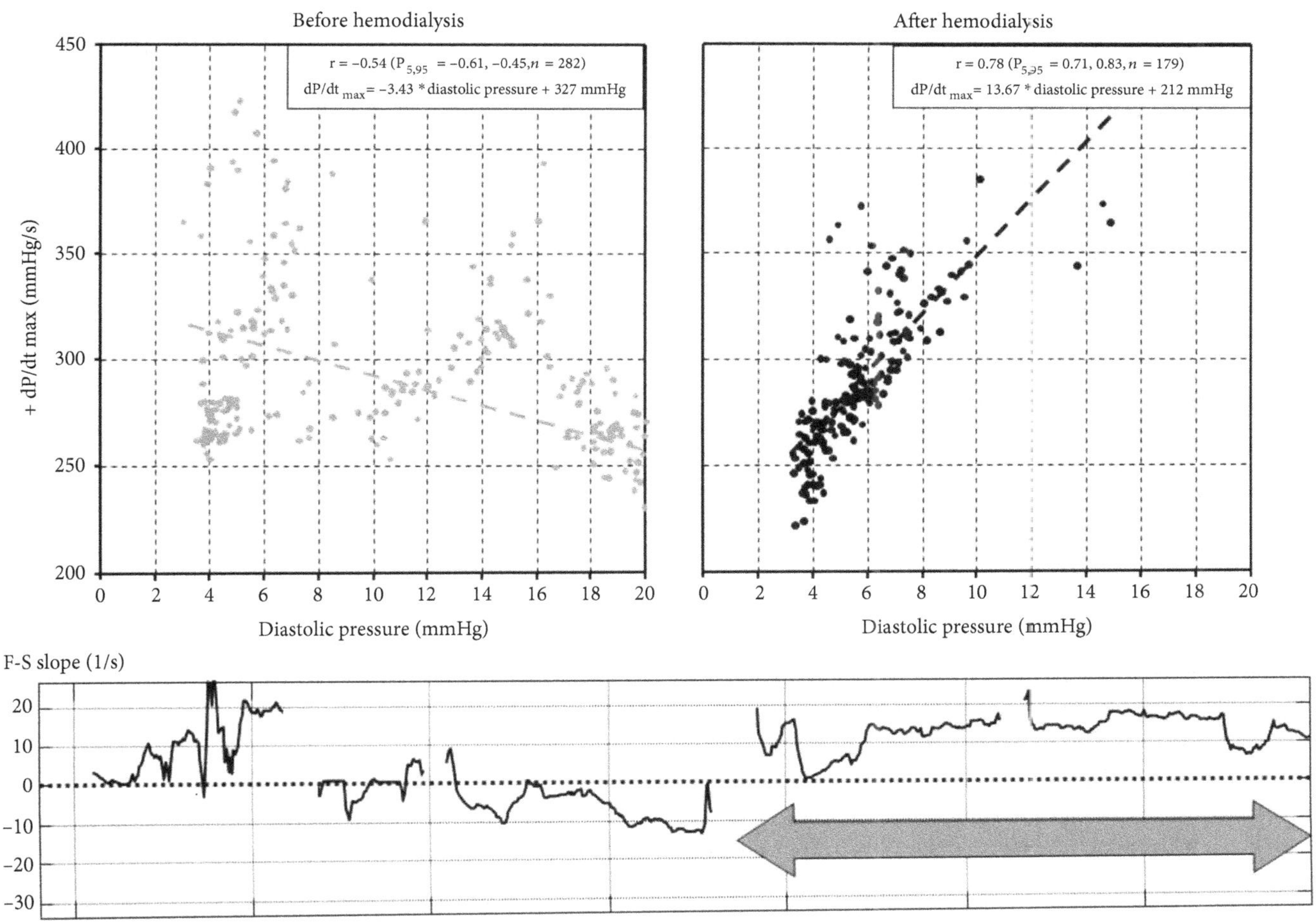

FIGURE 4: (a, b) Relation between maximum positive right ventricular dP/dt and diastolic pressure (ePAD). Two scatter diagrams show the relation between RV diastolic pressure (mmHg) and maximum dP/dt (mmHg/s) before ((a), grey) and after hemodialysis ((b), black). (c) Slope of the Frank-Starling curve obtained within a sliding window of 30 days. A positive F-S slope indicates an increase in maximum RV dP/dt (mmHg/s) at higher RV diastolic pressures (mmHg). Dashed lines indicate missing ePAD data. The arrow indicates the time frame of hemodialysis.

Of note, the much tighter coupling between ePAD and intrathoracic impedance (Figure 3) after dialysis indirectly indicates that before the initiation of the renal replacement therapy, both the failing heart and dysfunctional kidneys contributed to the rise in impedance and that dialysis prompt restored the well-known inverse interaction between ePAD and impedance.

Furthermore, following start of dialysis, the correlation between RV dP/dt max and ePAD (Figure 4) became positive.

An inverse correlation between pressure and contractility as observed before dialysis is quite unusual in humans. However, the congestion was the result not only of impaired cardiac function but also from decreased water clearance secondary to end-stage renal failure. Therefore, we speculate that a mixture of both phenomena can explain the abnormal pressure/volume relationship. Unloading of the heart by hemodialysis favorably resulted in better hemodynamics by both a right and downwards shift in the individual Frank-starling relationship as well as by a better ventricular contractile performance ensuing in a higher dP/dt max for a similar ePAD (Figure 4).

These hemodynamic observations demonstrate that in this particular patient with both end-stage renal failure and heart failure, hemodialysis not only unloads the heart but also restores the blunted Frank-Starling response at least partially by bringing the heart back on the ascending limb of the curve and by improving its contractile performance.

4. Conclusion

In patients with moderate to severe HF, routine physical examination is often unable to detect early volume overload leading to overt acute heart failure episodes and costly HF hospitalizations. The continuous measurement of RV pressure and intrathoracic impedance by implantable sensors is able to prevent acute heart failure episodes, provides interesting insights in the pathophysiology, and offers a promising tool to optimize the management of these patients [9].

In this particular case, an inverse correlation between hemodynamic pressure data and intrathoracic impedance during episodes of decompensation was noted. Secondly, simultaneous monitoring of the pressure and intrathoracic impedance facilitated the correct adjustment of the HF medication and was not only able to predict but also to prevent acute HF episodes. Finally, information derived from the impedance and RV pressure measurements allowed us to unravel the close interaction between the kidney and heart in this particular patient and demonstrated how hemodialysis unloaded the heart and improved its frank-starling relationship. Long-term prospective randomized trials that establish the role of hemodynamic monitoring-guided care in patients with advanced HF and chronic kidney disease are warranted.

References

[1] S. Stewart, "Recognising the "other half" of the heart failure equation: are we doing enough for family caregivers?," *European Journal of Heart Failure*, vol. 7, no. 4, pp. 590-591, 2005.

[2] S. Stewart, A. Jenkins, S. Buchan, A. McGuire, S. Capewell, and J. J. McMurray, "The current cost of heart failure to the National Health Service in the UK," *European Journal of Heart Failure*, vol. 4, no. 3, pp. 361–371, 2002.

[3] J. G. Cleland, J. C. Daubert, E. Erdmann et al., "The effect of cardiac resynchronization on morbidity and mortality in heart failure," *The New England Journal of Medicine*, vol. 352, no. 15, pp. 1539–1549, 2005.

[4] M. A. Pfeffer, K. Swedberg, C. B. Granger et al., "Effects of candesartan on mortality and morbidity in patients with chronic heart failure: the CHARM-Overall programme," *Lancet*, vol. 362, no. 9386, pp. 759–766, 2003.

[5] M. Kobayashi, N. Machida, M. Mitsuishi, and Y. Yamane, "?-Blocker improves survival, left ventricular function, and myocardial remodeling in hypertensive rats with diastolic heart failure," *American Journal of Hypertension*, vol. 17, no. 12, pp. 1112–1119, 2004.

[6] S. J. Bennett, G. A. Huster, S. L. Baker et al., "Characterization of the precipitants of hospitalization for heart failure decompensation," *American Journal of Critical Care*, vol. 7, no. 3, pp. 168–174, 1998.

[7] L. W. Stevenson, "Tailored therapy to hemodynamic goals for advanced heart failure," *European Journal of Heart Failure*, vol. 1, no. 3, pp. 251–257, 1999.

[8] P. B. Adamson, A. Magalski, F. Braunschweig et al., "Ongoing right ventricular hemodynamics in heart failure: clinical value of measurements derived from an implantable monitoring system," *Journal of the American College of Cardiology*, vol. 41, no. 4, pp. 565–571, 2003.

[9] M. M. Givertz, L. W. Stevenson, M. R. Costanzo et al., "Pulmonary artery pressure-guided management of patients with heart failure and reduced ejection fraction," *Journal of the American College of Cardiology*, vol. 70, no. 15, pp. 1875–1886, 2017.

[10] R. C. Bourge, W. T. Abraham, P. B. Adamson et al., "Randomized controlled trial of an implantable continuous hemodynamic monitor in patients with advanced heart failure: the COMPASS-HF study," *Journal of the American College of Cardiology*, vol. 51, no. 11, pp. 1073–1079, 2008.

[11] P. B. Adamson, R. C. Bourge, W. T. Abraham, R. Taepke, Y. K. Cho, and T. Bennett, "Automated detection of hemodynamic changes to predict heart failure hospitalization," *Heart Rhythm*, vol. 2, no. 5, 5, Supplement 1, pp. S128–S129, 2005.

[12] J. A. Brinker, "Implantable hemodynamic monitors: success in the pursuit of failure?," *Pacing and Clinical Electrophysiology*, vol. 28, no. 8, pp. 743–746, 2005.

[13] M. Vanderheyden, R. Houben, S. Verstreken et al., "Continuous monitoring of intrathoracic impedance and right ventricular pressures in patients with heart failure," *Circulation. Heart Failure*, vol. 3, no. 3, pp. 370–377, 2010.

41

Acute Limb Ischemia in the Young: A Rare Case of Essential Thrombocytosis

Johanes Nugroho[1,2] **and Ruth Gunadi**[2]

[1]*Department of Cardiology and Vascular Medicine, Faculty of Medicine, Universitas Airlangga, Surabaya, Indonesia*
[2]*Dr. Soetomo General Hospital, Surabaya, Indonesia*

Correspondence should be addressed to Johanes Nugroho; j.nugroho.eko@fk.unair.ac.id

Academic Editor: Yigit Canga

Acute limb ischemia (ALI) is rarely observed in young populations. The hypercoagulable state is a notable cause of ALI other than artery disease progression and cardiac embolization. A hypercoagulable state occurs in essential thrombocytosis because of the overproduction of hematopoietic cells secondary to the mutation of the JAK2, CALR, or MPL genes. We report a rare case of a 37-year-old woman presenting with Rutherford IIA ALI in the left lower extremity. Laboratory data revealed she had a platelet count reaching up to 1.38 mil/μL, with other blood profiles being normal. A JAK2 mutation examination was later performed and proved positive. After careful management with catheter-directed thrombolysis, surgical thrombectomy, and cytoreductive therapy using hydroxyurea, the symptoms subsided and eventually restored the patient to physical activity in less than one month.

1. Introduction

Patients with peripheral arterial disease (PAD) are at risk for ischemic events, which can cause significant morbidity and reduce functional status and the quality of life. Acute limb ischemia (ALI), which results from a sudden decrease in limb perfusion, can cause tissue death and threaten limb viability [1]. Sudden decreased perfusion can be caused either by progressive arterial disease, cardiac embolization, hypercoagulable disease, or complications related to vascular procedures [2]. A part of the hypercoagulation spectrum is essential thrombocytosis (ET). The incidence of ET increases with age, with most patients presenting between the ages of 50 and 60 years [3]. There have been previous case reports of cardiovascular involvement with ET in the fourth decade but not ALI with ET [4]. Hence, a young woman presenting with a complication of ET is considered rare.

2. Case Presentation

A 37-year-old female patient presented with a chief complaint of pain in the toes of her left foot since approximately 1-week prior to hospitalization. She complained of persistent pain which was aggravated with mobilization. In addition, her left toes often felt numb accompanied by a tingling sensation, with a bluish and pale colorization. She denied any current use of medication or prior hospitalizations, and her past medical history was otherwise unremarkable. She had two biological children, both born per vaginam. On physical examination, she had tachycardia with an initial heart rate of 102 beats per minute. Left inferior extremity assessment revealed a weakened pulsation in her left femoral artery, an absence of distal pulsations, and dry, cold, and pale digits (first to fifth) (Figure 1). Motoric abilities were unimpaired, but sensory impairment (numbness) was observed in her left foot.

Electrocardiogram, chest radiograph, and transthoracic echocardiography revealed no abnormality or intracardiac thrombus. Doppler ultrasound of the lower extremity arteries revealed triphasic waves in the right superficial femoral artery. For the left inferior extremity, a thrombus was documented in the common femoral artery (CFA); hence, arterial flow from the CFA towards the distal end was difficult to evaluate.

The patient's initial platelet count was $812 \times 103/\mu$L, while other routine blood profiles were within normal limits. A blood smear test showed thrombocytosis with giant platelets, leukocytosis, and immature granulocytes. Subsequently,

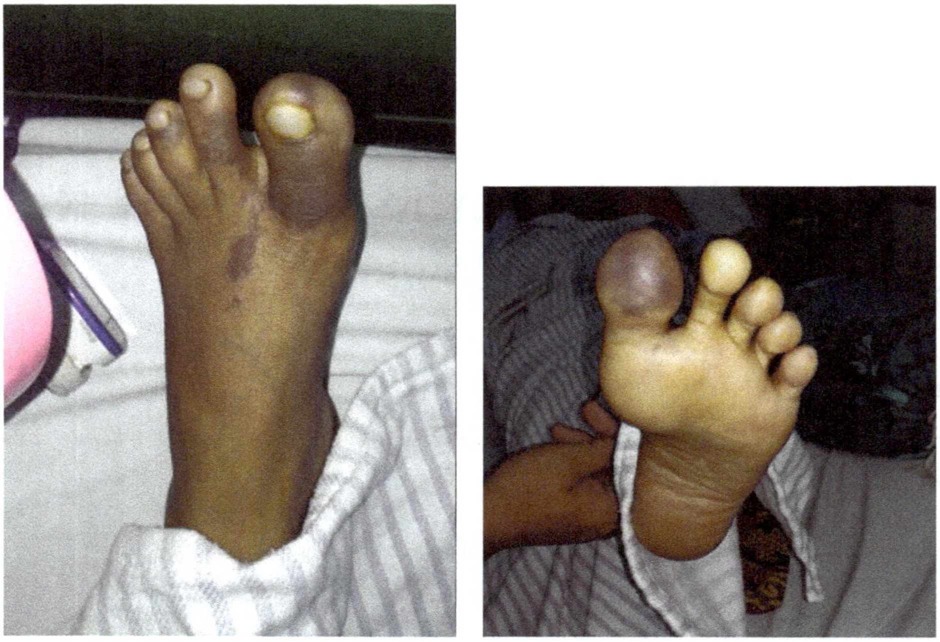

(a) (b)

Figure 1: Image of dorsal (a) and ventral (b) views of the left foot in the initial settings with bluish pale area mostly distributed in digits I and II.

a JAK-2 mutase examination was performed based on the suspicion of ET.

She then underwent an arteriography (Figure 2) with catheter-directed thrombolysis (CDT). A 6-French pigtail catheter was inserted through the right femoral artery and directed towards the left femoral artery. Digital subtraction cineangiography was performed using an injection of 10 mL of contrast with an anteroposterior projection. Arteriography revealed a thrombus that was as high as the left distal CFA. A total of 100,000 units of Fibrion (Streptokinase) was injected into the left femoral artery. No complications occurred during or after the procedure.

After the procedure, the patient was admitted to the intensive cardiac care unit and administered 100,000 units/hour of streptokinase via CDT, with hourly clinical evaluation and monitoring. At clinical evaluation 2 hours postarteriography, she complained of severe pain in her left lower leg. Accordingly, the patient was scheduled for emergency surgical thrombectomy. Antegrade and retrograde surgical thrombectomy of the posterior tibial artery was performed, with results of restored flow of the left popliteal artery and posterior tibial artery. During inpatient treatment, the platelet count increased drastically (from $812 \times 103/\mu L$ to $1.380 \times 103/\mu L$).

Once the diagnosis of ET was established, medical therapy was started immediately with hydroxyurea and clopidogrel once daily at doses of 1,000 mg and 75 mg, respectively. At the one-month follow-up, her platelet count had decreased by half to $434 \times 103/\mu L$ with improved clinical results. At the six-month follow-up, a marked reduction in cyanotic areas was observed throughout the first and second digits, with improved mobility and daily performance (Figure 3).

3. Discussion

Along with revascularization, etiological evaluation of ALI has become a priority, especially if the patient belongs to a young demographic, considering that the incidence of ALI occurs mostly in the elderly with various comorbidities. In the present case, the patient was a young woman who had no prior history of comorbidities; thus, an event such as ALI warrants considerations of etiologies beyond the more common ones.

Progressive arterial disease deemed unlikely due to her young age and no intracardiac thrombus on echocardiography. Hence, differential diagnoses include hypercoagulable states and myeloproliferative (MPN) disorders, which can manifest in thrombosis and symptoms of ALI in the young population. Since our patient's hematology data suggested high platelet levels in three separate occasions, with other hematology profile to be normal, our suspicion was focused on MPN disorders. According to recent observational studies, there were three common MPN disorders in the young: polycythemia vera (PV), essential thrombocytosis (ET), and primary myelofibrosis (PMF) [5, 6]. Since our patient's Hb and Hct levels were normal, PV became less suspicious. In PMF, although sharing a common JAK2, CALR, or MPL mutation, anemia is typically present and increases over time accompanied by mild to moderate leukocytosis, mild to marked thrombocytosis, abnormal cytokine expression, cachexia, and hepatosplenomegaly [7, 8]. With clinical signs and symptoms suggestive of ET, supported by positive JAK2 V617F mutation, the diagnosis of ET was established.

The incidence of ET varies from 1.0 to 2.5 per 100.000 individuals/year, with a prevalence of 38–57 per 100,000 individuals reported between 2008 and 2010, mostly among

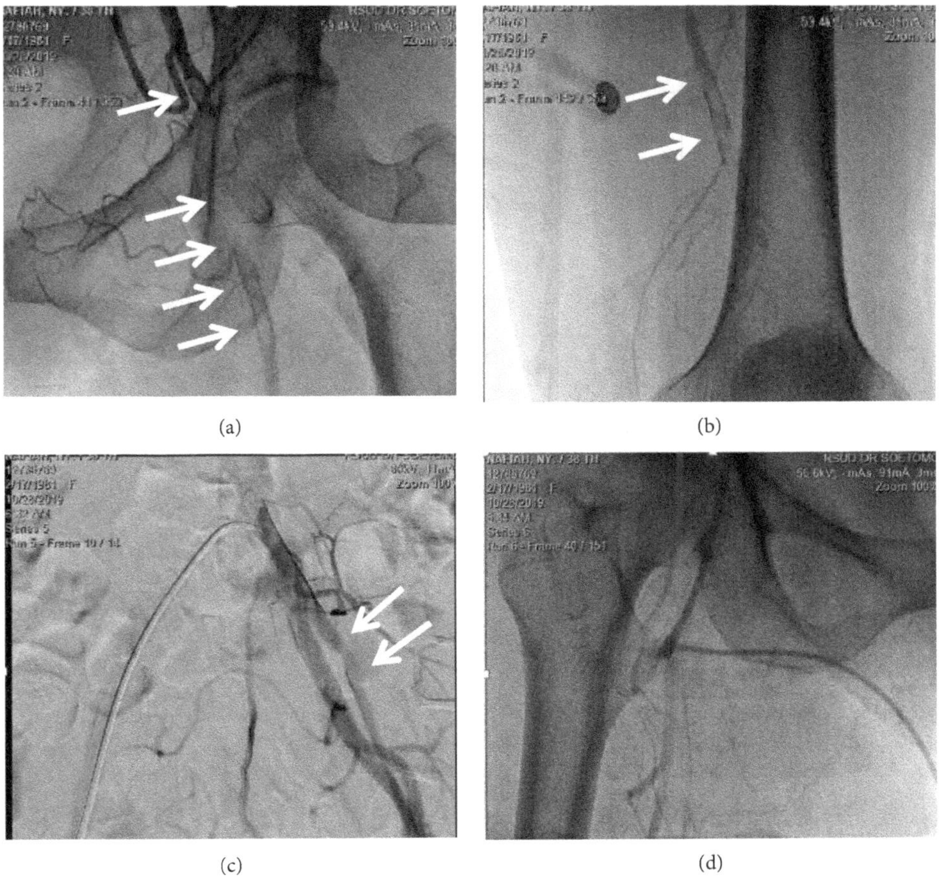

Figure 2: Arteriographic findings of the inferior extremities show that diffuse thrombus was visualized in the left common femoral artery (a) continuing until the superficial femoral artery and distal femoral artery (b). A thrombus appears on left external iliac artery (c). Contrast flow is normal in the right inferior limb (d).

women [3, 9]. According to the World Health Organization, ET is a disease that occurs when the platelet count is more than $450 \times 103/\mu L$ with proven mutations in Janus kinase 2 (JAK2) and calreticulin (CALR), or mutations in the oncogene leukemia myeloproliferative oncogene (MPL) virus, with exclusion of clonal disease or reactive causes [10]. Approximately 50% of patients with ET have JAK2 mutations [3].

Thrombosis is the most common cause of mortality and morbidity in patients with ET. The incidence of thrombosis is approximately 20%, followed by the incidence of bleeding (10%), and the estimated incidence of conversion (from thrombosis to hemorrhage) is less than 1% [9, 11]. In general, the management of ET includes control of cardiovascular risk factors and cytoreductive therapy, for example, hydroxyurea, in patients who are at high risk of thrombotic events [12]. Treatment with low-dose acetylsalicylic acid (aspirin) is crucial for the prevention of primary and secondary thrombosis in this patient group [13]. However, in patients with ALI, single antiplatelet therapy (SAPT) with clopidogrel is the preferred choice [2]. Hydroxyurea 500–1000 mg once daily is the first line of choice in most patients because of its effective thrombotic reduction profile with minimal side effects [14]. The aim of the treatment is to maintain a platelet count of $<400 \times 103/\mu L$ [13, 14]. Although the patient in the present case achieved a platelet count as low as $434 \times 103/\mu L$, the therapy target was not achieved due to poor regular intake of hydroxyurea, as the patient lived in a rural area and had limited access to cytoreductive drugs.

Long-term anticoagulant therapy may be combined with SAPT when a revascularization procedure is performed. Treatment using anticoagulants and SAPT can be considered for more than 1 month in patients with high ischemic risk or when there are other strong indications for long-term SAPT [2]. ET combined with ALI is classified in the high ischemic risk group; thus, it is advisable to administer SAPT and oral anticoagulants for >1 month, and doses should be monitored with a target International Normalized Ratio of 2.0–2.5 [2, 15]. Thus, our patient had increased mobile activity in less than two months after receiving proper revascularization and medication. ET is an indolent disease with a good prognosis. The reported life expectancy is 33 years, and in younger patients, it is 60 years [16]. Although indolent, ET patients have poorer life expectancy than the general population due to thrombotic events that may complicate the disease [17].

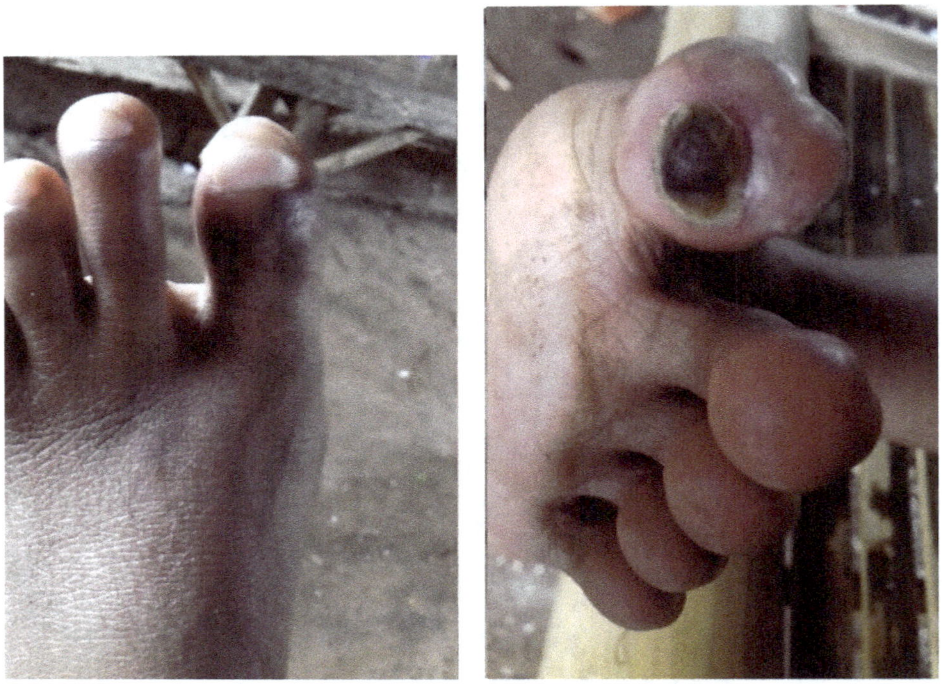

(a) (b)

Figure 3: Image of dorsal (a) and ventral (b) views of the left foot in the six-month follow-up, with significant clearing of cyanotic area.

In cases of ALI associated with neurological deficits, immediate revascularization is mandatory; investigations and imaging should not delay patient revascularization interventions [13]. Various revascularization modalities can be applied, including percutaneous CDT, percutaneous mechanical thrombus extraction or thrombus aspiration (with or without thrombolytic therapy), and surgical thrombectomy, bypass, and/or arterial repair. The choice of a revascularization strategy will depend on the presence of a neurologic deficit, duration of ischemia, localization, comorbidity, type of blood vessel (artery or graft), and therapy-related risk and outcome. Because of favorable morbidity and mortality rates, endovascular therapy is often preferred by clinicians, especially in patients with severe comorbidities [1, 18].

The modern concept of combined intraarterial thrombolysis and catheter-based clot removal can achieve an amputation rate of <10% within 6 months [1]. In the present case, due to a moderate neurological deficit, percutaneous CDT was performed immediately as soon as the ALI diagnosis was established. However, during follow-up, the patient's condition did not improve and prompted surgical thrombectomy. Subsequently, combined with adequate antithrombotic and hydroxyurea, her clinical condition and performance allowed her to be discharged after 10 days of hospitalization.

4. Conclusion

Cases of acute limb ischemia (ALI) in the young population are rare and should trigger investigations to determine the underlying cause. A frequently overlooked etiology of ALI is hypercoagulability, including essential thrombocytosis, which may cause extreme thrombocytosis, bleeding, or progressive arterial damage due to erythromelalgia. Revascularization interventions and medical therapy must be performed according to clinical protocols and indications. Long-term cytoreductive therapy with hydroxyurea is usually sufficient to control platelet count and prevent complications of thrombocytosis in patients with essential thrombocytosis.

Disclosure

This work did not receive specific funding but was performed as part of Johanes Nugroho's employment at the Department of Cardiology and Vascular Medicine, Universitas Airlangga/ Dr. Soetomo General Hospital, East Java, Indonesia.

References

[1] C. N. Hess, Z. Huang, M. R. Patel et al., "Acute limb ischemia in peripheral artery disease," *Circulation*, vol. 140, no. 7, pp. 556–565, 2019.

[2] V. Aboyans, J. B. Ricco, M. E. L. Bartelink et al., "2017 ESC guidelines on the diagnosis and treatment of peripheral arterial diseases, in collaboration with the European Society for Vascular Surgery (ESVS): document covering atherosclerotic disease of extracranial carotid and vertebral, mesenteric, renal, upper and lower extremity arteries endorsed by: the European Stroke Organization (ESO). The task force for the diagnosis and treatment of peripheral arterial diseases of the European Society of Cardiology (ESC) and of the European Society for Vascular Surgery (ESVS)," *European Heart Journal*, vol. 39, no. 9, pp. 763–816, 2018.

[3] J. Nangalia and A. R. Green, "Myeloproliferative neoplasms: from origins to outcomes," *Hematology 2014, the American Society of Hematology Education Program Book*, vol. 2017, no. 1, pp. 470–479, 2017.

[4] P. Sharma, S. Gupta, P. Patel, Y. Zhang, and S. Peles, "Acute ST-segment elevation myocardial infarction as the first manifestation of essential thrombocytosis," *Cureus*, vol. 11, no. 2, article e4032, 2019.

[5] Gruppo Italiano Studio Policitemia, "Polycythemia vera: the natural history of 1213 patients followed for 20 years," *Annals of Internal Medicine*, vol. 123, no. 9, pp. 656–664, 1995.

[6] A. Alvarez-Larrán, F. Cervantes, B. Bellosillo et al., "Essential thrombocythemia in young individuals: frequency and risk factors for vascular events and evolution to myelofibrosis in 126 patients," *Leukemia*, vol. 21, no. 6, pp. 1218–1223, 2007.

[7] L. A. Raedler, "Diagnosis and management of polycythemia vera," *American health & drug benefits*, vol. 7, 7 supplement 3, pp. S36–S47, 2014.

[8] A. Tefferi, "Primary myelofibrosis: 2019 update on diagnosis, risk-stratification and management," *American Journal of Hematology*, vol. 93, no. 12, pp. 1551–1560, 2018.

[9] B. Meier and J. H. Burton, "Myeloproliferative disorders," *Hematology/Oncology Clinics of North America*, vol. 31, no. 6, pp. 1029–1044, 2017.

[10] A. Tefferi, J. Thiele, A. Orazi et al., "Proposals and rationale for revision of the World Health Organization diagnostic criteria for polycythemia vera, essential thrombocythemia, and primary myelofibrosis: recommendations from an ad hoc international expert panel," *Blood*, vol. 110, no. 4, pp. 1092–1097, 2007.

[11] M. C. Soucy-Giguère, P. Y. Turgeon, and M. Sénéchal, "What cardiologists should know about essential thrombocythemia and acute myocardial infarction: report of two cases and advanced heart failure therapies considerations," *International medical case reports journal*, vol. 12, pp. 253–259, 2019.

[12] F. Cervantes, "Management of essential thrombocythemia," *Hematology. American Society of Hematology. Education Program*, vol. 2011, no. 1, pp. 215–221, 2011.

[13] N. Hiranuma, "TCTAP C-193 Critical Lower Limb Ischemia Due to Essential Thrombocytosis," *Journal of the American College of Cardiology*, vol. 71, no. 16, pp. S265–S266, 2018.

[14] C. N. Harrison, P. J. Campbell, G. Buck et al., "Hydroxyurea compared with anagrelide in high-risk essential thrombocythemia," *The New England Journal of Medicine*, vol. 353, no. 1, pp. 33–45, 2005.

[15] J. S. Bleeker and W. J. Hogan, "Thrombocytosis: diagnostic evaluation, thrombotic risk stratification, and risk-based management strategies," *Thrombosis*, vol. 2011, Article ID 536062, 16 pages, 2011.

[16] A. Tefferi, P. Guglielmelli, D. R. Larson et al., "Long-term survival and blast transformation in molecularly annotated essential thrombocythemia, polycythemia vera, and myelofibrosis," *Blood*, vol. 124, no. 16, pp. 2507–2513, 2014.

[17] L. Falchi, H. M. Kantarjian, and S. Verstovsek, "Assessing the thrombotic risk of patients with essential thrombocythemia in the genomic era," *Leukemia*, vol. 31, no. 9, pp. 1845–1854, 2017.

[18] E. A. Natelson, "Extreme thrombocytosis and cardiovascular surgery: risks and management," *Texas Heart Institute Journal*, vol. 39, no. 6, pp. 792–798, 2012.

42

A Rare Case of an Ectopic Liver Presenting as Right Atrial Mass

Adhirath Doshi,[1] Dhaval Shah,[1] Shradha Gupta,[2] Deepika Panday,[2] Arie Farji-Cisneros,[3] Eddison Ramsaran,[4] and Robert Bojar[5]

[1]*Division of Cardiology, St. Vincent Hospital, Worcester, MA, USA*
[2]*Department of Internal Medicine, St. Vincent Hospital, Worcester, MA, USA*
[3]*Department of Anesthesia, St. Vincent Hospital, Worcester, MA, USA*
[4]*Department of Cardiology, Reliant Medical Group, Worcester, MA, USA*
[5]*Division of Cardiothoracic Surgery, St. Vincent Hospital, Worcester, MA, USA*

Correspondence should be addressed to Robert Bojar; robert.bojar@stvincenthospital.com

Academic Editor: Takatoshi Kasai

Ectopic liver tissue is commonly observed in the abdominal cavity in adjacent organs. Extension of hepatic tissue into the intrathoracic cavity is rarely reported. We present the case of a 46-year-old woman with a 2.1 × 1.8 cm mass confirmed by transesophageal echocardiogram to be at the right atrial and inferior vena cava junction that was initially thought to be a myxoma which prompted surgical excision but subsequently identified as ectopic liver by histology.

1. Introduction

Primary cardiac tumors are rare with an autopsy frequency of 0.001-0.03% [1], whereas the incidence of secondary cardiac tumors is nearly 20 times higher [1–4]. The pathology of an intracardiac mass cannot always be determined by echocardiography, nearly always mandating surgical removal to prevent embolization and confirm the diagnosis. We herein report a rare case in literature of ectopic liver tissue presenting as two separate masses in the right atrium (RA) and inferior cava (IVC) [5–7].

2. Case

A 46-year-old woman with morbid obesity, hypertension, hyperlipidemia, active smoking, and bipolar disorder was evaluated for paroxysmal atrial fibrillation as an outpatient. A transthoracic echocardiogram showed a right atrial mass close to the RA-IVC junction. A transesophageal echocardiogram confirmed the presence of a pedunculated right atrial mobile bilobular mass measuring 2.1 × 1.8 cm, not arising from the interatrial septum with extension into the inferior vena cava (Figures 1–3). A secundum atrial septal defect was also identified. The patient was referred to cardiac surgery for resection of a presumed right atrial myxoma given the possibility of embolization. The intraoperative TEE suggested the presence of one bilobulated mass arising low in the right atrium.

Using aortic and bicaval cannulation, a right atriotomy was performed and a discrete 2 × 3 cm mass was removed from the IVC-RA junction near the Eustachian valve. The right atrium was closed and the patient weaned from bypass. The specimen did not appear to be a myxoma, so it was sent for frozen section and interpreted as being ectopic liver tissue. In the interim, a repeat TEE showed an additional discrete 2 × 2 cm mass in the IVC near the hepatic veins. Femoral venous cannulation was then performed to allow for visualization of the IVC below the pericardial reflection. Through the same right atriotomy and using additional suction directly in the IVC, the IVC mass

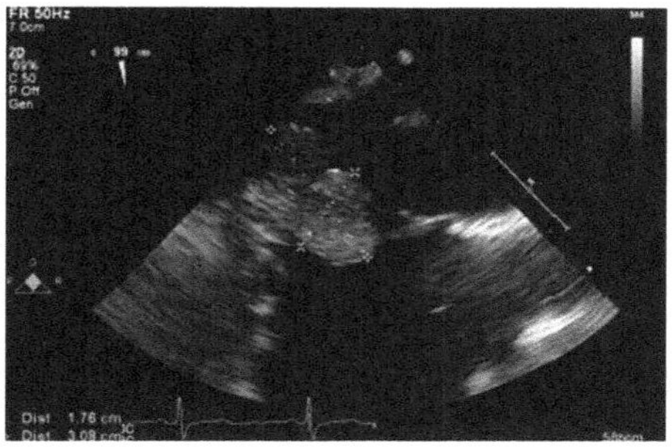

FIGURE 1: TEE showing the bilobed mass measuring 2.1×1.8 cm in the right atrium.

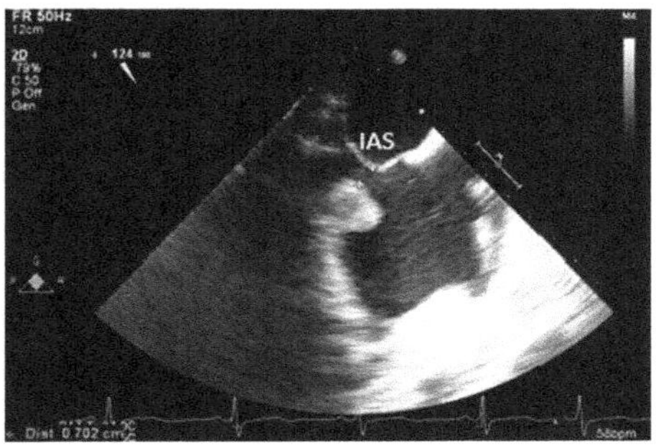

FIGURE 2: TEE showing the mass is not attached to the interatrial septum (IAS).

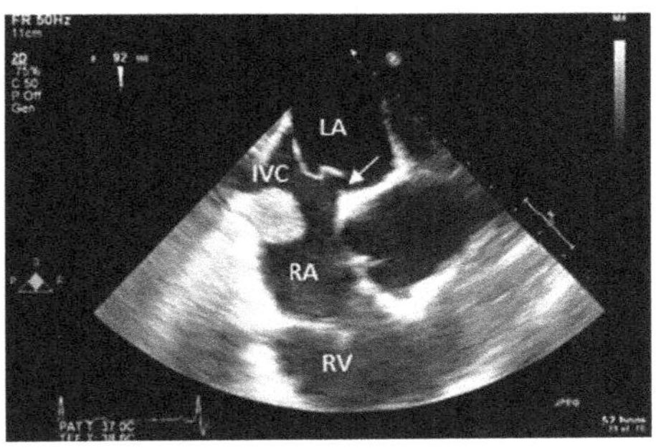

FIGURE 3: TEE showing extension of the mass into the IVC and a secundum ASD (white arrow). Left atrium: LA; right atrium: RA; right ventricle: RV.

was visualized and resected. Both specimens were interpreted as showing partially encapsulated liver parenchyma with mild steatosis, fibrosis, ductal proliferation, and periductal chronic inflammation, consistent with ectopic hepatic tissue (Figure 4).

Despite a brief period of cardiopulmonary bypass, the patient had persistent hypoxemic respiratory failure ascribed to her morbid obesity and underlying lung disease. She also developed extensive left lower extremity deep venous thrombosis from a presumed heparin-induced thrombocytopenia for which she was treated with argatroban and placement of an IVC filter. Because of chronic respiratory failure, she underwent tracheostomy and feeding tube placement, and she was placed on warfarin for intermittent atrial fibrillation due to her CHA_2DS_2-VASc score of 4. She gradually improved and was transferred to rehab where her tracheostomy tube and PEG tube were removed. A few months later, she looked quite well during an office visit.

3. Discussion

The differential diagnosis of intracardiac masses include benign tumors, primary or metastatic malignant tumors, and thrombus (Figure 5) [8]. The location, attachment site, size, shape, and underlying patient characteristics are helpful in prioritizing the diagnosis. Myxomas are the most common benign tumor located in the right atrium, and renal cell carcinoma is the most common tumor located at the RA-IVC junction [9]. Symptoms from the right atrial masses may result from obstruction of blood flow through the tricuspid valve mimicking tricuspid stenosis, distal embolization to the lungs, or in the case of an atrial septal defect, embolization to the systemic circulation.

The incidence of ectopic liver described by laparoscopic and autopsy studies is less than 0.5% [10–12]. In the absence of trauma, most cases of ectopic liver are believed to be congenital in origin. The liver develops from the ventral outgrowth of the foregut during the 4th week of gestation. The exact pathogenesis of ectopic liver is unclear and Trocciola et al. [5] offer the following hypotheses: (1) development from the second liver bud, (2) development from the original liver bud with migration of cells to form an accessory liver that is connected to the original liver by a stalk, (3) incomplete atrophy or regression of the developing liver lobes, and (4) migration of nests of hepatic cells outside the developing liver. Ectopic liver is usually found in an intraabdominal location but rarely in the intrathoracic cavity or heart. Ectopic liver is found to have increased neoplastic potential [13] and should be resected when identified, although rarely is the diagnosis suspected beforehand.

4. Conclusion

Isolated right atrial masses are rare and most are discovered incidentally on echocardiography or CT scanning. Imaging studies are useful to identify their size, mobility, and sites of attachment. Resection should be guided by symptoms and/or embolic potential of these masses. The location, attachment, texture, and consistency can provide a clue to the origin of these masses. Intracardiac ectopic liver is an extremely rare diagnosis, but an important one to make primarily due to an increased incidence of carcinogenesis in the ectopic tissue. In our patient, the presence of a separate tumor mass in the high inferior vena may have been a clue that this mass was not a myxoma or a renal cell carcinoma. Resection of caval tumors can be a technical challenge [14], depending on the extent of the tumor. In our patient, it was not immediately recognized that there were two masses, so the initial cannulation technique was inadequate to resect the IVC mass. Use of femoral venous cannulation was therefore required for better visualization.

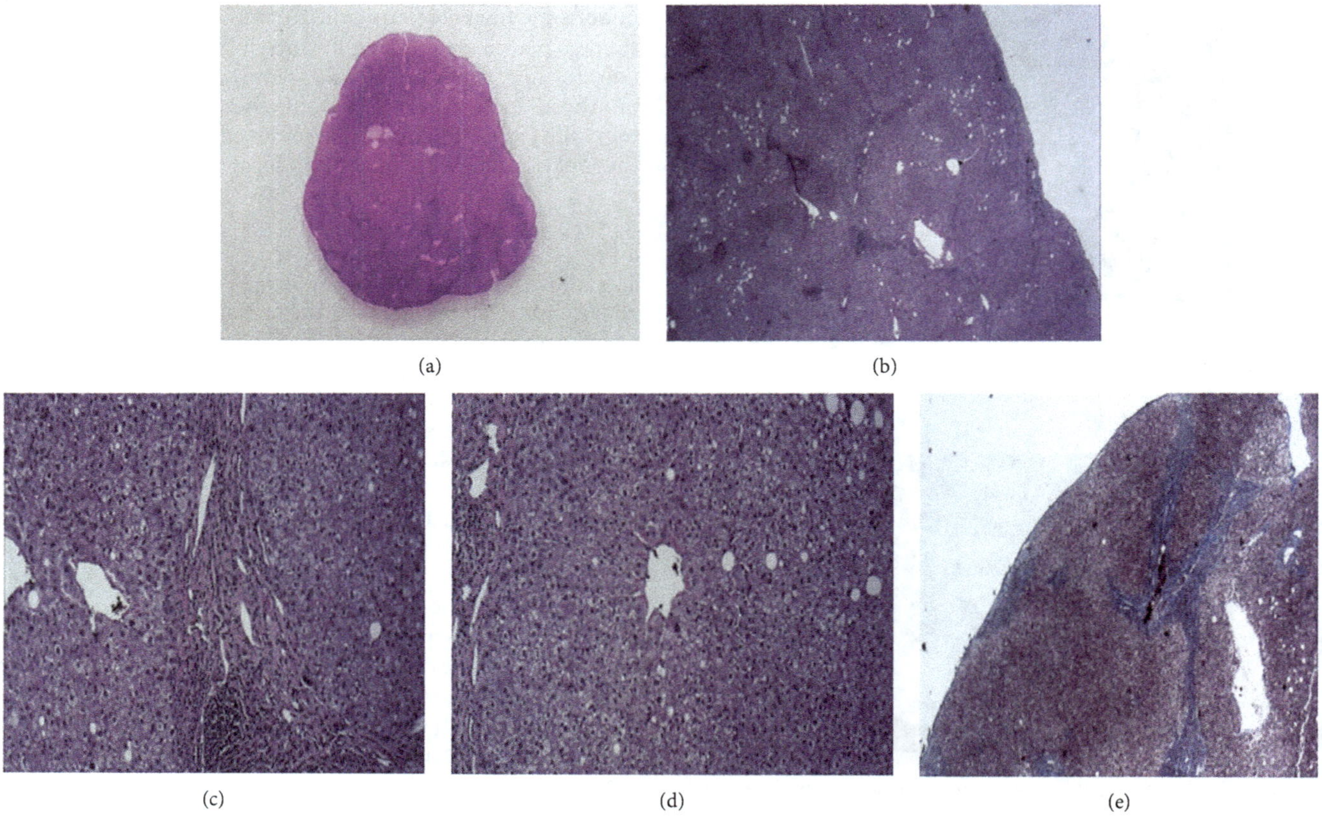

FIGURE 4: Histology of ectopic liver in the heart. (a) Photomicrograph with hematoxylin and eosin stain showing a 1.6 cm mass. (b) Normal liver parenchyma at 2x magnification. (c) Portal tract at 10x magnification with lymphocytic infiltration of parenchyma. (d) Central vein at 10x magnification. (e) Normal liver parenchymal architecture highlighted by trichrome stain at 2x magnification.

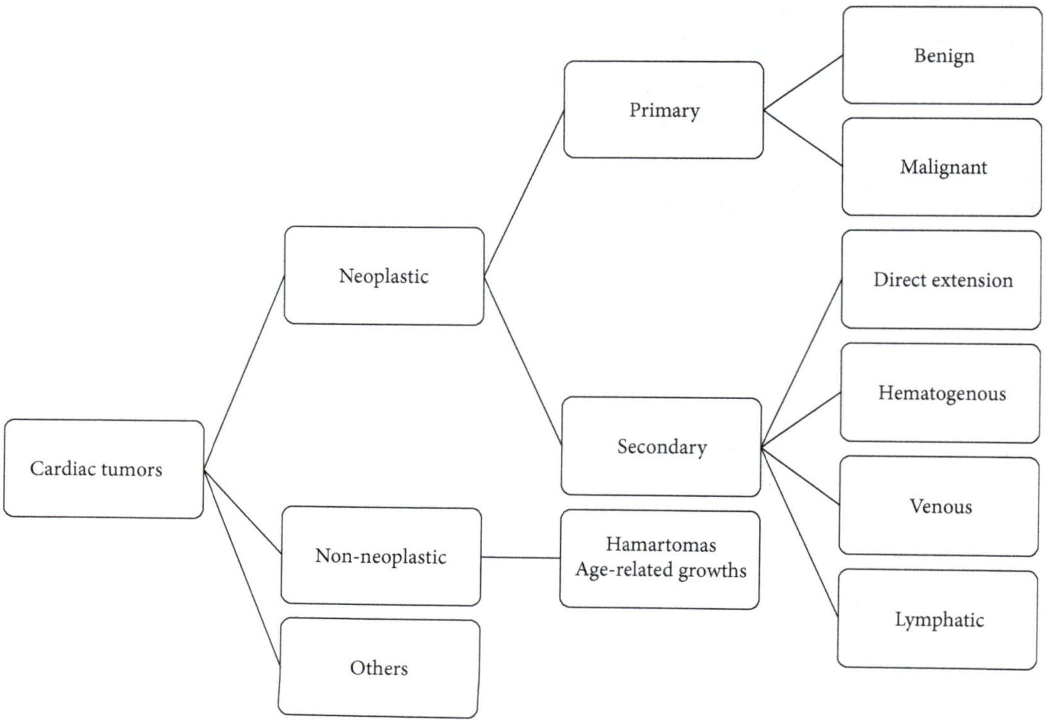

FIGURE 5

References

[1] K. Y. Lam, P. Dickens, and A. Chan, "Tumors of the heart. A 20-year experience with a review of 12,485 consecutive autopsies," *Archives of Pathology & Laboratory Medicine*, vol. 117, no. 10, pp. 1027–1031, 1993.

[2] H. A. McAllister and J. J. Fenoglio, "Tumors of the cardiovascular system," in *Atlas of Tumor Pathology, Second*, vol. - Fascicle 15, Armed Forces Institute of Pathology, Washington, DC, 1978.

[3] E. E. Salcedo, G. I. Cohen, R. D. White, and M. B. Davison, "Cardiac tumors: diagnosis and management," *Current Problems in Cardiology*, vol. 17, no. 2, pp. 77–137, 1992.

[4] F. Silvestri, R. Bussani, N. Pavletic, and T. Mannone, "Metastases of the heart and pericardium," *Giornale Italiano di Cardiologia*, vol. 27, no. 12, pp. 1252–1255, 1997.

[5] S. M. Trocciola, L. B. Balsam, H. Yee, E. Gianos, M. B. Srichai, and A. DeAnda Jr, "Ectopic liver: an unexpected finding in a right atrial mass," *The Annals of Thoracic Surgery*, vol. 92, no. 2, pp. 715–718, 2011.

[6] J. Chapman-Fredricks, R. Birusingh, M. Ricci, and M. Rodriguez, "Intracaval liver with cardiac extension. A new developmental anomaly?," *Fetal and Pediatric Pathology*, vol. 29, no. 6, pp. 401–406, 2010.

[7] L. Xu, J. Jeudy, and A. P. Burke, "Ectopic hepatic tissue presenting as right atrial mass," *Human Pathology*, vol. 43, no. 6, pp. 958–960, 2012.

[8] C. J. Bruce, "Cardiac tumours: diagnosis and management," *Heart*, vol. 97, no. 2, pp. 151–160, 2011.

[9] K. S. Dujardin, R. L. Click, and J. K. Oh, "The role of intraoperative transesophageal echocardiography in patients undergoing cardiac mass removal," *Journal of the American Society of Echocardiography*, vol. 13, no. 12, pp. 1080–1083, 2000.

[10] M. Watanabe, T. Matsura, Y. Takatori et al., "Five cases of ectopic liver and a case of accessory lobe of the liver," *Endoscopy*, vol. 21, no. 1, pp. 39–42, 1989.

[11] J. Asada, M. Onji, Y. Yamashita et al., "Ectopic liver observed by peritoneoscopy: report of a case," *Gastroenterological Endoscopy*, vol. 24, pp. 309–312, 1982.

[12] P. Eiserth, "Beiträge zur Kenntnis der Nebenlebern," *Virchows Archiv für Pathologische Anatomie und Physiologie und für Klinische Medizin*, vol. 307, no. 2, pp. 307–313, 1941.

[13] M. Matsuyama, S. Sugiura, A. Kakita, Y. Sato, and M. Kuroda, "Hepatocellular carcinoma arising from ectopic liver tissue in the spleen producing insulin-like growth factor II," *Pathology - Research and Practice*, vol. 207, no. 2, pp. 124–126, 2011.

[14] M. Gaudino, C. Lau, F. Cammertoni et al., "Surgical treatment of renal cell carcinoma with cavoatrial involvement: a systematic review of the literature," *The Annals of Thoracic Surgery*, vol. 101, no. 3, pp. 1213–1221, 2016.

Permissions

All chapters in this book were first published by Hindawi Publishing Corporation; hereby published with permission under the Creative Commons Attribution License or equivalent. Every chapter published in this book has been scrutinized by our experts. Their significance has been extensively debated. The topics covered herein carry significant findings which will fuel the growth of the discipline. They may even be implemented as practical applications or may be referred to as a beginning point for another development.

The contributors of this book come from diverse backgrounds, making this book a truly international effort. This book will bring forth new frontiers with its revolutionizing research information and detailed analysis of the nascent developments around the world.

We would like to thank all the contributing authors for lending their expertise to make the book truly unique. They have played a crucial role in the development of this book. Without their invaluable contributions this book wouldn't have been possible. They have made vital efforts to compile up to date information on the varied aspects of this subject to make this book a valuable addition to the collection of many professionals and students.

This book was conceptualized with the vision of imparting up-to-date information and advanced data in this field. To ensure the same, a matchless editorial board was set up. Every individual on the board went through rigorous rounds of assessment to prove their worth. After which they invested a large part of their time researching and compiling the most relevant data for our readers.

The editorial board has been involved in producing this book since its inception. They have spent rigorous hours researching and exploring the diverse topics which have resulted in the successful publishing of this book. They have passed on their knowledge of decades through this book. To expedite this challenging task, the publisher supported the team at every step. A small team of assistant editors was also appointed to further simplify the editing procedure and attain best results for the readers.

Apart from the editorial board, the designing team has also invested a significant amount of their time in understanding the subject and creating the most relevant covers. They scrutinized every image to scout for the most suitable representation of the subject and create an appropriate cover for the book.

The publishing team has been an ardent support to the editorial, designing and production team. Their endless efforts to recruit the best for this project, has resulted in the accomplishment of this book. They are a veteran in the field of academics and their pool of knowledge is as vast as their experience in printing. Their expertise and guidance has proved useful at every step. Their uncompromising quality standards have made this book an exceptional effort. Their encouragement from time to time has been an inspiration for everyone.

The publisher and the editorial board hope that this book will prove to be a valuable piece of knowledge for researchers, students, practitioners and scholars across the globe.

List of Contributors

Attila Frigy, Boglárka Belényi, Ádám Kirchmaier and Nándor Fekete
Department of Internal Medicine IV, G.E, Palade University of Medicine, Pharmacy, Science and Technology of Tirgu Mures, Tirgu Mures, Romania

István Adorján Szabó
Department of Physiopathology, G.E. Palade University of Medicine, Pharmacy, Science and Technology of Tirgu Mures, Tirgu Mures, Romania

A. Kalinskaya, D. Skrypnik, A. Kostin, E. Vasilieva and A. Shpektor
Moscow State University of Medicine and Dentistry Named After A.I. Evdokimov, Clinical Hospital Named After I.V. Davidovsky, Moscow, Russia

Soile Pauliina Salomäki
Department of infectious Diseases, Division of Medicine, Turku University Hospital, Turku, Finland
Faculty of Medicine, Department of Clinical Medicine, University of Turku, Turku, Finland
Turku PET Centre, University of Turku and Turku University Hospital, Turku, Finland

Antti Saraste
Faculty of Medicine, Department of Clinical Medicine, University of Turku, Turku, Finland
Turku PET Centre, University of Turku and Turku University Hospital, Turku, Finland
Heart Center, Turku University Hospital, Turku, Finland

Päivi Jalava-Karvinen and Ulla Hohenthal
Department of infectious Diseases, Division of Medicine, Turku University Hospital, Turku, Finland
Faculty of Medicine, Department of Clinical Medicine, University of Turku, Turku, Finland

Laura Pirilä
Department of infectious Diseases, Division of Medicine, Turku University Hospital, Turku, Finland
Department of Rheumatology, Division of Medicine, Turku University Hospital, Turku, Finland

Fernando Figueroa Rodriguez, Antonio Faieta Lasarcina and Francisco Davila Grijalva
Oakland University Beaumont Hospital, West 13 Mile Road, Royal Oak, MI 48073, USA

Stacy Willner, Zaid Imam and Ismail Hader
Beaumont, 3601 W 13 Mile Road, Royal Oak, MI 48073, USA

Mumtaz Zaman and Anthony Donato
Sidney Kimmel Medical College at Thomas Jefferson University, USA

Richard Loynd
Tower Health System, USA

Chris Pantsios, Zacharias-Alexandros Anyfantakis , Andrew Xanthopoulos, Ioannis Leventis, Spyridon Skoularigkis, Apostolos Dimos, Angeliki Bourazana, Michail Papamichalis, Grigorios Giamouzis , Filippos Triposkiadis and John Skoularigis
Department of Cardiology, General University Hospital of Larissa, Larissa, Greece

Alisha Alabre-Bonsu, Saurav Uppal, Ernest L. Mazzaferri Jr and Konstantinos Dean Boudoulas
Division of Cardiovascular Medicine, The Ohio State University, Columbus, Ohio, USA

Kanksha Peddi
Saba University School of Medicine, Saba, Dutch Caribbean, Netherlands

Alexander L. Hsu and Tomas H. Ayala
Department of Medicine, MedStar Harbor Hospital, Baltimore, MD, USA

Yuefeng Chen, Michael Amponsah and Cyril Nathaniel
Department of Cardiology, Conemaugh Memorial Medical Center, Johnstown, Pennsylvania 15905, USA

Seyedeh Maryam Hosseini and Muhammad Ajmal
University of Arizona College of Medicine, USA

Ranjith Shetty
Carondelet Medical Group, USA

Bashar Khiatah
Department of Internal Medicine, Community Memorial Hospital, 147 N Brent St, Ventura, CA 93003, USA

David Philips and Jonathan Dukes
Cardiology Associates Medical Group, Ventura, CA, USA

Amanda Frugoli
Department of GME Internal Medicine, Community Memorial Hospital, Ventura, CA, USA

Courtney R. Usry, Andrew S. Wilson and Kelvin N. V. Bush
Division of Cardiology, San Antonio Military Medical Center, 3551 Roger Brooke Dr. San Antonio, TX 78234, USA

Edgar Francisco Carrizales-Sepúlveda, Ángel Noé del Cueto-Aguilera, Raúl Alberto Jiménez-Castillo, Olga Norali de la Cruz-Mata, Mariana Fikir-Ordoñez, Raymundo Vera-Pineda and Dalí Alejandro Hernández-Guajardo
Internal Medicine Department, Hospital Universitario, Universidad Autónoma de Nuevo León, Monterrey, Nuevo León, Mexico

Ramiro Flores-Ramírez
Echocardiography Laboratory, Cardiology Service, Hospital Universitario, Universidad Autónoma de Nuevo León, Monterrey, Nuevo León, Mexico
1Internal Medicine Department, Hospital Universitario, Universidad Autónoma de Nuevo León, Monterrey, Nuevo León, Mexico

Alejandro Ordaz-Farías
Echocardiography Laboratory, Cardiology Service, Hospital Universitario, Universidad Autónoma de Nuevo León, Monterrey, Nuevo León, Mexico

Marko Perčić, Tea Friščić, Jasna Čerkez Habek, Dean Strinić and Jozica Šikić
Department of Cardiology, Clinic of Internal Medicine, "Sveti Duh" University Hospital, Zagreb, Croatia

Ninoslav Rudman
Department of Radiology, "Sveti Duh" University Hospital, Zagreb, Croatia

Weng-Chio Tam, U-Po Lam, Toi-Meng Mok, Tou Chang, Wa Ho and Mario Alberto De Brito Lima Evora
Department of Cardiology, Centro Hospitalar Conde São Januário, Macau, SAR, China

Bindu Gyawali, Bikash Baral and Sangam Shah
Maharajgunj Medical Campus, Institute of Medicine, Tribhuvan University, Maharajgunj, 44600, Nepal

Sutap Yadav
Department of Cardiology, Manmohan Cardiothoracic Vascular and Transplant Center, Nepal

Chandra Mani Poudel
Department of Cardiology, Manmohan Cardiothoracic Vascular and Transplant Center, Nepal
Maharajgunj Medical Campus, Institute of Medicine, Tribhuvan University, Maharajgunj 44600, Nepal

Nooraldin Merza, Assad Mohammedzein, Mazin Saadaldin and Tarek Naguib
Department of Internal Medicine, Texas Tech University Health Sciences Center, Amarillo, TX, USA

John Lung
School of Medicine, Texas Tech University Health Sciences Center, Amarillo, TX, USA

Taryn B. Bainum and Shanna James
Department of Pharmacy Practice, Texas Tech University Health Sciences Center Jerry H. Hodge School of Pharmacy, Amarillo, TX, USA

Connor C. Kerndt and Daniel F. Summers
Department of Internal Medicine, Spectrum Health Butterworth Hospital, Grand Rapids, Michigan, USA

John A. Bills and Zaid J. Shareef
Michigan State University College of Osteopathic Medicine, East Lansing, Michigan, USA

Alexander M. Balinski
Oakland University William Beaumont School of Medicine, Rochester, Michigan, USA

Jose M. Tan
Department of Internal Medicine, Spectrum Health Butterworth Hospital, Grand Rapids, Michigan, USA
Department of Cardiovascular Disease, Spectrum Health Butterworth Hospital, Grand Rapids, Michigan, USA

Rayyan Jadeed, Klaus Pethig and Dirk Böcker
Department of Cardiology, St. Marien Hospital, Hamm, Germany

S. Poddi, I. Tropea, G. Faggian and A. Rungatscher
Division of Cardiac Surgery, University of Verona Medical Center, Verona, Italy

S. De Feo
Division of Cardiovascular diseases, Pederzoli Hospital, Peschiera del Garda, Italy

M. Zordan
Division of Pathology, University of Verona Medical Center, Verona, Italy

Bdoor Bamousa and Taher Sbitli
Department of Medicine, Alfaisal University, Riyadh, Saudi Arabia

Tahir Mohamed and Ali Almasood
Heart Center, King Faisal Specialist Hospital & Research Center, Riyadh, Saudi Arabia

Khalid Al Johani
Cardiac Science Department, King Saud University, Riyadh, Saudi Arabia

Vidhushei Yogeswaran
Department of Medicine, University of California, San Francisco, CA, USA

Satvik Ramakrishna, John S. MacGregor, Lucas Zier and Nora Goldschlager
Department of Medicine, University of California, San Francisco, CA, USA
Division of Cardiology, Zuckerberg San Francisco General Hospital, San Francisco, CA, USA

Mohammad Altujjar, Ikram Ullah and Mohammad Tokir Mujtaba
Dartmouth Hitchcock Medical Center, Lebanon, USA

Feras Zaiem
Wayne State University, Detroit, USA

Erin Sheehan
Indiana University, Indianapolis, Indiana, USA

Willy Gan, Mohammed Mhanna and Waleed Khokher
University of Toledo, Toledo, USA

Sohab S. Radwan, Gauravpal Gill, Amre Ghazzal and Christopher Barnett
MedStar Washington Hospital Center, Washington, DC, USA

Awais Malik
MedStar Georgetown University Hospital, Washington, DC, USA

Muhammad H. Khan
Department of Internal Medicine, University of Cincinnati, USA

Obadah Aqtash, David M. Harris, Alexandru I. Costea and Myron C. Gerson
Department of Cardiovascular Medicine, University of Cincinnati, USA

Robyn Bryde
Department of Internal Medicine, Mayo Clinic Florida, 4500 San Pablo Road South, Jacksonville, Florida 32224, USA

Kevin Landolfo
Department of Cardiothoracic Surgery, Mayo Clinic Florida, 4500 San Pablo Road South, Jacksonville, Florida 32224, USA

Jordan C. Ray, Pragnesh Parikh and Carolyn Landolfo
Department of Cardiovascular Disease, Mayo Clinic Florida, 4500 San Pablo Road South, Jacksonville, Florida 32224, USA

Qihui "Jim" Zhai
Department of Pathology, Mayo Clinic Florida, 4500 San Pablo Road South, Jacksonville, Florida 32224, USA

Robby Singh and Marcel Zughaib
Providence Hospital, Michigan State University, USA

Santo Scarfone
Georgetown University, USA

Moaaz Baghal, Viralkumar Amrutiya, Bhoomi Patel, Rutwik Patel, Jonathan Hernandez, Mohamed Ahmed, Abraham Lo and Mark Gabelman
Hackensack Meridian Health Palisades Medical Center, Department of Internal Medicine, USA

Katia Bravo-Jaimes, Brian Walton, Poyee Tung and Richard W. Smalling
Division of Cardiology, University of Texas Health Science Center at Houston, Houston, Texas, USA

Ian Jackson, Yaman Alali and Abedel Rahman Anani
Department of Medicine, Creighton University School of Medicine, Omaha, NE, USA

Ali Nayfeh
Department of Pulmonary and Critical Care, Creighton University School of Medicine, Omaha, NE, USA

Arindam Sharma, Abhishek Thandra and Amjad Kabach
Department of Cardiology, Creighton University School of Medicine, Omaha, NE, USA

Ebubechukwu Ezeh and Maddie Perdoncin
Department of Internal Medicine, Marshall University, Huntington, WV, USA

Morgan K. Moroi
Pennsylvania State University, State College, PA, USA

Mohammad Amro
The Palestinian Ministry of Health and Higher Education, State of Palestine

Mohammed Ruzieh
University of Florida, Gainesville, FL, USA

Paul I. Okhumale
Cedar Valley Cardiovascular Center, Waterloo, IA, USA

Vitor Martinelli Batista Rolim and Pietro Dall'Orto Lima
Department of Cardiology, Santa Casa de Misericórdia de Vitória Hospital, Rua Dr. João dos Santos Neves, 143, Vila Rubim, 29025-023 Vitória, ES, Brazil

Eduardo Moreno Judice de Mattos Farina and Ramon Chiabai Moura
School of Medicine of Santa Casa de Misericórdia, Av. Nossa Sra. da Penha, 2190, Bela Vista, 29027-502 Vitória, ES, Brazil

Roberto Ramos Barbosa, Assad Miguel Sassine and Luiz Fernando Machado Barbosa
Department of Cardiology, Santa Casa de Misericórdia de Vitória Hospital, Rua Dr. João dos Santos Neves, 143, Vila Rubim, 29025-023 Vitória, ES, Brazil
School of Medicine of Santa Casa de Misericórdia, Av. Nossa Sra. da Penha, 2190, Bela Vista, 29027-502 -Vitória, ES, Brazil

Simran Gupta, Ricky Ayala, Aakash Desai, Viraj I. Modi, and Robert J. Nardino
Department of Internal Medicine, University of Connecticut School of Medicine, UCONN Health, Farmington, CT, USA

Josef Finsterer
Krankenanstalt Rudolfstiftung, Messerli Institute, Vienna, Austria

Claudia Stöllberger and Matthias Hasun
2nd Medical Department with Cardiology and Intensive Care Medicine, Krankenanstalt Rudolfstiftung, Vienna, Austria

Korbinian Riedhammer
Institute of Human Genetics, Germany
Department of Nephrology, Klinikum Rechts der Isar, School of Medicine, Technical University of Munich, Munich, Germany

Mathias Wagner
Institute of Human Genetics, Germany

Terumori Satoh, Masao Saotome, Kenichiro Suwa, Hayato Ohtani and Yuichiro Maekawa
Department of Cardiology, Internal Medicine 3, Hamamatsu University School of Medicine, Hamamatsu, Japan

Yasuyuki Nagata and Takaaki Ono
Department of Hematology, Internal Medicine 3, Hamamatsu University School of Medicine, Hamamatsu, Japan

Ying chi Yang and Thein Tun Aung
University of Iowa Hospitals and Clinics, Iowa City, IA, USA

Abdul Wase
Dayton Heart and Vascular Hospital, Dayton, OH, USA

Mohammad Ali Zakeri
Social Determinants of Health Research Center, Rafsanjan University of Medical Sciences, Rafsanjan, Iran
Non-Communicable Diseases Research Center, Rafsanjan University of Medical Sciences, Rafsanjan, Iran

Vahid Mohammadi
Department of Cardiology, Ali-Ibn Abi-Talib Hospital, School of Medicine, Rafsanjan University of Medical Sciences, Rafsanjan, Iran

Gholamreza Bazmandegan
Clinical Research Development Unit, Ali-Ibn Abi-Talib Hospital, Rafsanjan University of Medical Sciences, Rafsanjan, Iran
Department of Family Medicine, Ali-Ibn Abi-Talib Hospital, School of Medicine, Rafsanjan University of Medical Sciences, Rafsanjan, Iran

Maryam Zakeri
Physiology-Pharmacology Research Center, Research Institute of Basic Medical Sciences, Rafsanjan University of Medical Sciences, Rafsanjan, Iran

Marc Vanderheyden and Sofie Verstreken
Cardiovascular Center, Onze Lieve Vrouwziekenhuis, Aalst, Belgium

Richard Houben
2BMedical, Maastricht, Netherlands

Johanes Nugroho
Department of Cardiology and Vascular Medicine, Faculty of Medicine, Universitas Airlangga, Surabaya, Indonesia
Dr. Soetomo General Hospital, Surabaya, Indonesia

Ruth Gunadi
Dr. Soetomo General Hospital, Surabaya, Indonesia

Adhirath Doshi and Dhaval Shah
Division of Cardiology, St. Vincent Hospital, Worcester, MA, USA

Shradha Gupta and Deepika Panday
Department of Internal Medicine, St. Vincent Hospital, Worcester, MA, USA

Arie Farji-Cisneros
Department of Anesthesia, St. Vincent Hospital, Worcester, MA, USA

Eddison Ramsaran
Department of Cardiology, Reliant Medical Group, Worcester, MA, USA

Robert Bojar
Division of Cardiothoracic Surgery, St. Vincent Hospital, Worcester, MA, USA

Index

www.ingramcontent.com/pod-product-compliance
Lightning Source LLC
LaVergne TN
LVHW082224200926
848484LV00008B/2301